The Global HIV Epidemics among Men Who Have Sex with Men

Chris Beyrer, Andrea L. Wirtz, Damian Walker, Benjamin Johns, Frangiscos Sifakis, and Stefan D. Baral

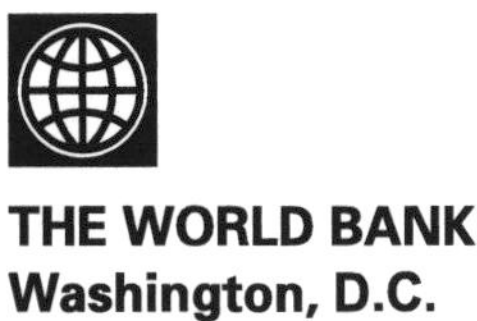

THE WORLD BANK
Washington, D.C.

1818 H Street NW
Washington DC 20433
Telephone: 202-473-1000
Internet: www.worldbank.org

1 2 3 4 14 13 12 11

ISBN: 978-0-8213-8726-9
eISBN: 978-0-8213-8727-6
DOI: 10.1596/978-0-8213-8726-9

Library of Congress Cataloging-in-Publication data has been requested

Cover painting: "Untitled" by Raimundo Rubio, 1998. Oil on canvas, 52 by 52 in., World Bank Art Collection.
Cover design: Naylor Design.

The Global HIV Epidemics among Men Who Have Sex with Men

Contents

Box

Figures

Tables

Acknowledgments

Foremost, the World Bank would like to thank and acknowledge the excellent work of the authors of this study from the Center for Public Health and Human Rights at the Johns Hopkins Bloomberg School of Public Health, expertly led by Chris Beyrer: Andrea L. Wirtz, Damian Walker, Benjamin Johns, Frangiscos Sifakis, and Stefan D. Baral. This work was undertaken in close partnership with the United Nations Development Programme (UNDP), and the Bank thanks Jeffrey O'Malley, Sam Avrett, and Cheikh Traore for their support and guidance. In addition, the Bank thanks Ying-Ru Lo from the World Health Organization (WHO) and Michael Bartos from the Joint United Nations Programme on HIV/AIDS (UNAIDS) for formative consultations and collaboration over the two years of this study, and especially congratulates WHO on the development of *Guidance for the Prevention and Treatment of HIV and Other Sexually Transmitted Infections among Men Having Sex with Men and Transgender People*, which will be a landmark contribution to health and human rights. The Bank thanks the Chinese and Thai governments for their hospitality in hosting meetings of communities and stakeholders that have informed this work.

Within the World Bank, the quality of this work has been greatly enhanced by the kind contributions of the peer reviewers, Gayle Martin and Christopher Thomas, and of David Wilson, Keith Hansen, Joy de Beyer, Mariam Claeson, Marelize Gorgens, Tony Thompson, and Kees Kostermans, as well as by the guidance of Cristian Baeza.

The authors would like to thank the Futures Institute, particularly Lori Bollinger and John Stover, for sharing the Goals Model with the group from the Center for Public Health and Human Rights at the Johns Hopkins Bloomberg School of Public Health, mentoring us all in its use and providing their expertise gratis in this effort.

Numerous individuals and organizations have significantly contributed to this effort and are acknowledged by region. The authors would like to especially acknowledge the Kenya Medical Research Institute research team for providing baseline data for modeling the HIV epidemic in Kenya, the Cayetano team in Peru, and the U.S. Centers for Disease Control and Prevention team for providing the data for Thailand.

Global: The Foundation for AIDS Research (amfAR) MSM Initiative, MSM GF (the Global Forum on MSM and HIV), Jack Beck, George Ayala, Evelyn Gonzales, Kristin Lauer, the Population Council, Patrick Sullivan, Kent Klindera, Chris Collins, Kevin Frost, Michael Cowing, Jirair Ratevosian, Tonia Poteat, Priya Mehra, Jen Johnsen, John Macauley, Ken Mayer, Cary Alan Johnson, the International Gay and Lesbian Human Rights Commission (IGLHRC), and Mandeep Dhaliwal

Africa: Charles Gueboguo, Angus Parkinson, Cesnabmihilo Aken, Most at Risk Populations Initiative–MARPI, (Uganda), Gift Trapence, Wiseman Chibwezo, Friedel Dausab, Ian Swartz, Scott Geibel (Population Council), Paul Semugoma, Ifeanyi Orazulike, Alliance Rights Nigeria, Shivaji Bhattacharya (UNDP), Association for the Defence of Homosexuals (ADEFHO, Cameroon), Alternatives-Cameroon, Sean Casey, Dawie Nel, Georges Kanuma, David Kuria, Sébastien Mandeng, Steave Nemande, Gays and Lesbians Coalition of Kenya, Gays and Lesbians of Zimbabwe, Samuel Matsikure, Heartland Alliance, Fatou Maria Drame, Daouda Diouf, CEDEP: Centre for the Development of People (Malawi), Darrin Adams, Sexual Minorities Uganda (SMUG), Frans Viljoen, Earl Burrell, Linda-Gail Bekker, and Tim Lane

Asia: David Lowe, Shale Ahmed, Bandhu (Bangladesh), Dennis Altman, Joseph Miletti, Sunil Solomon, Shruti Mehta, Wessam El Beih, Shiv Khan, National Foundation for India, HIV/AIDS Alliance India, Kyaw Myint, Frits van Griensven, Thomas Guadamuz, Phunlerd Piyaraj, Maninder Setia, and Wipas Wimonsate

Eastern Europe and Central Asia: AIDS Infoshare Russia, Alena Peryshkina, Vladimir Molgyini, Irina Deobald, Konstantin Dyakonov, Amulet Kazakhstan, Denis Efremov, Ludmila Kononenko, and Marije Klep

Latin America and the Caribbean: Carlos Cáceres, Caleb Orozco, Joel Simpson, Ken Morrison, Christian Rumu, Lilia Rossi, Kelika Konda, Luis Squiquera, Lorenzo Vargas, and David Richardson Santana

Middle East and North Africa: Helem (Lebanon), Matthew French, Myrieme Zniber, Nadia Rafif, and Salma Mousallem

This work was supported by a World Bank task team led by Robert Oelrichs and including Ndella Njie, Anderson Stanciole, Fazu Mansouri, and Iris Semini. Special thanks go to Martin Lutalo and Aziz Gökdemir for their careful supervision of the production of this volume.

Abbreviations

AIDS	acquired immune deficiency syndrome
aOR	adjusted odds ratio
ART	antiretroviral therapy
ARV	antiretroviral
BC	bisexual concurrent
BSS	National Behavioural Surveillance Survey
CCM	Country Coordinating Mechanism
CDC	U.S. Centers for Disease Control and Prevention
CHPI	combination HIV prevention intervention
CI	confidence interval
CPOL	community popular opinion leader
CT	conversion therapy
FSW	female sex worker
GDP	gross domestic product
GFATM	Global Fund to Fight AIDS, Tuberculosis and Malaria
GRADE	Grading of Recommendations Assessment, Development and Evaluation
GUD	genital ulcerative disease
HAART	highly active antiretroviral therapy
HASTE	Highest Attainable STandard of Evidence

HAV	hepatitis A virus
HBV	hepatitis B virus
HIV	human immunodeficiency virus
HPV	human papillomavirus
HR	hazard ratio
HSV-2	herpes simplex virus 2
IDU	injecting drug user
iPrEx	Preexposure Prophylaxis Initiative
KEMRI	Kenya Medical Research Institute
LGBT	lesbian, gay, bisexual, and transgendered
LMICs	low- and middle-income countries
MACS	Multicenter AIDS Cohort Study
MENA	Middle East and North Africa
MOH	ministry of health
MSM	men who have sex with men
MSW	male sex worker
N-9	nonoxynol-9
NACO	National AIDS Control Organisation
NGO	nongovernmental organization
OR	odds ratio
PEP	Promotores Educadores de Pares
PEPFAR	U.S. President's Emergency Plan for AIDS Relief
PLWHA	people living with HIV/AIDS
PSI	Population Services International
RR	relative risk
STI	sexually transmitted infection
TG	transgendered
UAI	unprotected anal intercourse
UN	United Nations
UNAIDS	Joint United Nations Programme on HIV/AIDS
UNDP	United Nations Development Programme
UNGASS	United Nations General Assembly Special Session
VCT	voluntary counseling and testing
WHO	World Health Organization
Int$	international dollar
US$	U.S. dollar

Executive Summary

Men who have sex with men (MSM) are currently at marked risk for HIV infection in low- and middle-income countries (LMICs) in Asia, Africa, Latin America and the Caribbean, and in Eastern Europe and Central Asia. Estimates of HIV prevalence rates have been consistently higher among MSM than for the general population of reproductive-age men virtually wherever MSM have been well studied. Although scarce, HIV incidence data support findings of high acquisition and transmission risks among MSM in multiple contexts, cultural settings, and economic levels.

Research among MSM in LMICs has been limited by the criminalization and social stigmatization of these behaviors, the safety considerations for study participants, the hidden nature of these populations, and a lack of targeted funding. Available evidence from these countries suggests that structural risks—social, economic, political, or legal factors—in addition to individual-level risk factors are likely to play important roles in shaping HIV risks and treatment and care options for these men.

Services and resources for populations of MSM remain markedly low in many settings. They have limited coverage and access to HIV/AIDS prevention, treatment, and care services—with some estimates suggesting that fewer than 1 in 10 MSM worldwide have access to the most basic package of preventive interventions.

To improve LMIC responses to HIV/AIDS, services for MSM must expand, and exclusion from key emerging interventions, such as expanded voluntary counseling and testing (VCT), earlier access to treatment, and treatment-as-prevention modalities, must be addressed. This book seeks to inform these responses by posing and attempting to answer several key questions:

- What fraction of the burden of HIV disease in selected countries is attributable to gay, bisexual, and other behaviors of MSM? How does this fraction vary by scenario and across the representative states?
- Where are these selected countries in 2010 in terms of coverage for prevention, treatment, and care for MSM?
- What would constitute a minimum acceptable package of evidence-based and human rights–affirming services for prevention, treatment, and care of MSM?
- What resources, political will, and novel approaches would be necessary to reach acceptable coverage levels of MSM in the targeted countries with this essential minimum package of services? How might resources be maximized to ensure acceptable coverage of populations of MSM by the prevention and treatment packages?

To answer these and related questions, a several-stage analysis was conducted of the global epidemics of HIV among MSM in LMICs. First, the available data on MSM were reviewed—including taxonomies; HIV epidemiology; risk factors; and access to prevention, treatment, and care—in nine selected countries: Brazil, India, Kenya, Malawi, Peru, the Russian Federation, Senegal, Thailand, and Ukraine.

Then, the existing literature on HIV preventive interventions and strategies among MSM was reviewed. These data were analyzed using a novel adaptation of the Grading of Recommendations Assessment, Development and Evaluation (GRADE) system for public health interventions to generate an essential package of HIV prevention services.

In collaboration with the Futures Institute, the Goals Model for MSM was then adapted. One country was selected for each scenario (Kenya, Peru, Thailand, and Ukraine), and the modified Goals Model and the data on preventive interventions were used to model the effects of HIV prevention services on the epidemic among MSM in these countries. A costing exercise was done to estimate the costs and cost-effectiveness of these programs.

Finally, a policy and human rights assessment was done using these findings to evaluate the effect of enabling policy environments on these HIV epidemics.

Epidemic Scenarios and Focus Countries

The emerging regional epidemics in Africa, Asia, Latin America, and Eastern Europe among MSM are occurring in contexts of diverse HIV epidemics that vary with respect to factors such as predominant modes of spread; epidemic level and stage; gender and age distribution; and levels of prevention, treatment, and care services. This great diversity means regional approaches to epidemics among MSM must be situated within their wider epidemic contexts to develop informed and appropriate responses. A critical component of HIV risk in all the regions explored is the intersection of HIV epidemics among MSM and substance use, which includes both injection drug use risk and noninjection risks.

Systematic searches were conducted of databases including PubMed, EMBASE, EBSCO, and the *Cochrane Database of Systematic Reviews* until January 1, 2010. Articles and citations were downloaded, organized, and reviewed using the QUOSA v8 information management software package. A total of 133 prevalence studies from 130 unique reports describing data from 50 countries were identified and used for this analysis.

An Algorithmic Approach to Characterizing Epidemics among MSM

An algorithmic approach was developed to characterize epidemics among MSM and the wider contexts in which they occur. The development of the algorithm began with the standard Joint United Nations Programme on HIV/AIDS (UNAIDS) definition of a concentrated HIV epidemic, which is greater than 5 percent HIV prevalence in any high-risk group, such as MSM, injecting drug users (IDUs), or male or female sex workers.

The algorithm proceeds to the ratio of HIV prevalence among MSM to that among the general population and dichotomizes this categorization into a ratio of (a) less than 10 or (b) greater than or equal to 10. The basis for the selection of a ratio of 10 as the cutoff value builds on prior work by the authors, which indicated that the adjusted odds ratio for MSM compared to other men in medium-HIV-prevalence countries was 9.6 (95 percent confidence interval, 9.0–10.2). Assuming the prevalence ratio will approximate the odds ratio, one uses the upper level of that

Figure ES.1 Algorithm Describing the Development of the Epidemic Scenarios

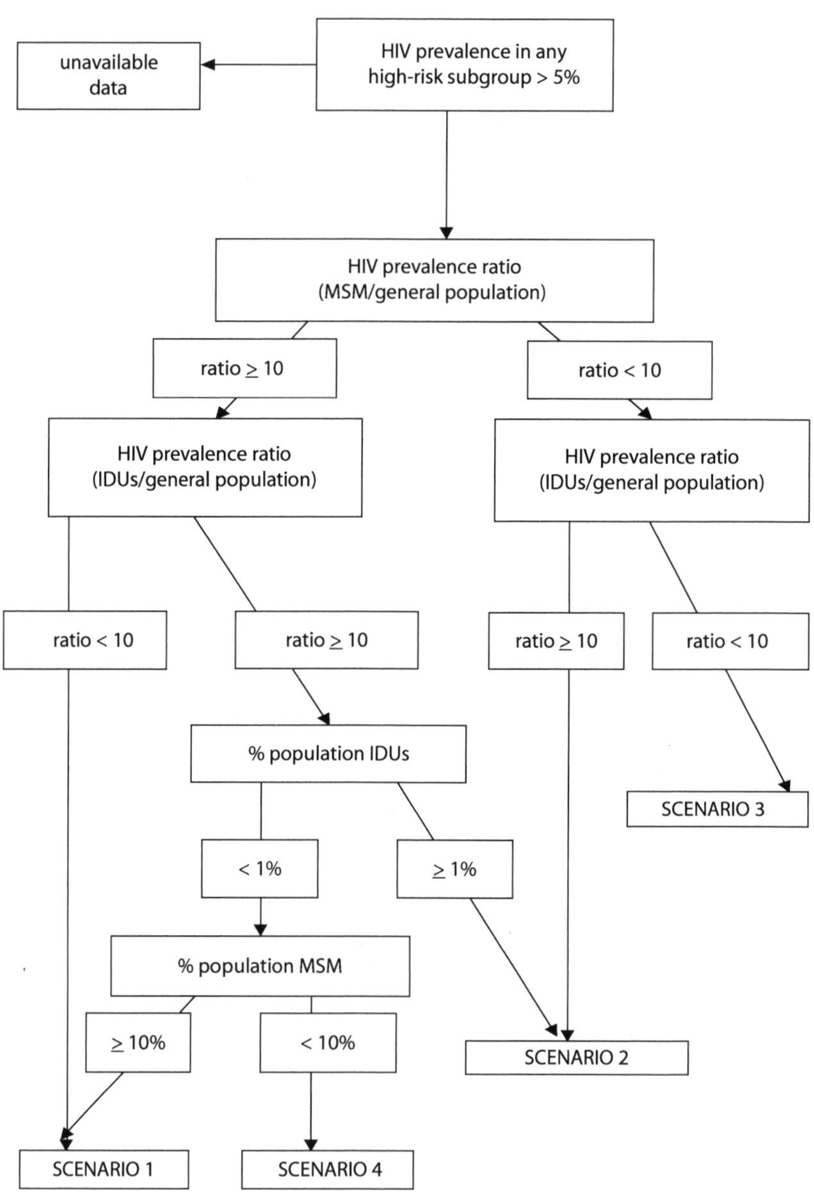

Source: Beyrer et al. 2010.

interval to guide the differentiation between countries whose HIV prevalence among MSM is substantial compared to the general population. The algorithm then takes into account the ratio of HIV infection prevalence among IDUs to the general population, again dichotomized into ratios of (a) less than 10 or (b) greater than or equal to 10. A parallel rationale is used to that regarding MSM, applying the same cutoff value of 10 for the ratio of HIV prevalence among IDUs over that of the general population. The final step is the categorization by proportion of the adult male population engaging in injecting drug use behavior, dichotomized by less than 1 percent and greater than or equal to 1 percent, and categorization by proportion of the adult male population with a history of ever engaging in MSM behavior, again dichotomized. Incorporation of denominator estimates for MSM and IDUs points to the extent of the HIV burden in a given country. Figure ES.1 illustrates the algorithm, and a detailed explanation for the algorithms yielding each of the four scenarios is available in appendix A.

In all, 1,612 citations were identified from published reports, and 819 from international conferences until January 1, 2010. After exclusion of duplicates and exclusion for lack of data, including biological measures of HIV, 178 citations and 61 conference reports were retrieved and reviewed. A total of 133 prevalence studies from 130 unique reports met all inclusion criteria. These data describe HIV prevalence among MSM in a total of 54 LMICs.

Using the algorithm with available country-level data yields the following four epidemic scenarios:

Scenario 1: Risks among MSM are the predominant exposure mode for HIV infection in the population. This scenario is seen across most of South America and in multiple settings in high-income countries. Here, HIV prevalence among MSM is generally over 10 percent; the ratio of MSM to the general population is very high; the prevalence among IDUs is variable, but the population prevalence of injecting drug use risks is well under 1 percent of adults; and the proportion of men reporting a lifetime history of sex with another man is well under 10 percent of adults.

Scenario 2: Risks among MSM occur within established HIV epidemics driven by injecting drug use. This scenario is the predominant epidemic context in Eastern Europe and Central Asia. Here, the HIV rate is highest among IDUs; the prevalence ratio for HIV infection among MSM compared to the general population is less than 10, but the same ratio for IDUs compared to the general population is well over 10; and the proportion of the adult population with a lifetime history of ever injecting

Figure ES.2 HIV Epidemic among MSM in LMICs According to Epidemic Scenario

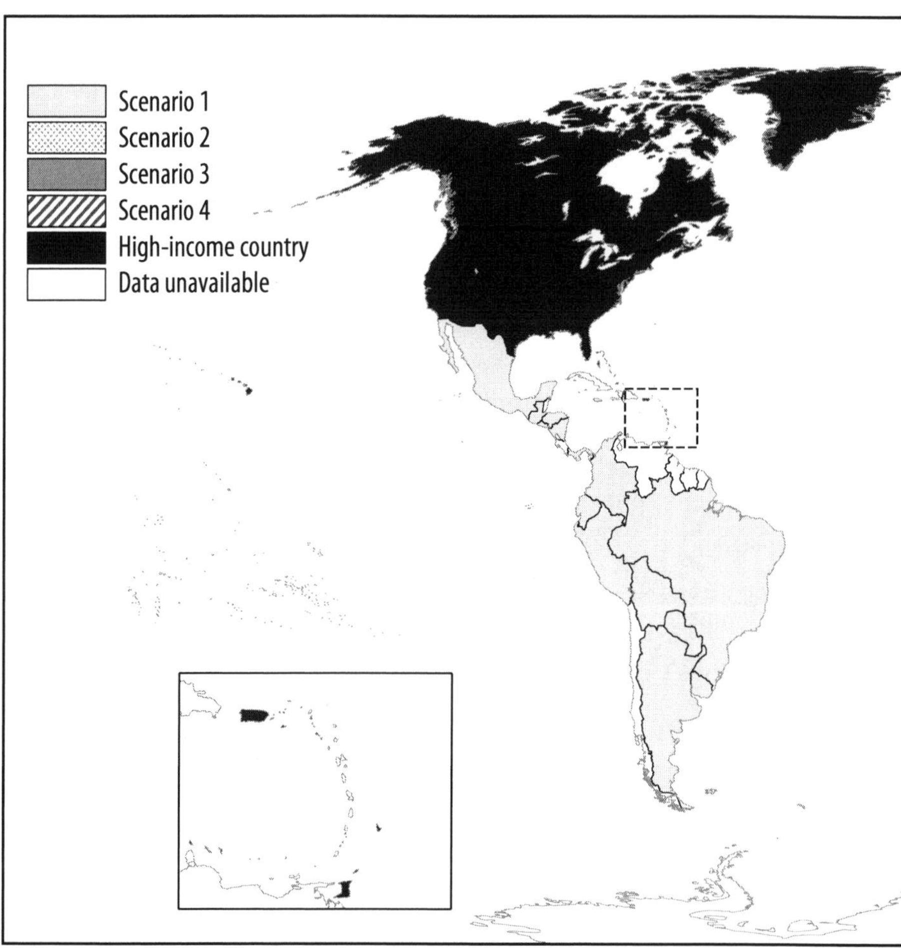

Source: Authors.
Note: Following the algorithm and based on available data, Senegal would also be assigned to scenario 4 and Ghana to scenario 1; both are somewhat outliers in these categories, and both have some uncertainties in risks and prevalence of HIV among female sex workers, IDU, and MSM, which make characterization difficult. In both cases, and there are doubtless others, more refined epidemiologic studies will likely be required to characterize these dynamics epidemics among MSM and others at risk.

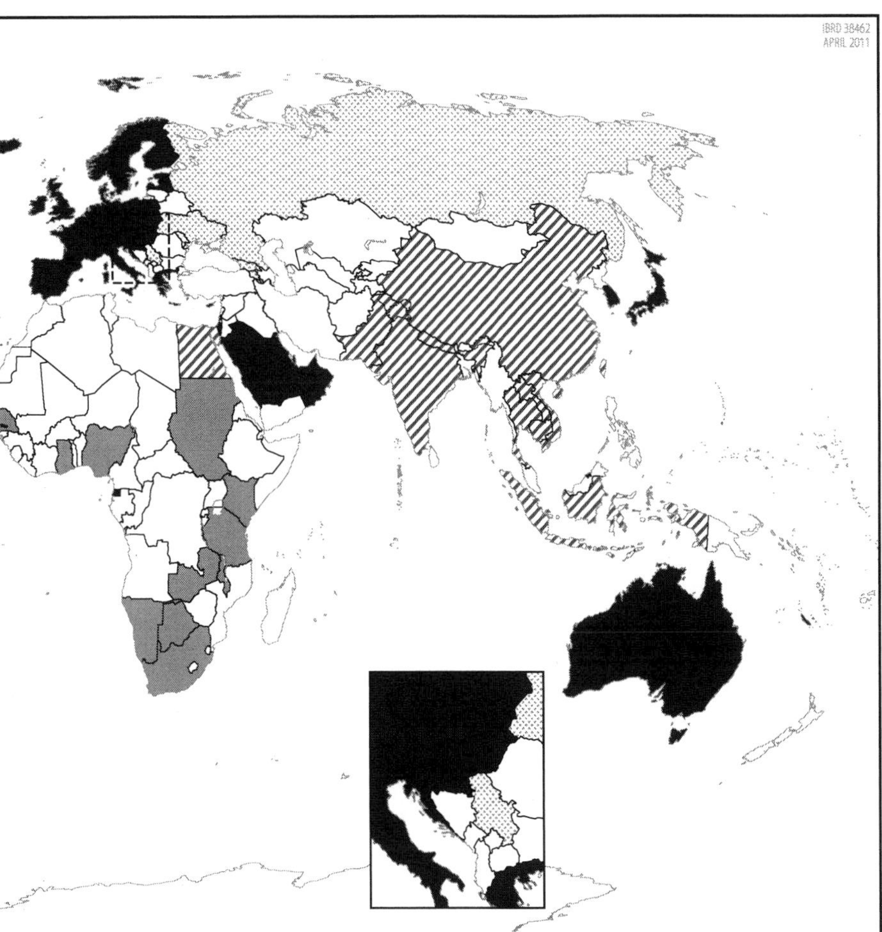
IBRD 38462
APRIL 2011

drugs is over 1 percent, the highest categorization stratum used by Mathers and colleagues (2008).

Scenario 3: Risks among MSM occur in the context of mature and widespread HIV epidemics among heterosexuals. This scenario is the prevailing context across Sub-Saharan Africa with particular relevance for the high-prevalence zones of East Africa and Southern Africa. Here, rates in heterosexuals are high, so the ratio of MSM to general population samples is well under 10, as is the ratio among IDUs compared to heterosexuals.

Scenario 4: Transmissions among MSM, IDUs, and heterosexuals all contribute significantly to the HIV epidemic. This scenario is the complex context of much of south, southeast, and northeast Asia. Finally, in this algorithm the same conditions prevail as in scenario 1, but the proportion of men with a history of same-sex behavior is markedly higher.

These scenarios are illustrated in figure ES.2.

Combination HIV Prevention Interventions for MSM: An Overview of the Evidence and Recommendations

Although increasing data highlight risk among MSM in low- and middle-income settings, the data set describing best practices for prevention, treatment, and care for this at-risk population remains limited. In assessing the evidence for this book, a series of systematic reviews were conducted of the published literature; extensive searches of the gray literature were done with support from an array of community, United Nations (UN) agencies, and civil society partners; and with support from the United Nations Development Programme, a global consultation for community best practices was then conducted in January 2010.

The literature supports the contention that to respond to multiple levels of HIV risk among MSM, combination HIV prevention interventions (CHPIs) must be used at multiple levels and presented through multiple modes to maximize potential effectiveness. The implementation of a single mode of HIV prevention will not provide effective control of the HIV epidemic at a population level and, moreover, has the potential to increase risk at the individual level secondary to treatment optimism. To date, condoms and lubricants are the best-evidenced biomedical HIV prevention tools; other biomedical strategies have so far failed to demonstrate efficacy, especially among MSM, or have not been evaluated in these men. An exception is antiretroviral therapy (ART), which has recently been demonstrated to have potent effects for HIV prevention (greater than 92 percent efficacy) among discordant couples. While this book was being written, the results of the iPrEx (Preexposure Prophylaxis Initiative) study, a randomized controlled trial of the safety and efficacy of daily oral preexposure chemoprophylaxis with Truvada (an antiviral combination of the drugs tenofovir DF and emtricitabine) for the prevention of HIV infection among MSM and transgendered women were announced (Grant et al. 2010).

The iPrEx study found an overall reduction in risk of HIV infection of some 44 percent (95 percent confidence interval, 15–63, P = 0.005). Efficacy was notably higher among those men and transgendered women who had greater adherence to the study protocol as determined by blood levels of drug. A landmark multicountry study that enrolled 2,499 subjects in Brazil, Ecuador, Peru, South Africa, Thailand, and the United States, iPrEx is the first major prevention trial to include African MSM. Should further studies support the findings of the iPrEx study, oral chemoprophylaxis may become an accepted addition to HIV prevention options.

Assessing the Quality of Evidence

The Highest Attainable STandard of Evidence (HASTE) system was used to evaluate evidence. The HASTE system developed by our team is specific to HIV interventions among most at-risk populations and focuses on three main characteristics with equal importance: efficacy data; implementation science data; and biological and public health plausibility. The system may be adaptable to other public health areas and disciplines. The inclusion of a review of efficacy data is a common denominator across all systems evaluating levels of evidence. However, the response to preventing HIV infection has differed from most other clinical conditions in that the implementation of these preventive measures is generally managed by civil society and not-for-profit nongovernmental institutions rather than health care facilities. Notably, with increasing evidence of effective biomedical interventions to prevent HIV infection including circumcision and topical and oral chemoprophylaxis, this balance may eventually change. Though peer-reviewed data from these implementers is often unattainable, these interventions constitute a predominant majority of HIV prevention services in low- and middle-income countries. Thus, our group considered capturing these implementation science data crucial in informing the optimal package of services for MSM.

To review the evidence for effective interventions to prevent HIV among MSM, this study used a process first proposed by the Community

Preventive Services Task Force of the U.S. Centers for Disease Control and Prevention when developing an evidence-based guide to public health interventions. This process included the following steps:

- Forming a multidisciplinary team
- Developing an approach to assessing the evidence for interventions
- Selecting which interventions would be included in the review
- Developing systematic search strategies for each intervention
- Implementing these search strategies
- Assessing and summarizing the quality of evidence using a modified GRADE process
- Translating this evidence into a set of recommendations for interventions to be included in CHPIs

Finally, through the global consultation of community-led initiatives supporting the needs of MSM in LMICs, information and data outside the realm of effectiveness were considered and research gaps were identified and summarized.

A derivative of the GRADE process targeting public health interventions has been proposed by investigators from the World Health Organization. The system proposed by Tang et al. (2008) focuses on three main causality criteria: strong association, consistency of results, and biologic plausibility. The HASTE system builds upon Tang et al.'s method and further integrates the lessons learned from implementation science of public health interventions. Four levels of HASTE are used, depending on the amount of peer-reviewed data as well as community-based data sources available (table ES.1):

- Strong (HASTE 1)
- Conditional (HASTE 2)
- Insufficient (HASTE 3)
- Inappropriate (HASTE 4)

HASTE includes four grades of evidence including Strong (Grade 1), Conditional (Grade 2), Insufficient (Grade 3), and Inappropriate (Grade 4) depending on the amount of peer-reviewed and implementation data available, as well as the plausibility of these interventions (table ES.1). Grade 1 or strong recommendations are given when there are available data showing that the desirable effect of an intervention clearly outweighs the potential risks or there are data showing that the intervention

Table ES.1 Four HASTE Levels of Evidence for Public Health Interventions

HASTE level	*Strength of recommendation*	*Explanation*
Grade 1	Strong	• Efficacy is consistent. • Intervention is biologically plausible. • Implementation data are available.
Grade 2a	Probable	• Efficacy data are limited. • Intervention is biologically plausible.
Grade 2b	Possible	• Efficacy is inconsistent. • Intervention is biologically plausible. • Consensus exists from implementation science data.
Grade 2c	Pending	• Definitive trials are ongoing. • Intervention is biologically plausible.
Grade 3	Insufficient	• Data are inconsistent. • Biologic plausibility is undefined.
Grade 4	Inappropriate	• Consistent data demonstrate lack of efficacy. • Consensus exists from implementation data of inappropriate intervention.

Source: Stefan Baral, Chris Beyrer, and Andrea Wirtz.

addresses a known causal risk factor of HIV risk among MARPS. Grade 2 or conditional recommendations are given when there is potential efficacy for an intervention, but further research is required. Conditional recommendations may be given when there has been only one or a few studies evaluating a particular intervention, but a strong association has been shown. Alternatively, there may be limited efficacy data, with strong plausibility in the context of strong consensus and experience from implementation or programmatic research, showing that this particular intervention constitutes an important component of comprehensive HIV interventions for MARPS. In either of these scenarios, the intervention would be defined as Grade 2a or probable. If data on efficacy are inconsistent, but they are biologically plausible and there is consensus from reviews of implementation science, the intervention would be called Grade 2b or possible. A grade of possible or Grade 2b can be given if the intervention in question has limited data, but has public health plausibility in being a component, causal pathway of another intervention of demonstrated value. Pending or Grade 2c recommendations are given when there are definitive trials among MARPS ongoing. Insufficient or Grade 3 is applied when there is inconsistent evidence for the efficacy of a particular intervention, the causal pathway is unclear or not well defined, and there is limited consensus from community experience about a particular intervention. A grade of inappropriate or Grade 4 is given when there is evidence of no efficacy or effectiveness of an intervention, where risks outweigh potential benefits, or where there is consensus from implementation data that this is an inappropriate intervention.

Findings: Targeting Individual-Level Risk

Individual-level risk reduction remains a key component of all HIV preventive interventions.

Condoms and water- or silicone-based lubricant access and distribution. Community-driven evidence has highlighted the need to effectively distribute condoms in ways that ensure MSM have access to condoms and lubricant when needed. No experimental studies have compared distribution systems for condoms, but community-driven experience strongly suggests that the free provision of condoms in settings ranging from bathhouses to service centers for MSM has advantages over making condoms available for purchase in the private sector. Given (a) this community-driven evidence and plausibility for the effective provision of condoms, (b) the efficacy data around the use of condoms in preventing HIV, and (c) the fact that all available experimental data are consistent with the need for effective distribution of condoms and lubricants, this intervention is given a Grade 1, or strong, recommendation for inclusion in CHPIs.

Interventions to decrease unprotected anal intercourse. On the basis of not only largely observational data and modest effect from randomized, controlled trials, but also on the plausibility of the need for sustained interventions, the recommendation that interventions focused on decreasing unprotected anal intercourse for MSM in CHPIs be sustained is given a strong, or Grade 1, recommendation.

Conversion or reparative therapy. Conversion therapy, also known as reparative therapy or reorientation therapy, refers to a set of interventions or treatments designed to change the sexual orientation of homosexual or bisexual persons to that of heterosexuals. An overwhelming body of evidence supported by the international community of professional organizations who have reviewed the extant literature on the efficacy of conversion therapy has rejected it as ineffective, unnecessary, potentially harmful, and ethically controversial. On the basis of expert consensus in combination with a lack of biologic plausibility and efficacy data, reparative or corrective therapy is given a Grade 4, or inappropriate, recommendation for inclusion in CHPIs.

ART as primary and secondary prevention. Highly active antiretroviral therapy for secondary prevention is given a Grade 1, or strong, recommendation for inclusion in CHPIs.

Post- and preexposure prophylaxis with antiretrovirals. With one trial (iPrEx) providing evidence of efficacy and other trials ongoing in other at-risk populations, primary prevention of HIV with antiretrovirals, chemoprophylaxis, or preexposure prophylaxis is given a Grade 2b, or probable, recommendation for inclusion in CHPIs.

Voluntary counseling and testing. Given that VCT provides an important engagement point between MSM and health care providers in the context of a plausible prevention strategy and moderate efficacy data, VCT is given a Grade 1, or strong, recommendation for inclusion in CHPIs for MSM.

Circumcision. Although the data from observational studies in MSM are not as compelling as those for heterosexual men, some benefit may exist for MSM who are predominantly insertive and for those who also have female sexual partners. In this population of MSM, a shared biologic basis for protection exists and arguably supports the need for an interventional trial of circumcision in MSM. Because circumcision has proven efficacious in three trials among heterosexual men, an argument can be made for a trial among MSM in the context of CHPI services. Given the current status of efficacy results among MSM as well as a lack of community experience with this prevention strategy, circumcision is given a Grade 2b, or possible, recommendation.

Syndromic STI treatment. Using the available data, one cannot conclude that syndromic sexually transmitted infection (STI) surveillance and treatment is sufficient to curb HIV spread among MSM. However, given the consistently demonstrated causal role of STIs in HIV acquisition and transmission, effectively managing these infectious diseases should constitute a component of CHPIs. These infections are an important component of sexual and reproductive health in their own right. Moreover, treating symptomatic STIs provides an opportunity for engagement and the provision of risk reduction counseling, which have been shown to decrease high-risk sexual practices. Thus, treating STIs is given a Grade 2a, or probable, recommendation for inclusion in CHPIs for MSM in LMICs.

Vaccination. Although no research is yet available on the role of human papillomavirus (HPV) vaccination in preventing HIV infection, HPV's role in promoting HIV acquisition and transmission among MSM creates an expectation that the HPV vaccine may have a significant role in comprehensive HIV prevention for MSM. Further research among MSM is needed, but the HPV vaccine may be an important component of primary HIV prevention among populations practicing receptive anal intercourse, such as MSM. As such, HPV vaccination has been designated a Grade 2a, or probable, intervention for MSM.

Rectal microbicides. Given the lack of current efficacy data, rectal microbicides are given a Grade 2c, or pending, recommendation for inclusion in CHPIs.

Findings: Targeting Structural Risk

All the individual interventions described so far, both biomedical and behavioral, have one thing in common: they are designed to address the needs of high-risk individuals rather than to target the population as a whole. In contrast, structural interventions are intended to target the entire population in a community or country by attempting to modify social, economic, political, and environmental factors.

An important example from an LMIC was the development of the policy "Brazil without Homophobia," which was sponsored by the Brazilian government and focused on decreasing population-based stigma targeting lesbian, gay, bisexual, and transgendered (LGBT) populations. It included a school-based component to decrease homophobia in the public schools and aimed at increasing self-esteem and self-efficacy for LGBT youth as an HIV preventive intervention.

Although convincing efficacy data are absent, a growing body of literature links structural risk with increased rates of individual risk for HIV infection among MSM. Moreover, plausibility exists that improving contexts for MSM will facilitate provision of HIV services and service uptake among them. Last, consistent consensus in community groups of MSM indicates that structural interventions are an important component of CHPIs for MSM in LMICs. Therefore, structural interventions are collectively given a strong, or Grade 1, recommendation for inclusion (table ES.2).

Table ES.2 Strength of Recommendations for Inclusion of Specific Prevention Components in CHPI Package for MSM

Intervention	*Components*	*GRADE level*	*Strength of recommendation*
Condoms and water- or silicone-based lubricants	Effective distribution	Grade 1	Strong
	Counseling and education about condoms and lubricants	Grade 1	Strong
	Thicker condoms	Grade 2b	Possible
	Female condoms	Grade 2b	Possible
Behavioral interventions	Individualized risk-reduction counseling	Grade 2a	Probable
	Conversion or reparative therapy	Grade 4	Inappropriate
	Didactic teaching	Grade 2b	Possible
	Brief client-focused counseling	Grade 2a	Probable
Intervention characteristics	Sustained interventions	Grade 1	Strong
	Community-level interventions	Grade 1	Strong
Highly active ART and ARV agent–based prevention modes	Method of secondary prevention	Grade 1	Strong
	Primary prevention	Grade 2b	Possible
	Address substance use and mental health disorders to increase adherence	Grade 2a	Probable
	Chemoprophylaxis (preexposure prophylaxis)	Grade 2a	Probable
VCT	HIV testing	Grade 1	Strong
	Rapid testing for HIV	Grade 2a	Probable
	LGBT sensitization	Grade 1	Strong
Circumcision	n.a.	Grade 2b	Possible
Syndromic STI treatment	Herpes simplex virus-2 suppression	Grade 4	Inappropriate
	Screening and treatment of all genital ulcerative diseases	Grade 2a	Probable
Vaccination	HPV	Grade 2a	Probable
Rectal microbicides	n.a.	Grade 2c	Pending
Structural interventions	Decriminalization, government-sponsored antihomophobia policy, mass media engagement, male engagement programs, community systems strengthening, health sector interventions	Grade 1	Strong

Source: Stefan Baral, Chris Beyrer, and Andrea Wirtz.
Note: Recommendations generated here employed the HASTE system described in chapter 8. n.a. = not applicable.

Modeling MSM Populations, HIV Transmission, and Intervention Impact

Developing an evidence-based response to the HIV epidemic requires understanding of a country's epidemic features, assessment of available resources and costs for various response options, and knowledge of appropriate and effective interventions. Understanding the proportions of HIV attributable to same-sex practices among men by country and region is important to understanding and responding to the HIV epidemic because MSM as a group constitute a significant portion of the HIV epidemic in many LMICs. Such calculations can then be used in tandem with mathematical models and cost estimates to assess and estimate appropriate interventions to meet public health priorities at the country level. For HIV interventions, mathematical models and cost analysis can be used to inform national and local programming by providing estimates of resources and funding necessary to reach targets, identify effective combinations or alternative interventions, and identify potential achievements with available resources.

Adapting and Using the Goals Model to Estimate HIV Prevalence and Incidence

In collaboration with the Futures Institute, the Goals Model was adapted to estimate HIV prevalence and incidence with and without one or more interventions delivered at different levels of coverage. In recognition of the social and behavioral variations that exist among MSM, a collaborative effort was undertaken with the Futures Institute to revise the Goals Model to allow the input of epidemiologic data relating to four risk categories among MSM. These risk categories are now defined as follows:

- High-risk MSM, who are male sex workers
- Medium-risk MSM, who are men with more than one male sexual partner in last 12 months
- Low-risk MSM, which includes men with no or one male sex partner in last 12 months (stable relationship)
- MSM IDUs, who are MSM who also inject drugs

The adapted program now accommodates estimates of the proportion of the male population that falls into each of these four risk groups as well as HIV and STI prevalence estimates, and behavioral inputs of each MSM risk group among the heterosexual male populations. The Goals Model was further adapted to include the distribution of condoms with water-based lubricants, community-based behavioral interventions, and access to ART to provide insight into the effects of proven interventions and possible combinations for reaching national targets.

Methods for the Models

The Goals Model has been widely used for program planning and projection purposes.

Inputs and assumptions for goals. The Goals Model is deterministic and requires data in three main areas to project HIV prevalence and incidence: national data for MSM and the general population on demography, sexual behavior, and HIV and STI prevalence. MSM-specific data were collected by communicating with country experts, whereas information specific to the general population, including HIV and STI prevalence percentages, intervention coverage, and other country background data, were collected from UNAIDS, annual country reporting data to the UN General Assembly Special Session on HIV/AIDS, the U.S. Agency for International Development, and country ministry of health reports. Working with in-country experts to collect MSM-specific data allowed issues specific to the modeling work to be addressed, such as variability in definitions, in recall periods, and in the data that are collected and their accessibility. Such collaborations helped ensure the accuracy and validity of country-specific data. Where MSM-specific data were not available from local experts, UNAIDS reports and peer-reviewed publications provided missing information. Other assumptions of transmission multipliers, intervention effectiveness, and time in infection stages were preloaded into the Goals Model from previous work, and these assumptions can be found in appendix A of this report.

Regarding inputs in general epidemiology to the Goals Model, the work conducted by the Futures Institute for the consortium aids2031 contributed to the majority of inputs on transmissibility, infectiousness, and intervention effectiveness, and the item "infectiousness when on ART" was updated with the most recent findings reported by Donnell and colleagues (2010), who reported a 92 percent reduction in HIV transmission after ART was initiated. The consortium aids2031 also contributed to the matrices used in the Goals Model detailing the effect of exposure to a prevention intervention on (a) the reduction in nonuse of condoms; (b) the reduction in nontreatment of STIs; (c) the reduction in number of partners; and (d) the rise in age at first sex for the high-, medium-, and low-risk heterosexual and IDU populations. Because two new interventions for MSM were added, the effects of exposure to MSM-targeted prevention interventions were derived through the systematic review of HIV prevention interventions for MSM. The results of the systematic review were added to the impact matrix for each MSM risk group.

Estimating the attributable fraction. Estimation of the total fraction of new HIV-positive cases attributable to MSM behavior is nested in the overall Goals Model analyses for each of the case countries. The number of new HIV infections used for the baseline was estimated by the Goals Model in each country's current state (that is, without any additional interventions to those currently in place). The HIV transmission probability for MSM was assumed to be zero, to use the counterfactual to estimate the number of new HIV infections *not* attributed to MSM behavior. The numerator, in turn, for the attributable fraction was calculated as the number of new HIV cases not attributed to MSM subtracted from the total number of new HIV cases; the denominator was the number of total new HIV cases. The fraction is presented for year 2015 for each case country.

Estimating effect. MSM-specific interventions to prevent HIV infections were assessed using multiple intervention scenarios with the outcome being total new infections. These interventions include the individual interventions of distribution of condoms with water-based lubricants with partner reduction counseling as well as community-based behavioral interventions. The interventions were modeled in three scenarios:

1. Null: current coverage drops to zero after 2007 for MSM-specific interventions only, all other interventions remaining constant.
2. Current: coverage remains current for MSM-specific community-based behavioral intervention and individual interventions, all other interventions remaining constant.
3. Coverage of 100 percent for MSM: community-based behavioral interventions and individual interventions increase to 100 percent from the 2007 coverage level, and ART coverage increases by a percentage sufficient to cover the estimated population of MSM living with HIV by 2015.

The Goals program currently does not target ART coverage for specific risk groups; therefore, this component was calculated by using current ART coverage data and then estimating the percentage of those on ART who may be HIV-positive MSM. The proportion of MSM with unmet need for ART was then added to the current coverage level; for this exercise only, the increase in ART is assumed to go strictly to the HIV-positive MSM population. This third scenario can be used to estimate the effect of a supportive environment in which interventions for MSM are fully provided and HIV-positive MSM have full access to ART.

For countries with an HIV epidemic among IDUs (Thailand and Ukraine), a fourth scenario was modeled that assessed an increase in coverage of services by 2015 to reach 100 percent coverage of interventions for MSM (scenario 3) plus 60 percent coverage of services for IDUs, including substitution therapy, harm reduction, and counseling services. Sensitivity analyses were performed using upper and lower bounds of impacts of MSM-specific interventions determined by the systematic review described previously.

Results. Impact assessments were performed for the four focus countries: Kenya, Peru, Thailand, and Ukraine. The results for Peru are shown in figure ES.3. These projections from the Peru data show that if coverage of interventions for MSM and ART remains constant, the number of new HIV infections in the general population will increase to reach almost 20,000 by 2015. Much higher coverage of interventions for MSM will be needed to change the trajectory of HIV in Peru. Increasing MSM-specific interventions to 100 percent coverage and providing HIV-positive MSM full access to ART, however, could effect a decrease in the epidemic or at least a stabilization.

Figure ES.3 Projections of the Number of New HIV Infections with Implementation of Three Intervention Scenarios for MSM, Peru, 2008–15

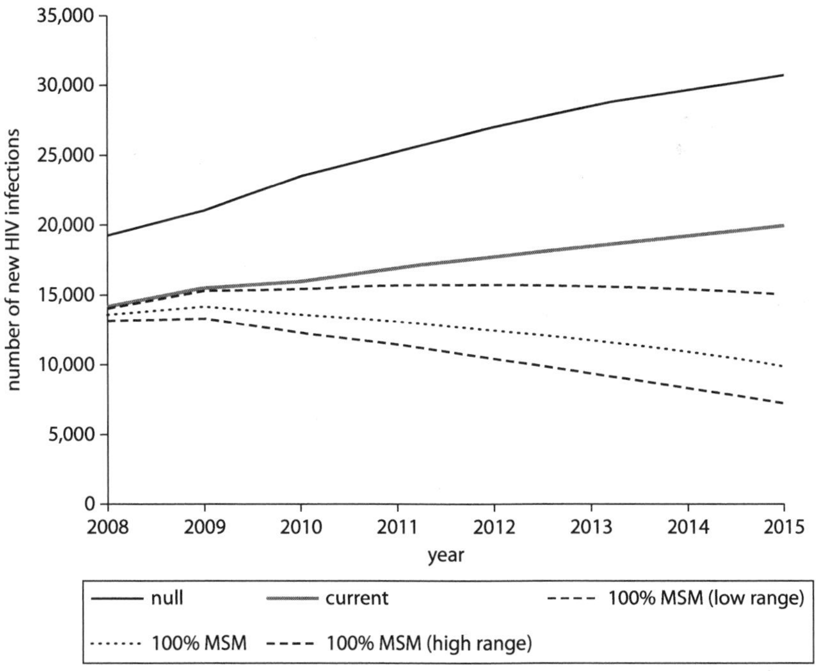

Source: Authors with L. Bollinger.

Modeling Cost and Cost-Effectiveness

In this section, the effects and costs of interventions for MSM in selected LMICs are demonstrated, modeled with varying coverage levels and combinations of interventions. These modeling and costing exercises were performed to demonstrate the utility of the Goals Model to inform strategic planning and the variation in results observed across epidemic scenarios and environments.

Methods

Coverage of selected interventions plays an important role in estimating impacts and costs. ART coverage is also a critical input and still varies substantially across LMICs.

Estimating effect: MSM-specific interventions and coverage scenarios. The effect of interventions on the HIV epidemic among MSM can be assessed by varying levels of access to ART among the general population. Predictions are based on rollout of preventive interventions. The number of HIV infections is estimated with five scenarios, assuming all other intervention coverage remains at current levels:

1. Null, or no MSM-specific intervention
2. Community-based behavioral intervention
3. Community-based behavioral intervention plus an individual intervention package of condoms with lubricant and partner reduction counseling
4. Community-based behavioral intervention plus an individual intervention package of condoms with lubricant and partner reduction counseling plus expanding ART coverage
5. Expanding ART coverage alone

The null intervention scenario is calculated by setting the current coverage of the two interventions for MSM at zero, as if all such interventions were suddenly removed. Then, the other combinations of interventions are tested at current coverage levels (assuming 30 percent coverage from 2008 through 2015 for both the community-based behavioral intervention and the individual intervention package of condoms with lubricant and partner reduction counseling, based on variations between 20 and 40 percent reported for intervention coverage). These combinations were then modeled to observe effects if 60 percent coverage were reached gradually by 2015. Finally, to estimate the effect of an optimally supportive environment, combinations in which interventions for MSM and ART reach 100 percent were modeled.

Estimating the costs of interventions. To estimate the costs of interventions for MSM, a comprehensive review was conducted. Data on the location in the country (for example, urban or rural), setting of the intervention (primary health care, hospital, community), target population, numbers in the target population, numbers treated or served, methods used in costing, costing perspective, and items included in the costing were also extracted. Data relating to the costing methods used and the cost data reported converted to 2008 U.S. dollars and international dollars (to reflect differences in purchasing power) were collected. Overall, 93 studies of relevance were found in the first phase of the literature search, and 74 additional studies of relevance were found in the second phase (or 167 total studies).

Results

Table ES.3 provides the total infections averted and average cost-effectiveness of various single interventions to control HIV/AIDS among

Table ES.3 Total Costs, Total Infections Averted, and Average Cost-Effectiveness of Various Single Interventions to Control HIV/AIDS among MSM Compared to No Intervention in Peru, 2007–15

Intervention	*Coverage level (%)*	*Total cost (2008 US$)*	*Total infections averted*	*Average cost per HIV infection averted (2008 US$)*
Promotion and distribution of condoms with lubricants	30	33,676,446	16,465	2,045
Promotion and distribution of condoms with lubricants	30–60	49,764,315	25,252	1,971
Promotion and distribution of condoms with lubricants	100	111,621,982	53,276	2,095
Community level	30	131,857,534	30,068	4,385
Community level	30–60	194,567,912	45,455	4,280
Community level	100	435,288,819	92,307	4,716
ART	30	472,701,927	26,274	186,245
ART	60	950,443,131	59,781	164,583
ART	100	1,598,770,873	120,704	137,116

Source: Authors.

MSM in Peru (the full report contains the same analyses and findings for Kenya, Thailand, and Ukraine) for 2007 to 2015, compared to no intervention. The largest number of HIV infections is averted through ART for MSM, apart from the scenarios where the interventions are set at 30 percent coverage, in which case community-level behavioral interventions avert more infections. However, ART is consistently the most costly of the three interventions examined.

Total costs, infections averted, and cost-effectiveness are then calculated for each country. Again, Peru is used as the example (table ES.4).

Table ES.4 Total Costs, Total Infections Averted, and Incremental Cost-Effectiveness of Nondominated[a] Intervention Combinations to Control HIV/AIDS among MSM in Peru, 2007–15

Intervention package	*Details*	*Total costs (2008 US$)*	*Total infections averted*	*Incremental cost-effectiveness ratio (2008 US$)*
P1	Promotion and distribution of condoms with lubricants, 30–60% coverage	49,764,315	25,252	1,971
P2	Promotion and distribution of condoms with lubricants, 100% coverage	111,621,982	53,276	2,207
P3	Promotion and distribution of condoms with lubricants, 100% coverage + community-level MSM, 60% coverage	306,189,894	98,731	4,280
P4	Promotion and distribution of condoms with lubricants, 100% coverage + community-level MSM, 100% coverage	546,910,801	145,583	5,138
P5	Promotion and distribution of condoms with lubricants, 100% coverage + community-level MSM, 100% coverage + ART, 100% coverage	2,145,681,674	266,287	13,245

Source: Authors.

a. Excludes interventions that were more costly but less effective than others (dominated interventions) and those with higher incremental cost-effectiveness ratios than more effective options (weakly dominated interventions).

Finally, these numbers are used to graphically depict the expansion path for interventions in Peru (figure ES.4).

Across countries, robust differences are seen in HIV intervention costs and intervention effects on HIV infections relating to MSM. In reducing HIV infections among MSM, promotion and distribution of condoms with lubricants is generally the most cost-effective use of resources, followed by community-level behavioral interventions, and then ART. ART may be comparatively less cost-effective than condom and lubricant distribution for the effect of reducing overall HIV infections among MSM, but ART is usually already implemented as a strategy with other multiple aims and cost-effectiveness measures. By World Health Organization benchmarks of cost-effectiveness, comparing costs of interventions per disability-adjusted life year averted against per capita gross national income, all of the assessed interventions provide value for money.

Discussion of Costs

In general, the main finding from this literature search and analysis is that few data are reported in the public literature on the costs of providing HIV/AIDS interventions to MSM. The literature search revealed only 18 studies specific for MSM. Thus, without additional primary data collection, assessing the costs or the cost-effectiveness of interventions

Figure ES.4 Expansion Path for Incremental Addition of Interventions in Peru

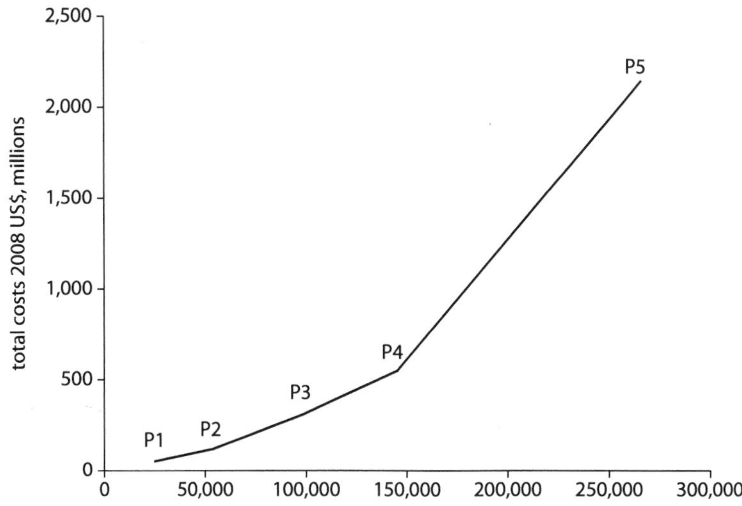

Source: Authors.

targeting MSM will remain uncertain. In this study, the choice has been made to rely on data for interventions targeting other groups that may be somewhat similar to MSM-targeted programs, but the results in this book should be interpreted as tentative, order-of-magnitude unit costs. The uncertainty ranges tend to reflect this conclusion.

The models for the outreach intervention show that different target populations (for example, male only compared with female only, or male only compared with both sexes) significantly ($p < 0.05$) affect unit costs. This finding reinforces the notion that further research into the costs of interventions and programs for MSM is needed. Such research can define not only the extent to which these programs have different costs from other types of programs, but also the reason they have different costs, which will help make results more generalizable. (An initial hypothesis may postulate that the outreach techniques needed for different programs, the number of contacts that peer outreach workers can establish in one location, and the need for lubricants could all influence the unit costs.)

Policy and Human Rights

The international community is at a critical period in the HIV response. HIV infections continue to rise in a number of subpopulations, resources for continuing the response are threatened, and an array of struggles over the human rights and social and political standing of MSM are the subject of intense public, media, political, and public health debate. Major advances in the legal standing of sexual minorities, most notably the repeal of India's sodomy laws and the end of criminalization of same-sex relations and diverse gender identities in Nepal, have been tempered by sharp rises in homophobic attacks and discriminatory legislative efforts in a number of countries.

Yet, as this book demonstrates, the epidemics among MSM in many LMICs are a severe, expanding, and underappreciated component of global HIV. Access to essential services for these men remains grossly under-resourced, challenging to access, and insufficient in scale and scope to address these expanding epidemics and to provide services for the growing number of MSM in need.

The nine countries investigated for this book broadly cover the spectrum of legal and policy environments for MSM in LMICs. They include countries with long-standing legal protection for MSM (Brazil and Peru), recent decriminalization (most recently India, and in the early 1990s, Russia and Ukraine), acceptance—if not tolerance—with no prior history of criminalization (Thailand), and active discrimination against MSM and laws against homosexuality (Kenya and Senegal). The most fundamental policy recommendations drawn from these reviews follow:

- Criminalization of same-sex behavior has profound implications across the spectrum of policies, issues, and programs for MSM: criminalization matters.
- Responses to HIV epidemics among MSM in these highly disparate political and human rights environments have to be context specific: one size will not fit all.
- Mainstreaming of programs and services for MSM into public sector health systems may improve rights contexts in some settings but may be harmful in others, making HIV programs targets of public attack: mainstreaming must be carefully evaluated and cannot be assumed to be an improvement in rights or care.
- Community participation in every step of program development and implementation for MSM is crucial: the community is *the* key partner for this population.
- Laws and policies that promote universal access and gender equality in principle may fail for MSM in practice where homophobic cultural, religious, or political forces are active: good policies for HIV do not guarantee good outcomes for MSM and other sexual minorities.
- Epidemiologic and cost-effectiveness findings are consistent with the rights argument, not counter to it: responding to MSM with high rates of coverage has positive effects for overall HIV trajectories in all four scenarios studied.
- Although quantification of the effect of structural interventions is important, action is mandated to decrease human rights abuses against MSM on social justice and human dignity grounds alone.

The role of governance in the AIDS response is relevant because in only a limited number of diseases other than HIV are the social drivers of risk much more predictive of disease burden than endogenous susceptibility. To effectively respond to social drivers of risk, governments should adopt evidence-based interventions mitigating the effects of the risk environment. In the context of MSM, many governments have done the opposite and have potentiated the risk environment by limiting the availability of service provision and preventing the uptake of whatever services are available. Moreover, although the majority of the laws criminalizing same-sex practices in these settings are national laws, they are implemented and enforced by municipal and regional tiers of government. This factor is relevant to the international community because all of the countries that criminalize same-sex practices are UN member states and signatories to a number of conventions that include legislated protections for sexual minorities. Separate from the issue of governance decisions related to politicians is the concept of public health governance. Whereas public health is global in that (a) infectious diseases know no boundaries and (b) international institutions, including UN agencies, provide technical support and guidance to all UN member states, the protection of the public's health is still implemented and operationalized at a local or regional level. The public health practitioner is mandated to develop comprehensive health protection and promote programming for all populations at risk for a disease. For HIV, that mandate includes MSM in the vast majority of the settings where HIV has been studied.

References

Adam, P. C. G., J. B. F. de Wit, I. Toskin, B. M. Mathers, M. Nashkhoev, I. Zablotska, R. Lyerla, and D. Rugg. 2009. "Estimating Levels of HIV Testing, HIV Prevention Coverage, HIV Knowledge, and Condom Use among Men Who Have Sex with Men (MSM) in Low-Income and Middle-Income Countries." *Journal of Acquired Immune Deficiency Syndromes* 52 (Suppl. 2): S143–51.

Beyrer, C., S. D. Baral, D. Walker, A. L. Wirtz, B. Johns, and F. Sifakis. 2010. "The Expanding Epidemics of HIV Type 1 among Men Who Have Sex with Men in Low- and Middle-Income Countries: Diversity and Consistency." *Epidemiologic Reviews* 32 (1): 137–51.

Donnell, D., J. M. Baeten, J. Kiarie, K. K. Thomas, W. Stevens, C. R. Cohen, J. McIntyre, J. R Lingappa, and C. Celum for the Partners in Prevention HSV/HIV Transmission Study Team. 2010. "Heterosexual HIV-1 Transmission after Initiation of Antiretroviral Therapy: A Prospective Cohort Analysis." *Lancet* 375 (9731): 2092–98.

Grant, R., J. Lama, P. Anderson, V. McMahan, A. Y. Liu, L. Vargas, P. Goicochea, M. Casapía, J. V. Guanira-Carranza, M. E. Ramirez-Cardich, et al. 2010. "Preexposure Chemoprophylaxis for HIV Prevention in Men Who Have Sex with Men." *New England Journal of Medicine* 363 (27): 2587–99.

Mathers, B. M., L. Degenhardt, P. Adam, I. Toskin, M. Nashkhoev, R. Lyerla, and D. Rugg. 2009. "Estimating the Level of HIV Prevention Coverage, Knowledge and Protective Behavior among Injecting Drug Users: What Does the 2008 UNGASS Reporting Round Tell Us?" *Journal of Acquired Immune Deficiency Syndromes* 52 (Suppl. 2): S132–42.

Tang, K. C., B. C. K. Choi, and R. Beaglehole. 2008. "Grading of Evidence of the Effectiveness of Health Promotion Interventions." *Journal of Epidemiology and Community Health* 62 (9): 832–34.

CHAPTER 1

Introduction

HIV/AIDS first emerged among populations of gay men and other men who have sex with men (MSM[1]) in Western Europe, North America, and Australia in the early 1980s. This reality shaped early responses to the epidemic and has had lasting effects on the stigma associated with HIV/AIDS. More than a quarter century later and in an increasingly broad range of countries, contexts, and development levels, emerging data show that epidemics of HIV among MSM are no longer limited to the high-income countries in which they were initially described. Recent evidence from a wide range of sources suggests that MSM are at marked risk for HIV infection in low- and middle-income countries (LMICs) in Asia, Africa, Latin America and the Caribbean, and in Eastern Europe and Central Asia (Baral et al. 2007; Smith et al. 2009; van Griensven et al. 2009). HIV prevalence rates have been consistently higher among MSM than estimates of such rates for the general population of reproductive-age men almost wherever MSM have been well studied, and HIV incidence data, although markedly scarcer, generally have supported high acquisition and transmission risks among MSM in multiple contexts, in varied cultural settings, and across economic levels.

Research among MSM in LMICs has been limited by the criminalization and social stigmatization of these behaviors, the safety considerations for study participants, the hidden nature of these populations, and a lack of targeted funding. Because these men are so hidden, behavior of MSM is generally underreported in population-based surveys, and work has been limited on the kinds of surveillance necessary to characterize these men and the emerging epidemics affecting them. Most available data evaluating determinants of HIV risk among MSM are derived from high-income country samples. Available evidence from these countries suggests that structural risks—social, economic, political, or legal factors—are likely as important as individual-level risk factors in shaping HIV risks and HIV/AIDS treatment and care options for these men. These same factors may profoundly influence how HIV epidemics in MSM affect wider populations.

MSM are notably underserved and underresourced populations in many settings. They have limited coverage and access to HIV/AIDS prevention, treatment, and care services—with some estimates suggesting that fewer than 1 in 10 MSM worldwide have access to the most basic package of preventive interventions (Global HIV Prevention Working Group 2007). Stigma, discrimination, and criminalization limit these men's access to what services are available. Nevertheless, considerable evidence shows that HIV preventive interventions at individual, community, and population levels have been effective and need to be greatly expanded to control the global epidemic of HIV among MSM and mitigate its impact.

Improving LMIC responses to HIV/AIDS requires expanding services for MSM and addressing their exclusion from key emerging interventions, such as expanded voluntary counseling and testing, earlier access to treatment, and treatment-as-prevention modalities. This book seeks to inform these responses by posing and attempting to answer several key questions:

- What fraction of the burden of HIV disease in selected countries is attributable to gay, bisexual, and other behaviors of MSM? How does this proportion vary by scenario and across the representative states?
- Where are these selected countries in 2010 in terms of coverage for prevention, treatment, and care for MSM?
- What would constitute a minimum acceptable package of evidence-based and human rights–affirming services for prevention, treatment, and care of MSM?
- What resources, political will, and novel approaches would be necessary to reach acceptable coverage levels of MSM in the targeted countries with this essential minimum package of services? How might

resources be maximized to ensure acceptable coverage of populations of MSM by the prevention and treatment packages?

Although a global response is called for, most country-specific epidemics among MSM have both common and unique features when compared to those in other LMICs. To answer these and related questions, a several-stage analysis has been conducted of the global epidemics of HIV among MSM in LMICs. First, the available data on MSM—including taxonomies, HIV epidemiology, risk factors, and access to prevention, treatment, and care—were reviewed in nine selected countries: Brazil, India, Kenya, Malawi, Peru, the Russian Federation, Senegal, Thailand, and Ukraine. A global review of the epidemiologic literature was conducted, and these data were used to generate an algorithmic approach to characterizing HIV epidemics among MSM. This effort yielded four scenarios for HIV epidemics among MSM.

For the second component of this assessment, the existing literature on HIV prevention among MSM was reviewed. These data were analyzed using a novel system to evaluate HIV interventions called the Highest Attainable STandard of Evidence (HASTE) to generate an essential package of HIV prevention services.

In collaboration with the Futures Institute, the Goals Model was then adapted for MSM. One country was selected for each scenario (Kenya, Peru, Thailand, Ukraine) to use the modified Goals Model and the data on preventive interventions to model the impact of HIV prevention services on the epidemic of MSM. A costing exercise was done to estimate the costs and cost-effectiveness of these programs.

Finally, a policy and human rights assessment was done based on these findings to evaluate the impact of enabling policy environments on these HIV epidemics.

Note

1. MSM is a technical phrase intended to be less stigmatizing than culturally bound terms such as gay, bisexual, or homosexual. It describes same-sex behaviors between men rather than identities, orientations, or cultural categories. Therefore, the term MSM includes gay men, bisexuals, MSM who do not identify as gay or bisexual despite their behaviors, male sex workers, some biologically male transgendered persons, and a range of culture- and country-specific populations of MSM. MSM belonging to these diverse populations may have both individual- and network-level risks, and these groups may have diverging HIV epidemic dynamics.

References

Baral, S., F. Sifakis, F. Cleghorn, and C. Beyrer. 2007. "Elevated Risk for HIV Infection among Men Who Have Sex with Men in Low- and Middle-Income Countries 2000–2006: A Systematic Review." *PLoS Medicine* 4 (12): e339.

Global HIV Prevention Working Group. 2007. *Bringing HIV Prevention to Scale: An Urgent Global Priority.* http://www.globalhivprevention.org/pdfs/PWG-HIV_prevention_report_FINAL.pdf.

Smith, A. D., P. Tapsoba, N. Peshu, E. J. Sanders, and H. W. Jaffe. 2009. "Men Who Have Sex with Men and HIV/AIDS in Sub-Saharan Africa." *Lancet* 374 (9687): 416–22.

van Griensven, F., J. W. de Lind van Wijngaarden, S. Baral, and A. Grulich. 2009. "The Global Epidemic of HIV Infection among Men Who Have Sex with Men." *Current Opinion in HIV and AIDS* 4 (4): 300–307.

PART I

Epidemic Scenarios and Focus Countries

CHAPTER 2

Introduction to the Epidemic Scenarios

Key themes:

- HIV epidemics among men who have sex with men (MSM) in low- and middle-income countries (LMICs) occur in highly diverse contexts of other affected risk groups, availability and access to HIV prevention and care, and social and political commitment to addressing HIV among MSM.
- Despite the contextual heterogeneity, MSM in LMICs uniformly bear a disproportionate burden of HIV infection when compared to the general population.
- In many countries, because same-sex behavior is socially stigmatized or even illegal, the epidemiology of HIV among MSM is based on very limited data.
- In an effort to align HIV epidemiology with a robust response to the HIV epidemic in these countries, four epidemic scenarios were developed to provide granularity to the United Nations definition of concentrated epidemic states.
- Categorization of countries in these scenarios, which take into account the social and HIV transmission contexts within which HIV epidemics among MSM occur, is not static. As HIV epidemics change, an algorithmic approach allows policy makers to match epidemiologic state with pertinent HIV prevention approaches.

The emerging regional epidemics among MSM in Africa, Asia, Latin America, and Eastern Europe are heterogeneous in themselves but are occurring in regional contexts of diverse HIV epidemics that vary with factors including predominant modes of spread, epidemic level and stage, gender and age distribution, and levels of prevention, treatment, and care services (Beyrer 2007). Sub-Saharan Africa, for example, remains by far the most affected region—and the only part of the world where generalized epidemics affecting more than 10 percent of all reproductive-age adults have been seen (UNAIDS 2008). Even within Africa, only among a cluster of contiguous countries in the southern region are multiple states with HIV prevalence greater than 15 or 20 percent seen among all adults of reproductive age. HIV prevalence rates in West and Central Africa have long been lower than those of the south, although the evidence suggests these epidemics are among the world's oldest. North Africa has largely been spared. The MSM component of Africa's epidemics is arguably the least studied, most hidden, and least understood of any region. Asia has not only had several quite severe HIV epidemics, most notably in Cambodia, Myanmar, and Thailand, but has also seen states with very low and seemingly stable HIV rates, including Japan, the Philippines, and the Republic of Korea. South America has multiple HIV epidemics that are highly concentrated among MSM. Fortunately, early predictions that Asia or Latin America might suffer "Africa-like" epidemics of HIV have not been supported by available evidence, and it is now clear that "Africa-like" epidemics have really only been seen in Africa. This great diversity suggests that regional approaches to epidemics among MSM must be clearly situated within their wider epidemic contexts to be understood and to develop informed and appropriate responses.

This book seeks to advance epidemiologic specificity in characterizing outbreaks among MSM in relation to the wider epidemic contexts in which they occur. To do so, a comprehensive review using systematic methodologies was conducted of the recent HIV/AIDS literature, and an algorithmic approach was developed to assist in understanding epidemics among MSM and the populations in which such epidemics are occurring. The algorithm classifies these epidemic scenarios based on select criteria relevant to the global HIV epidemic. This study then selected one representative country from each epidemic scenario to describe key features and responses.

Summaries from each example country begin by presenting a description of typologies of MSM and transgendered individuals used in epidemiologic studies. Inclusion of such descriptions is necessary because the taxonomy of male sexual orientation and gender identity is culturally bound, can be complex, and has important implications for HIV programming. The evidence for the various populations of MSM in each country has been reviewed, and differential risks of HIV, risk practices, and differing barriers to accessing health care and prevention services were ascertained if possible. Additionally, a critical component of HIV risk in all the regions explored is the intersection of HIV epidemics among MSM and substance use. This includes both injecting drug use risk and noninjection risks, such as those associated with noninjecting use of methamphetamine and cocaine and synthetic club drugs among MSM in many settings. This factor is critically important for MSM in injecting drug use–driven HIV epidemics but relevant across all regions. A recent study found that injecting drug use behavior was common among MSM in Botswana, Malawi, and Namibia, and substance use has been a prominent feature of outbreaks among MSM in Brazil and Thailand. Country summaries conclude with descriptions of the sexual and network dynamics, acknowledging that the sexual behaviors, patterns, and networks of MSM with female sex partners are highly diverse, complex, and important for understanding HIV spread among these men and in the populations of which they are a part. Because marriage and fatherhood are both so normative for men in most societies, and so highly socially valued and enforced, the great majority of MSM in many settings are married to women.

Methods

Search Strategies

The methods used in developing search strategies, abstracting data, and generating aggregate estimates of HIV disease burden among MSM and the general population have been previously described (Baral et al. 2007). In brief, systematic searches were conducted of databases including PubMed, EMBASE, EBSCO, and the *Cochrane Database of Systematic Reviews* up until January 1, 2010. Articles and citations were downloaded, organized, and reviewed using the QUOSA v8 information management software package (QUOSA [computer program], Version 8.05, Waltham, MA).

Medical Subject Heading terms from the U.S. National Library of Medicine were used as keywords in searching Google Scholar. In addition, databases, including Scopus and Web of Science, that link articles on the basis of complex algorithms were used to assess the validity of the search strategies. Both online and CD-based volumes of abstracts were searched from the International AIDS Conference; the Conference on HIV Pathogenesis, Treatment, and Prevention; and the Conference on Retroviruses and Opportunistic Infections with similar restrictions using Boolean logic (figure 2.1).

Figure 2.1 Search Protocol and Results: Systematic Review of Published and Unpublished Literature on the HIV Epidemic among MSM in LMICs

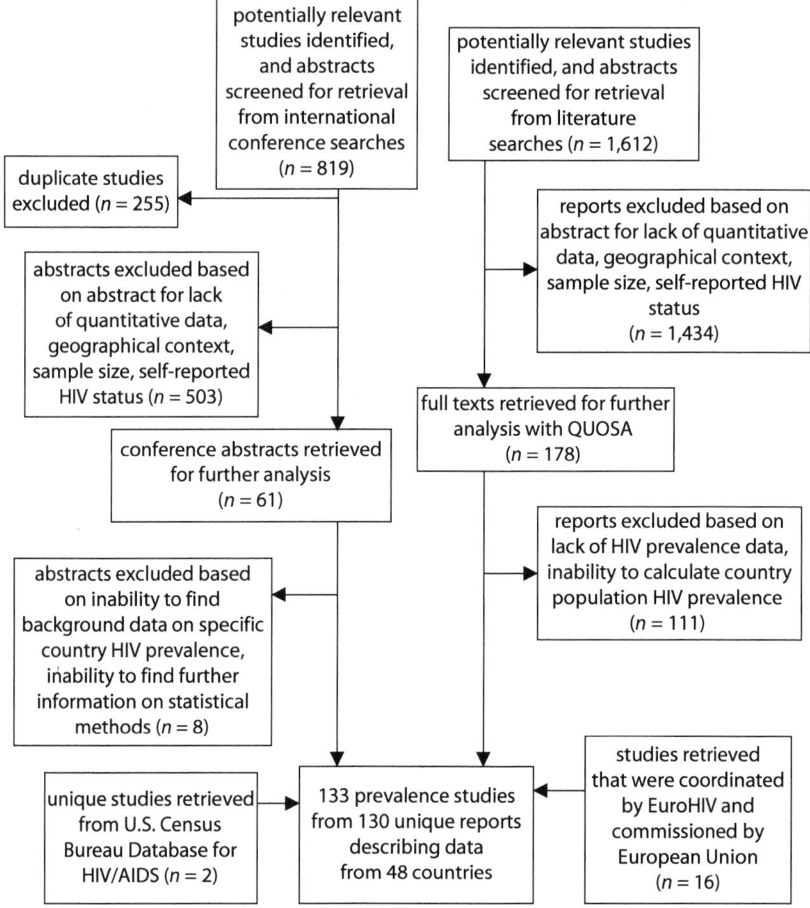

Source: Beyrer et al. 2010.

An Algorithmic Approach to Characterize Epidemics among MSM

The development of the algorithm begins with the standard Joint United Nations Programme on HIV/AIDS definition of a concentrated HIV epidemic, which is greater than 5 percent HIV prevalence in any high-risk group, such as MSM, injecting drug users (IDUs), or female or male sex workers (UNAIDS and WHO 2000).

The algorithm proceeds to the ratio of HIV prevalence among MSM to that among the general population, and dichotomizes this categorization into a ratio of (a) less than 10 or (b) greater than or equal to 10. The basis for the selection of a ratio of 10 as the cutoff value builds on prior work (Baral et al. 2007), which indicated that the adjusted odds ratio for MSM compared to other men in medium-HIV-prevalence countries was 9.6 (95 percent confidence interval: 9.0, 10.2). Assuming the prevalence ratio will approximate the odds ratio, this book uses the upper level of that interval to guide the differentiation between countries whose HIV prevalence among MSM is substantial compared to that of the general population. The algorithm then takes into account the ratio of HIV infection prevalence among IDUs to the general population, again dichotomized into ratios of (a) less than 10 or (b) greater than or equal to 10. Following a parallel rationale to that regarding MSM and because of a lack of a similar analysis for IDUs, this study uses the same cutoff value of 10 for the ratio of HIV prevalence among IDUs over that of the general population. The final step is the categorization by proportion of the adult male population engaging in injecting drug use behavior, dichotomized by (a) less than 1 percent and (b) greater than or equal to 1 percent, and categorization by proportion of the adult male population with a history of ever engaging in MSM behavior, again dichotomized (Mathers et al. 2008). Incorporation of denominator estimates for MSM and IDUs points to the extent of the HIV burden in a given country. Figure 2.2 illustrates the algorithm, and a detailed explanation for the algorithms that have yielded each of the four scenarios is available in appendix A.

LMIC Definitions

Economies are divided by the World Bank (2009) according to their 2008 gross national income per capita, calculated using the Atlas method (Sanchez et al. 2007). The groups are

- Low income, US$975 or less
- Lower-middle income, US$976–US$3,855

Figure 2.2 Algorithm Describing the Development of the Epidemic Scenarios

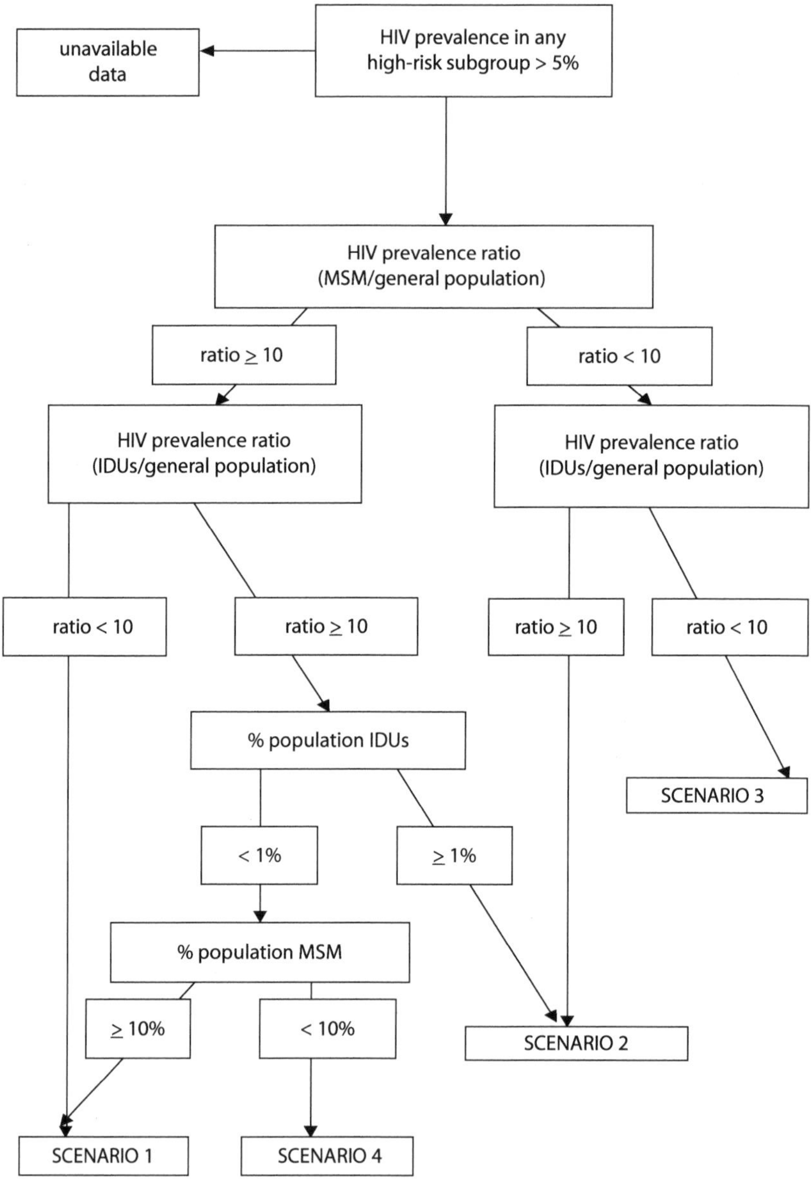

HIV prevalence in any high-risk subgroup > 5%

unavailable data

HIV prevalence ratio (MSM/general population)

ratio ≥ 10

ratio < 10

HIV prevalence ratio (IDUs/general population)

HIV prevalence ratio (IDUs/general population)

ratio < 10

ratio ≥ 10

ratio ≥ 10

ratio < 10

% population IDUs

SCENARIO 3

< 1%

≥ 1%

% population MSM

≥ 10%

< 10%

SCENARIO 2

SCENARIO 1

SCENARIO 4

Source: Beyrer et al. 2010.

- Upper-middle income, US$3,856–11,905
- High income, US$11,906 or more

Results

Search Findings

In all, 1,612 citations were identified from published reports, and 819 from international conferences after January 1, 2000 (see figure 2.1). After exclusion of duplicates and exclusion for lack of data, such as biological measures of HIV, 178 citations and 61 conference reports were retrieved and reviewed. A total of 133 prevalence studies from 130 unique reports met all inclusion criteria. These data describe HIV prevalence among MSM in a total of 48 LMICs.

Epidemic Scenarios and Representative Countries

Table 2.1 shows the MSM and general population HIV prevalence for the 48 countries. Figure 2.3 maps those countries in each of the regions where the available data suggest epidemics among MSM can be best characterized by one of the scenarios generated through use of the algorithm.

Use of the algorithm with available country-level data yields the following four epidemic scenarios:

- **Scenario 1:** Risks among MSM are the predominant exposure mode for HIV infection in the population. This scenario is seen across most of Latin and South America and in multiple settings in high-income countries. Here, HIV prevalence among MSM is generally over 10 percent; the ratio of MSM to the general population is very high (odds ratio is 33.5 in Baral et al. 2007); the prevalence among IDUs is variable, but the population prevalence of risks among IDUs is well under 1 percent of adults; and the proportion of men reporting a lifetime history of sex with another man is well under 10 percent of adults.

- **Scenario 2:** Risks occur among MSM within established HIV epidemics driven by injecting drug use. This scenario is the predominant epidemic context in Eastern Europe and Central Asia. Here, the HIV rate is highest among IDUs; the HIV prevalence ratio for HIV infection among MSM compared to the general population is less than 10, but the same ratio for IDUs compared to the general population is well over 10; and the proportion of the adult population with a lifetime history of ever injecting drugs is over 1 percent, the highest categorization stratum used by Mathers and colleagues (2008).

Table 2.1 HIV Prevalence Rates for MSM and General Population in 48 Countries

Country	*Sample size*	*Aggregate prevalence of HIV among MSM % (95% CI)*	*Women (15+) HIV prevalence*	*Men (15+) HIV prevalence*	*Population (15+) prevalence of HIV*	*Prevalence ratio: MSM vs. all*	*Prevalence ratio: MSM vs. women*	*Prevalence of IDU among population*	*HIV prevalence among IDU*	*Prevalence ratio: IDU vs. all*
Scenario 1. Risks among MSM are the predominant exposure mode for HIV infection in the population										
Ecuador	916	15.10 (12.8–17.4)	0.15	0.39	0.27	55.9	100.7	0.59	28.8	106.6
Peru*	22,284	13.80 (13.4–14.3)	0.21	0.53	0.37	37.3	65.7	0.59	13	35.1
Bolivia	520	21.20 (17.6–24.7)	0.07	0.20	0.13	163.1	302.9	0.59	28.8	221.3
Uruguay	736	18.90 (16.1–21.7)	0.20	0.56	0.38	49.7	94.5	0.59	28.8	75.7
Argentina	2,410	12.10 (10.8–13.4)	0.21	0.61	0.40	30.3	57.6	0.29	49.7	124.3
Colombia	1,274	19.40 (17.2–21.6)	0.29	0.75	0.51	38.0	66.9	0.59	1	2.0
Paraguay	92	13 (6.2–19.9)	0.28	0.68	0.48	27.1	46.4	0.59	9.4	19.5
Brazil*	1,937	8.20 (6.9–9.4)	0.33	0.68	0.50	16.4	24.8	0.67	48	96.0
Honduras	1,182	9.80 (8.1–11.5)	0.32	0.82	0.57	17.2	30.6	0.59	28.8	50.5
Panama	235	10.60 (6.7–14.6)	0.48	1.18	0.83	12.8	22.1	0.59	28.8	34.7
Guatemala	165	11.50 (6.7–16.4)	1.34	0.03	0.70	16.4	8.6	0.59	28.8	41.1
El Salvador	293	7.90 (4.8–10.9)	0.42	1.16	0.77	10.3	18.8	0.59	28.8	37.4
Nicaragua	162	9.30 (4.8–13.7)	0.11	0.30	0.20	46.5	84.5	0.59	6	30.0
Mexico	9,422	25.60 (24.8–26.5)	0.14	0.39	0.26	98.5	182.9	0.59	3	11.5
Jamaica	201	31.80 (25.4–38.3)	0.79	2.01	1.38	23.0	40.3	0.73	12.9	9.3
Scenario 2. Risks among MSM occur within established HIV epidemics driven by injecting drug use										
Poland	424	5.40 (3.3–7.6)	0.03	0.09	0.06	90.0	180.0	1.50	8.9	148.3
Serbia	277	8.70 (5.4–12.0)	0.04	0.11	0.08	108.8	217.5	1.50	27	338.0
Armenia	108	0.90 (0.0–2.7)	0.04	0.17	0.10	9.0	22.5	0.10	13.4	134.0
Georgia	113	5.30 (1.2–9.4)	0.05	0.09	0.07	75.7	106.0	4.19	1.6	23.3
Moldova	118	1.70 (0.0–4.0)	0.14	0.37	0.24	7.1	12.1	0.14	17	70.8

Russian Federation*	1,939	3.40	(2.6–4.2)	0.36	1.28	0.78	4.4	9.4	1.78	37.2	47.6
Timor-Leste	110	1	(0.0–2.6)	n.a.	n.a.	0.20	5.0	n.a.	0.27	16.7	83.5
Ukraine*	408	10.60	(12.4–12.9)	0.88	1.35	1.09	9.7	12.0	1.16	41.8	38.3
Scenario 3. Risks among MSM occur in the context of mature and widespread HIV epidemics among heterosexuals											
Namibia	217	12.40	(8.1–16.8)	16.35	10.31	13.32	0.9	0.8	0.43	12.4	0.9
Botswana	117	19.70	(12.5–26.9)	26.01	17.06	21.56	0.9	0.8	0.43	12.4	0.6
South Africa	574	15.30	(12.4–18.3)	18.59	13.13	15.89	1.0	0.8	0.87	12.4	0.8
Zambia	641	32.90	(29.3–36.6)	17.79	13.61	15.72	2.1	1.8	0.43	12.4	0.8
Kenya*	1,333	15.20	(13.3–17.2)	8.88	6.09	7.49	2.0	1.7	0.73	42.9	5.7
Tanzania	509	12.40	(9.5–15.2)	6.74	4.99	5.88	2.1	1.8	0.43	12.4	2.1
Malawi*	201	21.40	(15.7–27.1)	13.31	9.60	11.46	1.9	1.6	0.43	12.4	1.1
Nigeria	1,961	13.50	(12.0–15.0)	3.42	2.36	2.88	4.7	3.9	0.43	12.4	4.3
Sudan	1,119	8.80	(7.1–10.4)	1.49	1.04	1.26	7.0	5.9	0.05	2.9	2.3
Ghana[t]	360	25	(20.5–29.5)	1.99	1.34	1.67	15.0	12.6	0.43	12.4	7.4
Senegal*[t]	1,227	24.30	(21.9–26.7)	1.04	0.72	0.88	27.6	23.4	0.43	12.4	14.1
Scenario 4. MSM, IDUs, and heterosexual transmissions all contribute significantly to the HIV epidemic											
Thailand*	1,221	23	(20.1–25.4)	0.96	1.40	1.18	19.5	24.0	0.38	42.5	36.0
Vietnam	1,965	6.20	(5.1–7.3)	0.21	0.67	0.42	14.8	29.5	0.25	33.9	80.6
Lao PDR	540	5.40	(3.5–7.2)	0.07	0.22	0.14	38.6	77.1	0.27	16.7	119.3
Cambodia	754	7.80	(5.9–9.7)	0.42	1.13	0.76	10.3	18.6	0.02	22.8	30.0
China	12,982	4.30	(4.0-4.7)	0.04	0.09	0.07	61.4	107.5	0.19	12.3	175.7
Indonesia	770	9	(6.9–11.0)	0.06	0.26	0.16	56.3	150.0	0.13	42.5	265.6
India*	3,790	14.50	(13.3–15.6)	0.23	0.36	0.30	48.3	63.0	0.02	11.2	37.2
Nepal	358	4.80	(2.6–7.0)	0.20	0.56	0.38	12.6	24.0	0.15	41.4	108.9
Pakistan	1,210	1.80	(1.1–2.6)	0.05	0.12	0.09	20.0	36.0	0.14	10.8	120.0
Egypt, Arab Rep.	340	5.30	(2.9–7.7)	0.01	0.02	0.02	265.0	530.0	0.05	2.9	147.0

(continued next page)

Table 2.1 *(continued)*

Country	*Sample size*	*Aggregate prevalence of HIV among MSM % (95% CI)*		*Women (15+) HIV prevalence*	*Men (15+) HIV prevalence*	*Population (15+) prevalence of HIV*	*Prevalence ratio: MSM vs. all*	*Prevalence ratio: MSM vs. women*	*Prevalence of IDU among population*	*HIV prevalence among IDU*	*Prevalence ratio: IDU vs. all*
Insufficient data											
Belarus	170	0	(0.0–0.0)	0.09	0.24	0.16	0.0	0.0	0.09	16.6	103.8
Kazakhstan	100	0	(0.0–0.0)	0.05	0.15	0.10	0.0	0.0	0.96	9.2	92.0
Kyrgyz Republic	101	0	(0.0–0.0)	0.06	0.17	0.11	0.0	0.0	0.74	8	72.7
Azerbaijan	7	42.90	(6.2–79.5)	0.04	0.22	0.12	357.5	1,072.5	5.21	13	108.3

Source: Authors.

Note: n.a. = not applicable. C.I.= confidence interval. Highlighted countries are countries selected to illustrate each epidemic scenario.

* Countries are selected focus countries for each Epidemic Scenario.

[t] Following the algorithm and based on available data, Senegal would also be assigned to scenario 4 and Ghana to scenario 1; both are somewhat outliers in these categories, and both have some uncertainties in risks and prevalence of HIV for female sex workers, IDU, and MSM which make characterization difficult. In both cases, and there are doubtless others; more refined epidemiologic studies will likely be required to characterize these dynamics epidemics among MSM and others at risk.

- **Scenario 3:** Risks among MSM occur in the context of mature and widespread HIV epidemics among heterosexuals. This scenario is the prevailing context across Sub-Saharan Africa, with particular relevance for the high-prevalence zones of East Africa and Southern Africa. Here, rates in heterosexuals are high, so the ratio of MSM to general population samples is well under 10, as is the ratio among IDUs compared to heterosexuals.

- **Scenario 4:** Transmissions among MSM, IDUs, and heterosexuals all contribute significantly to the HIV epidemic. This scenario is the complex context of much of South, Southeast, and Northeast Asia.

For the most part, scenarios followed geographic groupings by continent, with some exceptions. The Arab Republic of Egypt joined countries of the Asian continent in scenario 4 and Timor-Leste and Vietnam joined countries in Eastern Europe and Central Asia in scenario 2. Following the algorithm and based on available data, Senegal would also be assigned to scenario 4 and Ghana to scenario 1; both are somewhat outliers in these categories, and both have some uncertainties in risks and prevalence of HIV among female sex workers, IDU, and MSM, which make characterization difficult. In both cases, and there are doubtless others, more refined epidemiologic studies will likely be required to characterize these dynamics epidemics among MSM and others at risk. Finally, Azerbaijan, Belarus, Kazakhstan, and the Kyrgyz Republic lacked dependable data on HIV prevalence among MSM, so these countries were assigned to a default category with unavailable data.

The HIV pandemic is marked by enormous regional diversity, and this diversity is true of epidemics among MSM as well (Beyrer 2007). Generally, Sub-Saharan Africa remains by far the most affected region, and the only part of the world where generalized epidemics affected more than 10 percent of all reproductive-age adults (UNAIDS 2007). The MSM component of Africa's epidemics is arguably the least studied, most hidden, and least understood of any region, and not surprisingly, the least number of reports was found for this region. Asia has had several quite severe HIV epidemics, with high rates in several subgroups, including MSM, most notably in Cambodia, Myanmar, and Thailand, and a mixed picture with substantial spread among MSM, IDUs, and heterosexuals. South America has multiple HIV epidemics that are highly concentrated among MSM. This great diversity suggests approaches to MSM

Figure 2.3 HIV Epidemic among MSM in LMICs According to Epidemic Scenario

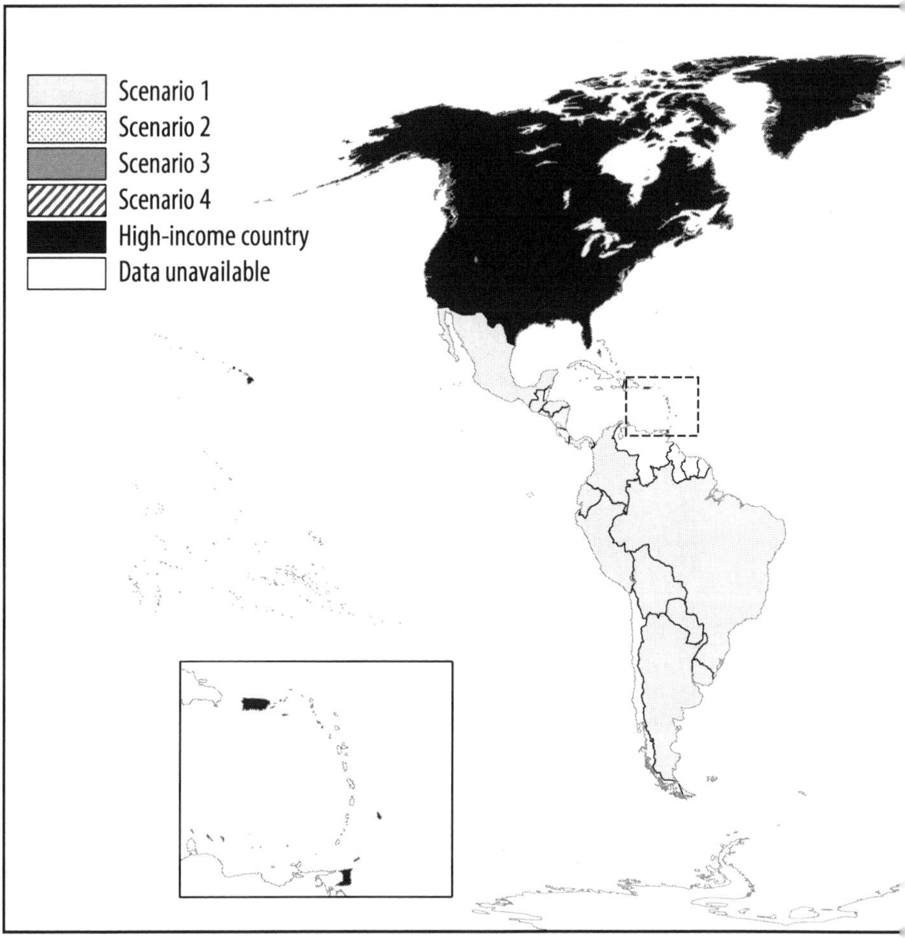

Source: Authors.

Note: Following the algorithm and based on available data, Senegal would also be assigned to scenario 4 and Ghana to scenario 1; both are somewhat outliers in these categories, and both have some uncertainties in risks and prevalence of HIV among female sex workers, IDU, and MSM, which make characterization difficult. In both cases, and there are doubtless others, more refined epidemiologic studies will likely be required to characterize these dynamics epidemics among MSM and others at risk.

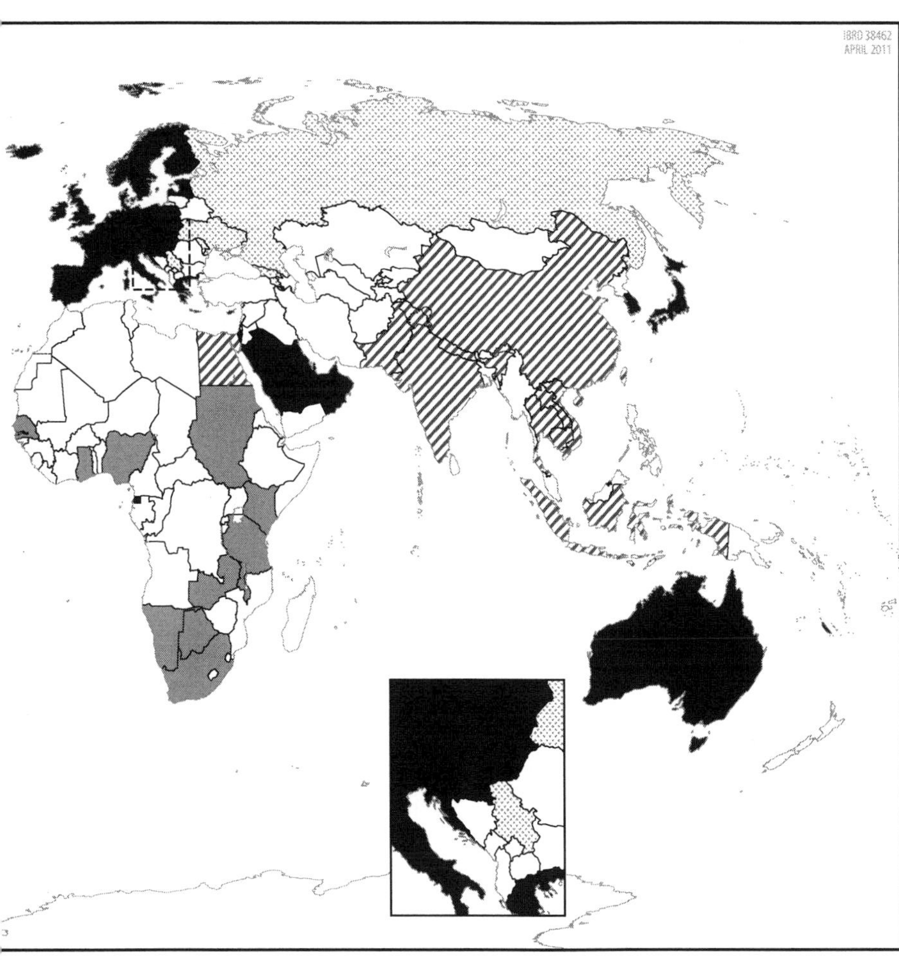
IBRD 38462
APRIL 2011

epidemics must be clearly situated in their wider national and regional epidemic contexts to be understood.

To explore these regional scenarios in some detail, this book describes at least two representative countries for each scenario based on the following criteria:

- Data were available on MSM.
- The countries were of significant size and regional importance so that findings would have relevance for their wider region.
- HIV/AIDS epidemics and responses to those epidemics were substantial enough in 2009 to make evaluation possible.

For scenario 1, the authors investigated Brazil and Peru; for scenario 2, the Russian Federation and Ukraine; for scenario 3, Kenya, Malawi, and Senegal; and for scenario 4, India and Thailand. Table 2.2 shows HIV prevalence from community-based samples of MSM in the representative countries for each scenario.

Because the taxonomy of male sexual orientation and gender identity is culturally bound, can be complex, and has implications for HIV programming, this book has attempted to characterize the typologies used for MSM and transgendered individuals in epidemiologic studies for each representative country. The evidence for the various populations of MSM has been reviewed, and differential risks of HIV have been ascertained where possible. This study also explored the intersection of HIV epidemics among MSM and substance use, both injecting drug use risk and noninjection risks, such as those associated with noninjecting use of methamphetamine and cocaine. Because sexual behaviors with female sex partners are also diverse, complex, and important for understanding HIV spread among these men, those domains were also investigated.

The Middle East and North Africa

A challenge to this scenario-based approach is the characterization of HIV epidemics in the Middle East and North Africa. This geographically defined set of states includes high-, middle-, and low-income countries. Cultural and political realities across much of this region have led to hidden populations of MSM and others at risk and have impeded epidemiologic characterization. Nevertheless, what evidence is available suggests that individuals, networks, and in some cases communities of MSM do exist throughout the region and that some may be at substantial risk for

Table 2.2 HIV Prevalence in Community-Based Samples of MSM in the Four Representative Countries

Source	*Location*	*Type of sample*	*Year*	*Number in sample*	*Number HIV positive*	*Prevalence (%)*
Peru (scenario 1)						
Sanchez et al. 2007; Tabet et al. 2002	Lima	Convenience	1996	444	82	18.50
Hierzholzer et al. 2002	Lima	Convenience	1998–2000	7,041	982	13.90
Hierzholzer et al. 2002	Other cities	Convenience	1998–2000	4,514	241	5.30
Sanchez et al. 2007	Lima	Convenience	1998–99	1,211	215	17.80
Sanchez et al. 2007	Lima	Convenience	2000	3,200	528	16.50
Sanchez et al. 2007	Lima	Convenience	2000	1,357	268	19.70
Sanchez et al. 2007	Lima	Convenience	2002	1,358	303	22.30
La Rosa et al. 2009; MINSA 2009; UNAIDS and WHO 2008b	Lima	Convenience	2002	893	198	22.20
La Rosa et al. 2009; MINSA 2009; UNAIDS and WHO 2008b	Sullana, Piura	Convenience	2002	732	59	8.10
La Rosa et al. 2009; MINSA 2009; UNAIDS and WHO 2008b	Arequipa	Convenience	2002	424	28	6.60
La Rosa et al. 2009; MINSA 2009; UNAIDS and WHO 2008b	Iquitos	Convenience	2002	285	34	11.90
La Rosa et al. 2009; MINSA 2009; UNAIDS and WHO 2008b	Pucallpa	Convenience	2002	266	18	6.76
Clark, Konda, Segura et al. 2008	Lima	Convenience	2007	559	124	22.20
Total				22,284	3,080	13.80 (95 CI: 13.4, 14.3)
Ukraine (scenario 2)						
Balakiryeva, Bondar, and Kasyanczuk 2008; UNAIDS and Ministry of Health of Ukraine 2008	Kyiv	Respondent-driven sampling	2007	90	4	4.40

(continued next page)

Table 2.2 *(continued)*

Source	*Location*	*Type of sample*	*Year*	*Number in sample*	*Number HIV positive*	*Prevalence (%)*
Balakiryeva, Bondar, and Kasyanczuk 2008; UNAIDS and Ministry of Health of Ukraine 2008	Kryviy Rig	Respondent-driven sampling	2007	100	8	8.00
Balakiryeva, Bondar, and Kasyanczuk 2008; UNAIDS and Ministry of Health of Ukraine 2008	Mykolayiv	Respondent-driven sampling	2007	100	10	10.00
Balakiryeva, Bondar, and Kasyanczuk 2008; UNAIDS and Ministry of Health of Ukraine 2008	Odessa	Respondent-driven sampling	2007	69	16	23.20
Total				359	38	10.60 (95 CI: 7.8, 14.2)
Kenya (scenario 3)						
Angala et al. 2006	National VCT centers	VCT-based	2006	780	83	10.60
Sanders et al. 2007	Mombasa, Kilifi	Convenience	2009	553	120	21.70
Total				1,333	203	15.20 (95 CI: 13.3, 17.2)
Thailand (scenario 4)						
van Griensven et al. 2009	Bangkok	Time location sampling	2007	400	123	30.80
CDC 2006	Bangkok	Time location sampling	2005	399	113	28.30
CDC 2006	Chang Mai	Time location sampling	2005	222	34	15.30
CDC 2006	Phuket	Time location sampling	2005	200	11	5.50
Total				1,221	281	23.00 (95 CI: 20.1, 25.4)

Source: Authors.
Note: CI = confidence interval; VCT = voluntary counseling and testing.

HIV infection. In most Middle Eastern and North African countries, the HIV epidemics are low-level epidemics, or very low HIV prevalence exists in the general population. Where most at-risk populations, including sex workers, IDUs, and MSM have been studied, they have generally been found to be at disproportionately high risk. For MSM, examples include Egypt and Sudan, where rates among MSM are high enough to characterize as concentrated epidemics. The majority of countries in the region use passive surveillance mechanisms for HIV reporting, however, which tends to underestimate the role of specific high-risk practices, such as same-sex practices, in driving HIV acquisition and transmission. Where directed studies have been completed, populations of MSM at high risk for HIV transmission, including those with high-risk sexual practices, low levels of condom usage, and low levels of HIV knowledge, have been observed.

Publicly available data characterizing the burden of disease of HIV among MSM in the Middle East and North Africa were reviewed, and identified risk factors for HIV infection among these men were explored. This book reviews the most recent United Nations General Assembly Special Session reports to characterize indicators describing reported levels of coverage for HIV preventive services for MSM. Finally, this book provides an overview of studies describing the human rights contexts for MSM, including assessing barriers to accessing preventive and health care services.

Bibliography

Ainsworth, M., C. Beyrer, and A. Soucat. 2003. "AIDS and Public Policy: The Lessons and Challenges of 'Success' in Thailand." *Health Policy* 64 (1): 13–37.

Aldridge, R. W., D. Iglesias, C. F. Cáceres, and J. J. Miranda. 2009. "Determining a Cost Effective Intervention Response to HIV/AIDS in Peru." *BMC Public Health* 9: 352.

Amjadeen, L. 2005. *Report on the Survey "Monitoring Behaviours of MSM as a Component of Second Generation Surveillance"* [in Ukrainian]. Kyiv: International HIV/AIDS Alliance in Ukraine.

Amjadeen, L., L. Andrushchak, I. Zvershkhovska, et al. 2005. *A Review of Work with Injecting Drug Users in Ukraine in the Context of the HIV/AIDS Epidemic.* Kyiv: National Academy of Sciences of Ukraine.

Angala, P., A. Parkinson, N. Kilonzo et al. 2006. Men who have sex with men (MSM) as presented in VCT data in Kenya. (Abstract MOPE0581). Presented at the XVI International AIDS Conference, Toronto, Ontario, Canada, August 13–18.

Balakiryeva, O. N., T. V. Bondar, M. G. Kasyanczuk, Z. R. Kis, Y. B. Leszczynski, and S. P. Sheremet-Sheremetyev. 2008. *Report on the Survey "Monitoring Behaviours of Men Having Sex with Men as a Component of Second Generation Surveillance."* Kyiv: International HIV/AIDS Alliance in Ukraine.

Baral, S., F. Sifakis, F. Cleghorn, and C. Beyrer. 2007. "Elevated Risk for HIV Infection among Men Who Have Sex with Men in Low- and Middle-Income Countries 2000–2006: A Systematic Review." *PLoS Medicine* 4 (12): e339.

Baral, S., G. Trapence, F. Motimedi, E. Umar, S. Iipinge, F. Dausab, and C. Beyrer. 2009. "HIV Prevalence, Risks for HIV Infection, and Human Rights among Men Who Have Sex with Men (MSM) in Malawi, Namibia, and Botswana." *PLoS One* 4 (3): e4997.

Beyrer, C. 2007. "HIV Epidemiology Update and Transmission Factors: Risks and Risk Contexts—16th International AIDS Conference Epidemiology Plenary." *Clinical Infectious Diseases* 44 (7): 981–87.

Beyrer, C., S. D. Baral, D. Walker, A. L. Wirtz, B. Johns, and F. Sifakis. 2010. "The Expanding Epidemics of HIV Type 1 among Men Who Have Sex with Men in Low- and Middle-Income Countries: Diversity and Consistency." *Epidemiologic Reviews* 32 (1): 137–51.

Beyrer, C., T. Sripaipan, S. Tovanabutra, J. Jittiwutikarn, V. Suriyanon, T. Vongchak, N. Srirak, S. Kawichai, M. H. Razak, and D. D. Celentano. 2005. "High HIV, Hepatitis C and Sexual Risks among Drug-Using Men Who Have Sex with Men in Northern Thailand." *AIDS* 19 (14): 1535–40.

Cáceres, C. F., K. Konda, M. Pecheny, A. Chatterjee, and R. Lyerla. 2006. "Estimating the Number of Men Who Have Sex with Men in Low and Middle Income Countries." *Sexually Transmitted Infections* 82 (Suppl. 3): iii3–9.

Cáceres, C. F., K. Konda, E. R. Segura, and R. Lyerla. 2008. "Epidemiology of Male Same-Sex Behaviour and Associated Sexual Health Indicators in Low- and Middle-Income Countries: 2003-2007 Estimates." *Sexually Transmitted Infections* 84 (Suppl. 1): i49–56.

Cáceres C. F., and W. Mendoza. 2009. "The National Response to the HIV/AIDS Epidemic in Peru: Accomplishments and Gaps—a Review." *Journal of Acquired Immune Deficiency Syndromes* 51 (Suppl. 1): S60–66.

CDC (U.S. Centers for Disease Control and Prevention). 2006. "HIV Prevalence among Populations of Men Who Have Sex with Men—Thailand, 2003 and 2005." *Morbidity and Mortality Weekly Report* 55 (31): 844–48.

Celentano, D. D. 2005. "Undocumented Epidemics of HIV Continue to Persist in the Twenty-First Century." *AIDS* 19 (5): 527–28.

Centre of Social Expertise at the Institute of Sociology of the National Academy of Sciences of Ukraine. 2004. *Analytical Report: Behavioural Monitoring of*

MSM as a Second Generation Surveillance Component. Kyiv: International HIV/AIDS Alliance in Ukraine.

Clark, J. L., K. A. Konda, C. V. Munayco, M. Pun, A. G. Lescano, S. R. Leon, J. Pajuelo, L. Suarez-Ognio, J. D. Klausner, T. J. Coates, et al. 2008. "Prevalence of HIV, Herpes Simplex Virus-2, and Syphilis in Male Sex Partners of Pregnant Women in Peru." *BMC Public Health* 8: 65.

Clark, J. L., K. A. Konda, E. R. Segura, H. J. Salvatierra, S. R. Leon, E. R. Hall, C. F. Cáceres, J. D. Klausner, and T. J. Coates. 2008. "Risk Factors for the Spread of HIV and Other Sexually Transmitted Infections among Men Who Have Sex with Men Infected with HIV in Lima, Peru." *Sexually Transmitted Infections* 84 (6): 449–54.

Csete, J., A. Gathumbi, D. Wolfe, and J. Cohen. 2009. "Lives to Save: PEPFAR, HIV, and Injecting Drug Use in Africa." *Lancet* 373 (9680): 2006–7.

Filipov, D. 2005. The Research of Risky Behaviour in the Context of HIV among MSM in Kyiv [in Russian]. *HIV/AIDS News* 3: 5.

Gálvez-Buccollini, J. A., S. DeLea, P. M. Herrera, R. H. Gilman, and V. Paz-Soldan. 2009. Sexual Behavior and Drug Consumption among Young Adults in a Shantytown in Lima, Peru." *BMC Public Health* 9: 23.

Geibel, S., N. King'ola, and S. Luchters. 2009. "Impact of Male Sex Worker Peer Education on Condom Use in Mombasa, Kenya." Presentation at the 5th IAS Conference on HIV Pathogenesis, Treatment and Prevention, Cape Town, South Africa, July 19–22.

Geibel, S., S. Luchters, N. King'ola, E. Esu-Williams, A. Rinyiru, and W. Tun. 2008. "Factors Associated with Self-Reported Unprotected Anal Sex among Male Sex Workers in Mombasa, Kenya." *Sexually Transmitted Diseases* 35 (8): 746–52.

Geibel, S., E. M. van der Elst, N. King'ola, S. Luchters, A. Davies, E. M. Getambu, N. Peshu, S. M. Graham, R. S. McClelland, and E. J. Sanders. 2007. "'Are You on the Market?': A Capture-Recapture Enumeration of Men Who Sell Sex to Men in and around Mombasa, Kenya." *AIDS* 21 (10): 1349–54.

Gouws, E., P. J. White, J. Stover, and T. Brown. 2006. "Short Term Estimates of Adult HIV Incidence by Mode of Transmission: Kenya and Thailand as Examples." *Sexually Transmitted Infections* 82 (Suppl. 3): iii51–55.

Gribanov, A., Z. Kis, A. Maimulakhin, L. Chorniy, et al. 2005. *Gay Rights Are Human Rights: Report about Discrimination on the Grounds of Sexual Orientation in Ukraine*. Kyiv: Nash Mir Gay and Lesbian Center. http://gay.org.ua/publication/report2005-e.pdf. Accessed June 4, 2008.

Guadamuz, T. E., W. Wimonsate, A. Varangrat, P. Phanuphak, R. Jommaroeng, P. A. Mock, J. W. Tappero, and F. van Griensven. 2009. "Correlates of Forced Sex among Populations of Men Who Have Sex with Men in Thailand." *Archives of Sexual Behavior*. doi: 10.1007/s10508-009-9557-8.

Hierholzer, J., S. Montano, M. Hoelscher, M. Negrete, M. Hierholzer, M. M. Avila, M. Gomez Carrillo, J. C. Russi, J. Vinoles, A. Alava, et al. 2002. "Molecular Epidemiology of HIV Type 1 in Ecuador, Peru, Bolivia, Uruguay, and Argentina." *AIDS Research and Human Retroviruses* 18 (18): 1339–50.

"HIV and Kenya's Homosexuals." 1998. *African Health* 20 (6): 48.

"HIV Prevalence among Populations of Men Who Have Sex with Men—Thailand, 2003 and 2005." 2006. *Morbidity and Mortality Weekly Report (MMWR)* 55 (31): 844–48.

Jackson, P. A., and N. M. Cook, eds. 1999. *Genders and Sexualities in Modern Thailand.* Chiang Mai, Thailand: Silkworm Books.

Joint United Nations Programme On HIV/AIDS. 2008. "Peru Epidemiological Fact Sheet on HIV and AIDS: Core Data on Epidemiology and Response." Geneva, December.

"Kenya: Halt Anti-Gay Campaign." 2010. *Human Righs Watch,* New York, NY, February 17.

Kiama, W. 1999. "Where Are Kenya's Homosexuals?" *AIDS Analysis Africa* 9 (5): 9–10.

Konda, K., J. L. Clark, E. R. Segura, H. J. Salvatierra, J. T. Galea, S. Leon, E. R. Hall, J. D. Klausner, C. Cáceres, and T. Coates. 2008. "Characterizing Sex Work among Male and Transgender STI Clinic Clients in Lima, Peru." Presentation at XVII International AIDS Conference, Mexico City, August 3–8.

Konda, K. A., A. G. Lescano, E. Leontsini, P. Fernandez, J. D. Klausner, T. J. Coates, and C. F. Cáceres. 2008. "High Rates of Sex with Men among High-Risk, Heterosexually-Identified Men in Low-Income, Coastal Peru." *AIDS and Behavior* 12 (3): 483–91.

Kruglov, Y. V., Y. V. Kobyshcha, T. Salyuk, O. Varetska, A. Shakarishvili, and V. P. Saldanha. 2008. "The Most Severe HIV Epidemic in Europe: Ukraine's National HIV Prevalence Estimates for 2007." *Sexually Transmitted Infections* 84 (Suppl. 1): i37–41.

Lane, T., J. McIntyre, and S. Morin. 2006. "High-Risk Sex among Black MSM in South Africa: Results from the Gauteng MSM Survey." Presentation at "AIDS 2006": XVI International AIDS Conference, Toronto, Canada, August 13–18.

Lane, T., H. F. Raymond, S. Dladla, J. Rasethe, H. Struthers, W. McFarland, and J. McIntyre. 2009. "High HIV Prevalence among Men Who Have Sex with Men in Soweto, South Africa: Results from the Soweto Men's Study." *AIDS and Behavior,* August 7 [Epub ahead of print].

Lane, T., S. B. Shade, J. McIntyre, and S. F. Morin. 2008. "Alcohol and Sexual Risk Behavior among Men Who Have Sex with Men in South African Township Communities." *AIDS and Behavior* 12 (Suppl. 4): S78–85.

La Rosa, A. M., J. R. Zunt, J. Peinado, J. R. Lama, T. G. Ton, L. Suarez, M. Pun, C. Cabezas, J. Sanchez, and Peruvian HIV Sentinel Surveillance Working Group. 2009. "Retroviral Infection in Peruvian Men Who Have Sex with Men." *Clinical Infectious Diseases* 49 (1): 112–17.

Mathers B. M., L. Degenhardt, B. Phillips, L. Wiessing, M. Hickman, S. A. Strathdee, A. Wodak, S. Panda, M. Tyndall, A. Toufik, and R. Mattick for the 2007 Reference Group to the UN on HIV and Injecting Drug Use. 2008. "Global Epidemiology of Injecting Drug Use and HIV among People Who Inject Drugs: A Systematic Review." *Lancet* 372 (9651): 1733–45.

MINSA (Ministerio de Salud del Perú). 2009. *Estadistica: Indicadores de Salud.* Lima: Ministerio de Salud del Perú.

Ministry of Health of Ukraine. 2006. *Ukraine: National Report on the Follow-up to the UNGASS Declaration of Commitment on HIV/AIDS—Reporting Period: January 2003–December 2005*. Kyiv: Ministry of Health of Ukraine.

Muhaari, A. 2009. "High HIV-1 Incidence in Men Who Have Sex with Men in Mombasa, Kenya." Presented at the MSM Satellite Meeting of the 4th Southern African AIDS Conference, Durban, South Africa, March 31–April 3.

Murray, S. O. 2004. "Africa: Sub-Saharan, Pre-Independence." In *glbtq: An Encyclopedia of Gay, Lesbian, Bisexual, Transgender, and Queer Culture,* ed. C. J. Summers. Chicago, IL: glbtq, Inc. http://www.glbtq.com/social-sciences/africa_pre.html.

NACC (National AIDS Control Council, Office of the President, Kenya), World Bank, and UNAIDS (Joint United Nations Programme on HIV/AIDS). 2009. *Kenya HIV Prevention Response and Modes of Transmission Analysis*. Nairobi: NACC.

NAPaA Committee (National HIV and AIDS Prevention and Alleviation Committee). 2007. *National Plan for Strategic and Integrated HIV and AIDS Prevention and Alleviation (2007–2011)*. Nonthaburi, Thailand: The National Committee for HIV and AIDS Prevention and Alleviation Drafting Working Group on National Plan for Strategic and Integrated HIV and AIDS Prevention and Alleviation 2007–2011.

Ndetei, D. 2004. *Study on the Assessment of the Linkages between Drug Abuse, Injecting Drug Abuse and HIV/AIDS in Kenya: A Rapid Situation Assessment.* Nairobi: United Nations Office on Drugs and Crime.

Nelson, K. E., D. D. Celentano, S. Eiumtrakol, D. R. Hoover, C. Beyrer, S. Suprasert, S. Kuntolbutra, and C. Khamboonruang. 1996. "Changes in Sexual Behavior and a Decline in HIV Infection among Young Men in Thailand." *New England Journal of Medicine* 335 (5): 297–303.

Odek-Ogunde, M., F. A. Okoth, W. Lore, and F. R. Owiti. 2004. "Seroprevalence of HIV, HBC and HCV in Injecting Drug Users in Nairobi, Kenya: World

Health Organization Drug Injecting Study Phase II Findings." Presentation at 15th International Conference on AIDS, Bangkok, Thailand, July 11–16.

Odek-Ogunde, M., and World Health Organization. 2004. Phase II drug injecting study: behavioural and seroprevalence (HIV, HBV, HCV) survey among injecting drug users in Nairobi. Nairobi, Kenya: WHO.

Okal, J., S. Luchters, S. Geibel, M. F. Chersich, D. Lango, and M. Temmerman. 2009. "Social Context, Sexual Risk Perceptions and Stigma: HIV Vulnerability among Male Sex Workers in Mombasa, Kenya." *Culture, Health, and Sexuality* 11 (8): 811–26.

Onyango-Ouma, W., H. Birungi, and S. Geibel. 2005. *Understanding the HIV/STI Risks and Prevention Needs of Men Who Have Sex with Men in Nairobi, Kenya.* Horizons Final Report. Washington, DC: Population Council.

———. 2006. "Understanding the HIV/STI Prevention Needs of Men Who Have Sex with Men in Kenya." Horizons Research Summary. Washington, DC: Population Council.

Piot, P., M. Bartos, H. Larson, D. Zewdie, and P. Mane. 2008. "Coming to Terms with Complexity: A Call to Action for HIV Prevention." *Lancet* 372 (9641): 845–59.

Sanchez, J., J. R. Lama, L. Kusunoki, H. Manrique, P. Goicochea, A. Lucchetti, M. Rouillon, M. Pun, L. Suarez, S. Montano, J. L. Sanchez, S. Tabet, J. P. Hughes, and C. Celum. 2007. "HIV-1, Sexually Transmitted Infections, and Sexual Behavior Trends among Men Who Have Sex with Men in Lima, Peru." *Journal of Acquired Immune Deficiency Syndromes* 44 (5): 578–85.

Sanders, E. J., S. M. Graham, H. S. Okuku, E. M. van der Elst, A. Muhaari, A. Davies, N. Peshu, M. Price, R. S. McClelland, and A. D. Smith. 2007. "HIV-1 Infection in High Risk Men Who Have Sex with Men in Mombasa, Kenya." *AIDS* 21 (18): 2513–20.

Sharma, A., E. Bukusi, P. Gorbach, C. R. Cohen, C. Muga, Z. Kwena, and K. K. Holmes. 2008. "Sexual Identity and Risk of HIV/STI among Men Who Have Sex with Men in Nairobi." *Sexually Transmitted Diseases* 35 (4): 352–54.

Tabet, S., J. Sanchez, J. R. Lama, P. Goicochea, P. Campos, M. Rouillon, J. L. Cairo, L. Ueda, D. Watts, C. Celum, et al. 2002. "HIV, Syphilis and Heterosexual Bridging among Peruvian Men Who Have Sex with Men." *AIDS* 16 (9): 1271–77.

UNAIDS (Joint United Nations Programme on HIV/AIDS). 2007. *Financial Resources Required to Achieve Universal Access to HIV Prevention, Treatment, Care and Support.* Geneva: UNAIDS.

———. 2008. *2008 Report on the Global AIDS Epidemic.* Geneva: UNAIDS.

UNAIDS and Ministry of Health of Ukraine. 2008. *Ukraine: National Report on Monitoring Progress towards the UNGASS Declaration of Commitment on HIV/AIDS. Reporting Period: January 2006–December 2007*. Kyiv: Ministry of Health of Ukraine.

UNAIDS (United Nations Joint Programme on HIV/AIDS) and WHO (World Health Organization). 2000. *Guidelines for Second Generation HIV Surveillance*. WHO/CDS/CSR/EDC/2000.5; UNAIDS/00.03E. Geneva: UNAIDS and WHO.

———. 2008a. *Sub-Saharan Africa: AIDS Epidemic Update Regional Summary*. Geneva: UNAIDS and WHO.

———. 2008b. "UNAIDS/WHO Epidemiological Fact Sheet on HIV and AIDS, Peru 2008 Update: Core Data on Epidemiology and Response." Geneva: UNAIDS and WHO.

———. 2009. *AIDS Epidemic Update 2009: November* UNAIDS/09.36E/JC1700E. Geneva: UNAIDS and WHO.

USAID (U.S. Agency for International Development)/Ukraine. 2008. "HIV/AIDS Profile: Ukraine."

Valverde, R., and R. Cabello. 2008. *Monitoring the Implementation of the UNGASS Declaration of Commitment: Country Report: Peru*. Lima: Organization Vía Libre.

van Griensven, F. 2007. "Men Who Have Sex with Men and Their HIV Epidemics in Africa." *AIDS* 21 (10): 1361–62.

van Griensven, F., S. Thanprasertsuk, R. Jommaroeng, G. Mansergh, S. Naorat, R. A. Jenkins, K. Ungchusak, P. Phanuphak, J. W. Tappero, and Bangkok MSM Study Group. 2005. "Evidence of a Previously Undocumented Epidemic of HIV Infection among Men Who Have Sex with Men in Bangkok, Thailand." *AIDS* 19 (5): 521–26.

van Griensven, F., A. Varangrat, W. Wimonsate, S. Tanpradech, K. Kladsawad, T. Chemnasiri, O. Suksripanich, P. Phanuphak, P. Mock, K. Kanggarnrua, et al. 2009. "Trends in HIV Prevalence, Estimated HIV Incidence, and Risk Behavior among Men Who Have Sex with Men in Bangkok, Thailand, 2003–2007." *Journal of Acquired Immune Deficiency Syndromes* 53 (2): 234–39.

Wade, A. S., C. T. Kane, P. A. Diallo, A. K. Diop, K. Gueye, S. Mboup, I. Ndoye, and E. Lagarde. 2005. "HIV Infection and Sexually Transmitted Infections among Men Who Have Sex with Men in Senegal." *AIDS* 19 (18): 2133–40.

Wadhams, N. 2009. "In Fight against AIDS, Kenya Confronts Gay Taboo." Time.com/Nairobi, November 7.

Weniger, B. G., K. Limpakarnjanarat, K. Ungchusak, S. Thanprasertsuk, K. Choopanya, S. Vanichseni, T. Uneklabh, P. Thongcharoen, and C. Wasi.

1991. "The Epidemiology of HIV Infection and AIDS in Thailand." *AIDS* 5 (Suppl. 2): S71–85.

Weniger, B., P. Takebe, and T. John. 1992. "The HIV Epidemic in Thailand, India, and Neighboring Nations: A Fourth Epidemiologic Pattern Emerges in Asia." Presentation at Eighth International Conference on AIDS, Amsterdam, the Netherlands, July 19–24.

World Bank. 2009. "Gross national income per capita 2008, Atlas method and PPP." World Development Indicators database, World Bank, October 7.

CHAPTER 3

Scenario 1 Country Studies: Brazil and Peru

Brazil: Early Interventions, Early Successes

Scenario: Risks among men who have sex with men (MSM) are the predominant mode of exposure for HIV in the population.

Key themes:

- Brazil's epidemic remains well controlled, with a population prevalence of HIV infection of some 0.6 percent of reproductive age adults (95 percent confidence interval [CI] 0.5–0.8) in 2007.
- Early prevention efforts; protection of human rights; and a focus on MSM, injecting drug users (IDUs), and sex workers helped Brazil avoid a potentially much larger HIV epidemic.
- Nevertheless, MSM remain at much higher risk for HIV infection than do other Brazilians. Compared to the general population of men age 15 to 49, MSM were 28.7 times more likely to have HIV infection (95 percent CI 24.8–33.3) in 2007.
- Brazil's focus on decreasing homophobia and stigma in clinical care settings, schools, and broader society is an outstanding example of human rights–based HIV prevention programming.

Brazil is South America's largest country, with a 2008 population estimated at 196 million citizens. It is a middle-income state by World Bank 2007 standards, with a gross domestic product per capita of US$8,300 (U.S. Department of State 2009). Brazil was one of the first countries to be affected by HIV/AIDS in the Western Hemisphere, with an initial outbreak in the early 1980s concentrated among MSM and IDUs in the urban centers of São Paulo and Rio de Janeiro. After a stalled early response under waning military rule, Brazil's Sistema Único de Saúde emerged in the early 1990s as a regional leader in HIV prevention for at-risk populations and in the protection of human rights. As HIV/AIDS treatments became available, Brazil became the first middle-income country to provide universal access to HIV/AIDS treatment (Gauri, Beyrer, and Vaillancourt 2007). Brazil's program was substantially supported by three rounds of five-year loans from the World Bank. Inclusion of gay men, bisexual men, and other MSM, including Brazil's substantial population of transvestites (the term most commonly used in Brazil) and male sex workers (MSWs), was a cornerstone of national response.

Brazil's HIV epidemic was estimated at just over 1 percent of reproductive-age adults in 1990 (Gauri, Beyrer, and Vaillancourt 2007). Further expansion has been limited, and the most recent estimates for overall HIV prevalence are that some 730,000 Brazilians (600,000–890,000) were living with HIV infection in 2007, of whom approximately 710,000 (580,000–870,000) were 15 years of age or older (UNAIDS 2008). This estimate is roughly half the disease burden predicted in the 1990s (Ministry of Health 2001). The adult burden of 710,000 persons living with HIV yields an overall estimated HIV prevalence among reproductive-age adults (15–49 years) of 0.6 percent (95 percent CI 0.5–0.8). Although trends toward more women have been seen among reported AIDS cases, male predominance continues with an estimated 1.96:1 male-to-female ratio (calculated from UNAIDS and WHO [2007] data). In 2001, the male-to-female ratio was 1.67:1, which evidences the increase in male predominance.

MSM and Transgender Typologies Used in Epidemiologic Studies in Brazil

Brazil generally categorizes MSM into gay men; bisexual men; transvestites and transsexuals; and MSWs, a significant proportion of whom are transgendered (TG) in identity or expression (de Andrade et al. 2007). An open and positively identified gay culture has been a strong feature of Brazilian society, particularly in urban areas. Gay men have long played leading roles in advocacy for HIV/AIDS programs in Brazil, for human rights for sexual minorities, and for universal access to antiretroviral therapy.

Other MSM in Brazil include bisexual men and hidden and married men. Estimates of the proportion of Brazilian men who have ever had sex with another man vary. Szwarcwald and colleagues (2005) estimated that between 2.4 percent and 3.5 percent of all Brazilian men age 15 to 54 had had sex with another man in their lifetime. Cáceres and colleagues (2008) produced a widely used estimate for Latin America based on data from five countries (which did not include Brazil) of a 4 percent lifetime history of sex with another man, with a range of 3 percent to 15 percent. This exercise also included an estimate of the proportion of MSM married to women in Latin America, some 5 percent, which is much lower than in other regions.

Male sex workers are a significant proportion of MSM in Brazil. A recent large study in Campinas (an urban area of the São Paulo metropolitan zone) found that MSWs were significantly more likely to be TG than other MSM—about 40.5 percent were TG, compared with 8.1 percent of MSM who were not sex workers (Tun et al. 2008). Overall, some 15 percent of men in this sample of 658 had engaged in exchange sex, and 8 percent identified themselves as commercial sex workers.

MSM Groups and Risks for HIV Infection

Data are available from four recent studies of HIV infection among MSM in Brazil. The study by Ferreira and colleagues (2006) is an outlier that found a 48 percent HIV prevalence among MSM who were IDUs, a subgroup discussed below. Using the three remaining references yields an overall HIV prevalence estimate among MSM of 8.2 percent (table 3.1).

Comparing prevalence of HIV among MSM to prevalence in the general population of all men age 15–49, Baral and colleagues (2007) found that MSM were some 28.7 times more likely to have HIV infection (95 percent CI 24.8–33.3).

Data are largely unavailable disaggregated by age, but reports from the Sistema Único de Saúde show that among MSM, the proportion of infections among the youngest group (age 13–24) accounted for 24.8 percent of new infections in 1996 but for 41.1 percent of new infections in 2006 (*Medical News Today* 2008).

Table 3.1 Three Prevalence Studies of HIV Infection among MSM in Brazil

Source	*Year*	*HIV+*	*HIV–*	*Total N*	*HIV prevalence (%)*
Carneiro et al. 2003	2003	61	560	621	9.8
Périssé et al. 2006	2006	51	597	648	7.8
Mello et al. 2008	2008	46	612	658	6.9
Total		158	1,769	1,927	8.2

Source: Authors.

Bisexual MSM and Relationships with Women

Samples of Brazilian MSM have consistently reported relatively higher rates of gay (homosexual) orientation and exclusive same-sex sexual activity than other Latin American reports. Sampaio and colleagues (2002) reported only 3.5 percent of a sample of MSM in Bahia having recent sex with a woman. Tun and colleagues (2008) found that whereas some 24 percent of MSM in a Campinas sample reported bisexual orientation, recent sex (within the last two months) with a woman was reported by only 5.6 percent of MSM overall. The subset of MSWs in this sample reported higher rates of recent sex with women, at 16.5 percent. Cáceres and colleagues (2008) report that in Latin American MSM (data that did not include Brazil) 25 to 64 percent of MSM have ever had sex with a woman; 8 to 30 percent have had sex with a woman in the past year; and 5 percent of MSM were married to a woman.

Male Sex Workers

Tun and colleagues (2008) reported on MSWs and non-MSWs in Brazil in a 2008 study of 658 MSM recruited through respondent-driven sampling in Campinas. They found that MSWs were significantly more likely to have practiced unprotected receptive anal intercourse (22.4 percent compared with 4.6 percent) than were other MSM. HIV rates were significantly higher among MSWs at 13.5 percent, compared to 5.8 percent among other MSM. MSWs were also much more likely to have ever injected drugs; 4.1 percent of MSWs reported this behavior, whereas only 0.7 percent of other MSM did so (Tun et al. 2008). MSWs in this study were significantly less likely than other MSM to report homosexual (gay) orientation: 52.1 percent of MSWs identified as gay compared with 72.5 percent of other MSM. They were more likely to state heterosexual identity (10.6 percent) and bisexual identity (32.1 percent) but were also about five times more likely to be TG, at 40.5 percent. The strength of these data allows them to be used as proxy population estimates for the proportions of interest by doing respondent-driven sampling and adjusting the findings of the sample for homophily.

IDUs among MSM

Samples of MSM in Brazil have generally reported low rates of injecting drug use among this population, but higher rates of substance use overall (Tun et al. 2008). Ferreira and colleagues (2006) investigated behaviors of MSM among a cohort of 709 male IDUs to assess their HIV rates and risks. Drug users were recruited through syringe exchange programs in six urban centers in Brazil. IDUs were asked about lifetime and recent (previous six months) sex with another man. Lifetime prevalence of MSM behavior was 26.4 percent of the sample; recent sex was reported by 20.2 percent. HIV rates were very high among all IDUs—36 percent of all men were HIV infected; but MSM IDUs were about twice as likely to have HIV than other IDUs (adjusted odds ratio 2.1; 95 percent CI 1.5–3.1). These authors called for interventions for IDUs focused on their sexual risks, including MSM risks.

Interventions

Brazil was the first low- or middle-income country to commit to universal access to antiretrovirals (ARVs). An estimated 83 percent of HIV-infected Brazilians who need treatment are currently receiving it—among the highest rate globally (CDC 2006). High rates of treatment access and ARV use have doubtless contributed to the sustained low HIV prevalence in Brazil, although this effect is arguably impossible to measure on population levels or for any subgroup. MSM have been actively included in treatment programs since their inception in Brazil, but ARV treatment program data are not available by risk exposure category.

Brazil has been a long-standing leader in targeted HIV prevention programs for persons at risk, including MSM (Gauri, Beyrer, and Vaillancourt 2007). Operating on both human rights principles of equality and dignity, and the participatory principle "nothing about us without us," Brazil demonstrates several key positive examples in best practices for HIV prevention. The national AIDS program reported that from 1999 to 2003, 486 HIV prevention programs were supported for MSM nationally (Gauri, Beyrer, and Vaillancourt 2007). These services were reported to have reached 3,074,980 MSM with prevention programs, an estimated coverage of 96 percent.

Despite these successes, homophobia has remained a feature of Brazilian society and in some health care settings (Araújo et al. 2009). The government has initiated a number of programs to combat homophobia and stigma—several with an explicit link to reducing homophobia as an approach to HIV prevention among MSM. The largest of these programs is "Brazil without Homophobia," which was launched in 2004. It is an effort to improve services for gay men, other MSM, and TG persons through state health institutions (UNAIDS 2009). "Brazil without Homophobia" included an affirmative agenda for gay men and other MSM and an affirmative agenda for transvestite and TG persons. In accordance with Brazilian policy, the program was conducted by lesbian, gay, bisexual, and transgendered (LGBT) groups; people living with HIV/AIDS groups; and civil society in partnership with government.

A more recent initiative has targeted HIV among young MSM, age 13–24 (*Medical News Today* 2008). This program has a mass media focus, including use of radio and television programs and train and bus venues, to promote social marketing of condoms and to deliver safe sex messages nationwide.

Brazil's focus on decreasing homophobia and stigma in clinical care settings, in schools, and in society more broadly is an example of human rights–based HIV prevention programming.

Peru: A Country with Complex Subgroups and Networks

Scenario: Risks among MSM are the predominant mode of HIV exposure for the population.

Key themes:

- The HIV epidemic in Peru is concentrated, and MSM bear a disproportionate burden of infection.
- The population of MSM is diverse with varying sexual practices, sexual and social risks, and identities, suggesting that HIV prevention programs should be targeted.
- Prevention efforts targeted to these men and clear policies to ensure rights of vulnerable populations in Peru provide an example of how human rights and community organizations can be integrated into national HIV strategies.
- Prevention programs must remain focused on the population of MSM to change the direction of the epidemic.

Classified by the World Bank as a middle-income county, Peru had an estimated gross national income (per capita) of US$3,990 in 2008 (World

Bank 2009). Similar to the general demographic trend in which 29 percent of the total population is concentrated in the capital, Lima, three-quarters of the estimated 20,000 cases of AIDS in Peru are also concentrated in Lima (Ministerio de Salud del Perú 2009). The first AIDS case was reported in 1983, and since then, the number of people living with HIV has grown and is estimated at between 20,000 and 79,000 (Cáceres and Mendoza 2009; Ministerio de Salud del Perú 2009; UNAIDS and WHO 2008). In 2002, Peru was selected to receive support from the Global Fund to Fight AIDS, Tuberculosis and Malaria (GFATM) of approximately US$80 million, the largest funding in the Latin American region for implementation from 2004 to 2012 (Cáceres and Mendoza 2009).

In Peru, however, the current HIV epidemic is concentrated among the population of MSM, whose population was last estimated at 620,978 in 2005 (Aldridge et al. 2009; Cáceres et al. 2007). Joint United Nations Programme on HIV/AIDS (UNAIDS) data from 2002 indicate that the greatest HIV prevalence among MSM has been observed in Lima, where estimates have ranged from 9.8 to 22.3 percent. This book's meta-analysis estimates a nationwide prevalence of 12.4 percent among MSM (95 CI, 11.9–12.8, n = 19,260), compared with a prevalence among reproductive-age adults of approximately 0.4 percent (UNAIDS and WHO 2008). Surveillance data from 2006 collected in Lima indicate the epidemic is more concentrated among the population of MSM, with a prevalence of 10.8 percent, than among any of the other high-risk groups, including female sex workers (FSWs) among whom the prevalence is 0.5 percent, for example (Cáceres et al. 2010; Ugarte Ubilluz et al. 2010). These figures stand in contrast, however, to 2006–08 reported prevention activities in which 54 percent of the sex worker population, compared to 21 percent of MSM, had been tested for HIV and knew their results (WHO, UNAIDS, and UNICEF 2009).

The national response to the HIV epidemic among MSM began in Lima in 1996 when HIV sentinel surveillance indicated an HIV prevalence of 18.5 percent among MSM with an annual incidence of 11.2 percent per year. As a result, HIV prevention strategies for MSM became a priority for national response. From then forward, such strategies began including MSM in HIV prevention activities for high-risk populations as well as providing gay-friendly clinics, free condom distribution, testing for sexually transmitted infections (STIs), and voluntary counseling and testing (VCT). To monitor changes in the epidemic, develop an "early warning system," and evaluate public HIV interventions, second-generation HIV sentinel surveillance was initiated at that time and was to be conducted biannually among MSM in Lima (Sanchez et al. 2007). Despite these national efforts to address the risk for HIV among MSM and other vulnerable populations, experts have argued that the national AIDS programs were not developed using a human rights framework and failed to address or prevent stigma or actively seek to improve access to services and reduce vulnerability of high-risk populations (Cáceres and Mendoza 2009). With the encouragement of community organizations, however, the national response gained momentum in the late 1990s and gradually recognized the rights of those affected by the epidemic; AIDS service organizations, such as Red SIDA Perú, pushed for government action on the HIV epidemic; LGBT communities became active in HIV prevention; and organizations for people living with HIV/AIDS (PLWHA), such as Peruanos Positivos, promoted legal changes in the provision of treatment for HIV. HIV research and academic centers have further enabled the characterization of the epidemic and an understanding of the populations, particularly subgroups of MSM, with the intent of informing HIV programming efforts. Such efforts have informed the development and implementation of interventions, programs, and policies and have led to national recognition of the rights of those affected by the epidemic. Provisions to ensure these rights were outlined in the second GFATM project and Peru's Multisectoral Strategic Plan (Cáceres and Mendoza 2009). Following an analysis of past GFATM programs, several strategic prevention areas were identified, notably including prevention for vulnerable populations such as MSM and sex workers (Visser-Valfrey, Cassagnol, and Espinel 2009).

MSM and Transgender Typologies Used for Epidemiologic Studies in Peru

In the late 1990s, a strong research environment developed in Peru and led to numerous ethnographic, behavioral, and epidemiologic studies of populations most at risk for HIV. The 2002 data from Lima suggest differential risk between subpopulations of MSM, with the highest prevalence rates among self-identified gay men (26.2 percent) and TG MSM (32.2 percent) and lower rates among bisexual men (13.3 percent) and heterosexual-identified MSM (12.1 percent) (Sanchez et al. 2007). Recognizing that the population of MSM is not homogeneous and exclusive but rather is diverse and nuanced by identities, sexual practices, and networks, research teams in Peru have devoted great efforts to study the risks of various subpopulations of MSM and to develop methods of reaching and providing preventive services that are acceptable and accessible for these men and their partners.

- *Homosexuals:* Second-generation HIV sentinel surveillance surveys among MSM in Peru found the majority of participants self-identifying as homosexual or gay (42 to 67 percent), as reported by Sanchez and colleagues (2007).
- *Transgendered individuals:* Research studies indicate the transgendered populations, represented by a variety of nomenclature and identities, often report some of the greatest risk behaviors, highest prevalence of HIV and STIs, and frequent incidents of discrimination and violence. A study by Tabet and colleagues (2002), conducted among more than 400 MSM in 2002, demonstrated that HIV and syphilis prevalence levels were 33.3 percent and 51.1 percent, respectively, among transgendered MSM ("cross-dressers") and were greater than levels observed among the sampled MSM population (18.5 percent and 16.0 percent, respectively). Using enzyme immunoassay tests to determine incidence, they found the estimated overall HIV seroincidence among MSM was 11.2 percent per year (95 percent CI, 4.8–23.6). Of the MSM who reported ever having sex with a woman, 12 percent were transgendered individuals (overall, 47 percent of MSM reported ever having sex with a woman; Tabet et al. 2002). As in the study by Tabet and colleagues, the biannual second-generation sentinel surveillance conducted among MSM in Lima found that the STI rates (herpes simplex virus 2 [HSV-2] at 80 percent and syphilis at 51 percent in 1996 but decreasing to 24 percent in 2002) were greatest among the 7.4 to 19.2 percent of MSM (1996–2002) who self-identified as "transvestites," compared to the other subpopulations (Sanchez et al. 2007).
- *Heterosexual and bisexual men:* Sentinel surveillance and other research efforts conducted among MSM in Peru indicate a small proportion of MSM self-identify as heterosexual and maintain sexual or romantic relationships with women. The proportion of sampled men who self-identified as heterosexual ranged from 6.3 to 31.9 percent and those as bisexual from 8.0 to 22.7 percent.

Having Sex with Women and Involvement in Concurrent Sexual Relationships

To many, the term MSM incorrectly implies homosexuality. However, as previously mentioned, same-sex behavior among men is complex, and research has attempted to explain networks and risks among MSM, women, and TG individuals. Although HIV prevalence is greatest among urban MSM, the decrease in the male-to-female case ratio from 17:1 in 1985 to 3:1 in 2000, at which level it has remained stable, has led to concern that heterosexual transmission was on the rise (Cáceres, Konda, Salazar et al. 2008).

Despite these debates, research has demonstrated "bridging" behavior in the MSM population. A study of male partners of pregnant women in coastal Peru found that previous sexual contact with another man was reported by 11 percent of the men enrolled, although fewer participants reported male sexual contacts in the previous year (2 percent) and unprotected sex with men during that time (0.9 percent of the total population). Of those who reported sexual contact with another man in the past year, 52 percent reported unprotected intercourse during those contacts, and 45 percent reported contact with an FSW in the last year as well (Clark, Konda, Munayco et al. 2008).

A study conducted in low-income areas of Peru (selected neighborhoods in Lima, Chiclayo, and Trujillo) sought to further explore the risk among urban poor populations as well as to understand the relationships among high-risk populations. This study included *homosexuales*, that is, men who self-identify as homosexual or TG, and men who frequently engage in transactional sex with homosexual men, called *esquineros* or "street corner men." The study identified two new high-risk populations that are included in the sexual networks of *homosexuales: esquineros*, who are often unemployed, associated with theft, gang activity, and substance use, and despite participating in sexual activity with *homosexuales*, do not self-identify as homosexual or bisexual; and *movidas*, or "active women," who often associate with *esquineros*. This study uncovered high rates of unprotected sex with a nonstable partner in the last three months (77 percent *esquineros*, 48 percent *homosexuales*, 16 percent *movidas*). Although exchange sex was socially considered to be a characteristic of the *movidas* group, it was most often reported among *homosexuales* and *esquineros* (26 and 15 percent, respectively) (Cáceres, Konda, Salazar et al. 2008). Forced sex in the last six months was also commonly reported by all groups: 16 percent of *esquineros*, 32 percent of *homosexuales*, and 28 percent of *movidas* ($p < 0.001$). Forced sex reported by *esquineros* was associated with greater numbers of sex partners in the last six months, recent unprotected sex act with a nonprimary partner (last six months), sex with a man (last six months), and alcohol and drug use prior to sex (Konda, Lescano, Sandoval et al. 2008). Of great importance to HIV prevention efforts, researchers noted that of these three groups participating in high-risk behaviors, only *homosexuales* would be considered MSM and therefore eligible for prevention services available to high-risk groups. Despite engaging with *homosexuales, esquineros*—who would be considered MSM by current research standards—and *movidas* who associate with these groups and also exhibit high-risk behaviors would be eligible for only limited services available to the general population; thus, the research team argued that prevention programs targeted toward MSM and led by the government were, in this scenario, unsuccessful (Cáceres, Konda, Salazar et al. 2008).

Self-identified bisexuality and heterosexuality were also reported but varied greatly among the MSM sampled in the six-year sentinel surveillance study conducted in Lima. Prevalence of HIV ranged from the lowest (6.4 percent) in 1996 to the highest (31.9 percent) in 2000 for those identifying as heterosexuals and from the lowest (8.0 percent) in 1998 to the highest (27.3 percent) among homosexual men in 2002. A substantial but wide range of MSM reported having sex with women (26.4 to 47.6 percent of MSM studied) (Sanchez et al. 2007). Those with frequent bisexual activity (MSM reporting two or more female partners in the last year) were defined as "bridgers" by Tabet and colleagues (2002), who recognized the added risk for this population associated with high-risk sexual practices with both male and female populations. Of the 400 MSM surveyed in Tabet's study, 27 percent were "bridgers," and 55 percent of the men reported having two or more female partners during the last year. Condom use among "bridgers" was less common during vaginal intercourse (17 percent used a condom in the last year) than for practices of insertive anal sex with men (25.5 percent) (Konda, Lescano, Leontsini et al. 2008; Tabet et al. 2002).

HIV-Positive Men

Although not necessarily a subpopulation of MSM, HIV-infected MSM have been found to engage in high-risk sexual activity, and such activities warrant special focus by HIV prevention programs. A study of sexual practices among 124 HIV-infected MSM in Lima showed evidence of continued high-risk behavior among infected men, even though 73 percent of the men were previously aware of their HIV infection. In comparing those with known HIV infection to those with unknown HIV infection, no difference was found in number of recent male partners (last six months) and frequency of unprotected anal intercourse. Furthermore, no suggestion occurred of changes in strategic positioning (insertive compared to receptive) or of serosorting. Unprotected anal intercourse was common among those men who were unaware of their HIV infection as well as those who were aware, but this practice could not be attributed to lack of knowledge about where to purchase condoms or to the cost of condoms. Following the revelation that high-risk practices continue among MSM infected with HIV, and particularly among MSM with a known HIV infection, Clark and colleagues (2007) suggested that discussions on strategic positioning and serosorting harm-reduction methods are warranted even if they are not proven methods for HIV prevention. Community and population-based approaches should be taken to address poverty that influences transactional sex, to decrease stigma against HIV-infected individuals as well as MSM that would encourage disclosure of HIV status, and to promote consideration of social norms that would potentially allow increased uptake of condom use (Clark, Konda, Segura et al. 2008).

Other Risk Factors

Low income and urban poverty. Although the poverty rate has declined in all areas of Peru except Lima, estimates from 2004 suggest that poverty continues to be a concern for the population, particularly those residing in rural areas (72.5 percent in poverty and 40.3 percent living in extreme poverty) and in Lima (36.6 percent in poverty and 3.4 percent living in extreme poverty) (Valverde and Cabello 2008). Poverty not only affects daily quality of life but has also been a factor in the HIV epidemic that first affected the upper middle class but quickly increased among the urban poor (Cáceres and Mendoza 2009). Low income and poverty may influence education and knowledge of HIV risks and prevention as well as access to appropriate prevention options and may lead to increased incidents of transactional sex. A study conducted among young adults (18–30 years) in a shantytown of Lima where the estimated annual income is significantly less than that of the rest of the country (US$2,100 compared with US$7,600) found high-risk behavior among men: 12 percent reported having sex with an FSW or with another man while under the influence of alcohol, and 2 percent reported doing so under the influence of illicit drugs. Furthermore, condom use was not routine; only 45 percent of the men studied used condoms with a casual partner, and 84 percent reported using them with sex workers. Interestingly, despite using condoms more frequently, women felt they could not access condoms (Gálvez-Buccollini et al. 2009).

The relationship of poverty and sexual risk is not always easily explained by traditional models, however, as the study by Cáceres,

Konda, Salazar, and colleagues (2008) among high-risk groups (*homosexuales*, *esquineros*, and *movidas*) demonstrates. Despite having higher rates of high school attendance (64 percent of *homosexuales* graduated high school compared with 47 percent of *esquineros* and 39 percent of *movidas*) and higher employment rates (85 percent), over a quarter of the men identifying as *homosexuales* had participated in transactional sex in the last three months, had reported forced sex (prevalence not reported), and reported the greatest prevalence of unprotected sex with a nonprimary partner (48 percent compared with 32 percent among *esquineros* and 16 percent among *movidas*). Unprotected sex was significantly associated with exchange sex and not having regular work. These risk factors among *homosexuales* are reflected in the prevalence of STIs, such as that of syphilis (29 percent), HSV-2 (72 percent), and HIV infection (10 percent). The significant association between unprotected sex with a nonprimary partner and exchange sex combined with the sexual networking among high-risk groups suggests social and economic factors may have added influence on the epidemiology of HIV and highlights that HIV interventions not only should target STI and HIV prevention among those identifying as MSM but also should seek to identify and provide services to sexual partners and consider other social and economic interventions (Cáceres, Konda, Salazar et al. 2008).

Transactional sex. Definitions of transactional sex and self-identity as a sex worker are variable among MSM, but such identities and behaviors were important for accessing prevention and care early in the epidemic because the national response provided HIV and STI services for sex workers (Valverde and Cabello 2008). At the last collection of second-generation sentinel surveillance (2002), 17.2 percent of the MSM surveyed self-reported as a sex worker, yet more than 30 percent of subjects reported receiving financial or material compensation for sexual activity with another man (Sanchez et al. 2007). Konda, Clark, and colleagues (2008) surveyed and tested a convenience sample of 547 MSM and TG individuals attending an STI clinic in Lima and found that 31 percent reported engaging in compensated sex, whereas 24 percent of the study population self-identified as a sex worker. Those reporting compensated sex were significantly less likely to have graduated high school and also reported greater perception of risk for HIV. Those reporting compensated sex were more likely to be TG individuals (51 percent) or self-identified as gay (23 percent). In the study of HIV-infected MSM in Lima (previously described in the section "HIV-Positive Men"), Clark, Konda, Segura, and colleagues (2008) found that 34 percent of infected MSM had provided compensated sex in the last six months and, upon further analysis, this rate remained consistent among those who were aware of their HIV status (31 percent). Other factors associated with compensated sex included alcohol use (49 percent), drug use (mostly marijuana and cocaine, 36 percent), and HSV (66 percent) and syphilis (32 percent) infection. Among those who identified as sex workers, participants reported the median age at which sex work began was 19 years and they had sex with an average 10 clients per week. These sex workers also reported a high prevalence of police abuse (40 percent), but few knew of organizations from which to seek assistance in the event of such abuse (17 percent) (Konda, Clark, et al. 2008).

Drug use. Risk associated with injecting drug use is not investigated among MSM because investigators state that no cases of HIV are reported among the population of injecting drug users as a whole, and the practice of injecting drug use is rare in Peru (Aldridge et al. 2009) although sterile, disposable syringes are widely distributed within the public health care settings and in markets (Valverde and Cabello 2008). Because injecting drug use is not considered a critical aspect of the HIV epidemic in Peru, drug use in general (injecting and noninjecting) has not historically been a priority of HIV research and only recently has begun to be assessed, often in studies conducted among lower-income communities in Peru. The study conducted by Cáceres, Konda, Salazar, and colleagues (2008) found that *esquineros* from Peruvian *barrios* reported significantly greater use of illegal drugs (assessed use of marijuana, cocaine, and cocaine-based drugs in last 30 days) compared to *homosexuales* and *movidas* in the study population and was a risk factor that was significantly associated with unprotected sex. Konda, Lescano, Sandoval, and colleagues' (2008) study of forced sex found that incidents were associated with illicit drug and alcohol use, and Gálvez-Buccolini and colleagues' (2009) study in the Limeño shantytown found high-risk behavior, including inconsistent condom use, associated with drug use.

Age. National and international estimates suggest the younger, adult male population (15–24 years) is particularly affected (UNAIDS and WHO 2008), and approximately 70 percent of those affected are of prime reproductive age (20–39 years) (Valverde and Cabello 2008) even though 55 percent of both genders demonstrate an understanding of HIV transmission (UNAIDS and WHO 2008). In the biannual second-generation sentinel surveillance conducted among MSM in Lima, no trend was seen in HIV prevalence among self-indentifying homosexual men 18–20 years of age across the study period (8 percent in 1996, 10 percent in 1998, and 13 percent in 2002), nor was a trend observed when the prevalence among a greater age range of 18–24 years was assessed (Sanchez et al. 2007). A review of data from 1999–2002 among South American MSM, however, demonstrated that Peruvian MSM 30 years or older had a greater prevalence of HIV (16.0 percent) compared with those in lower age categories (Bautista et al. 2004).

Interventions

Despite acknowledgment of the concentrated epidemic among the population of MSM and Peru's intention to reach these men, data suggest that focused efforts are still needed to improve prevention for MSM. Past interventions have been criticized for inadequate use of scientific evidence and lack of monitoring and evaluation, although early government response focused on provision of medical examinations and peer-promotion interventions targeted to FSWs and MSM as well as STI management and provision of free antibiotics for the general population (Cáceres, Konda, Salazar et al. 2008). Tellingly, recent UNAIDS data indicated that only 21 percent of the population of MSM had received an HIV test in the last year and were aware of their results, compared to the 54 percent of FSWs who had been tested and were aware of these results. Similarly, only 44 percent of MSM were reached by HIV prevention programs, compared to the 80 percent of FSWs reached by prevention programs (Cáceres, Konda, Salazar et al. 2008; UNAIDS and WHO 2008). HIV intervention strategies for the general population have been used individually or in combination in Peru and are often presumed to be accessible to MSM; these strategies include but are not limited to mass media campaigns, VCT, youth education targeting individuals between 10 and 18 years of age, distribution of condoms (male-type only), and STI treatment (including counseling and condom provision). Such prevention programs that may be available to the population as a whole, including MSM, may inadvertently exclude vulnerable populations that are unaware of the risks of transmission or who face stigma and discrimination when attempting to access "available" prevention, treatment, and sexual health services.

Counseling and treatment. VCT (using the enzyme-linked immunosorbent assay, or ELISA, test), including both pre- and posttest counseling, has been available in the public health sector since the establishment of the CONTRASIDA law in 1997 (Valverde and Cabello 2008). Specifically targeted to MSWs and FSWs, the national strategy developed and established the system Unidad de Atención Médica Periódica (regular medical care unit) for detection and treatment of STIs and HIV/AIDS. Nevertheless, the evaluation of the 2001–04 Strategic Plan for the Prevention and Control of HIV/AIDS in Peru found an increase in the prevalence of new STI cases, mostly among populations of sex workers and MSM, and further reported that only 48 percent of the MSWs and FSWs had completed six or more checkups, indicating that the majority did not have adequate follow-up procedures. In 2005, new regulations were developed to provide testing and counseling every six months for MSM, MSWs, and FSWs and were incorporated into the peer health educators (Promotores Educadores de Pares; PEP) strategy; however, these activities were required to be carried out in STI Reference Centers (Centro de Referencia de Enfermedades de Transmisión Sexual) or in the UAMP themselves and were mostly available in formal sex-trade districts and so may miss those informally involved or who move into and out of the sex trade (Valverde and Cabello 2008).

The early national response to the HIV epidemic initiated the use of community-based interventions aimed at decreasing HIV incidence and STI prevalence among MSM. PEPs from 15 cities in Peru were trained on the basic topics of STIs, including recognition of symptoms, risk factors for transmission, prevention, and where to access testing and treatment; methods for approaching individuals at risk in public venues; and methods for negotiating condom use and promoting personal health and self-esteem. In 1999, 208 PEPs distributed almost 2 million pamphlets and 1.5 million condoms and referred more than 6,900 MSM to gay-friendly health centers for STI testing and treatment (Escudero Panduro et al. 2000). Comparisons of the cost-effectiveness of providing this intervention to MSM with others, such as STI treatment, VCT, counseling and treatment for FSWs, prevention of mother-to-child transmission of HIV/AIDS, and provision of antiretroviral therapy (ART), indicated that the intervention for MSM was more costly (in terms of unit cost per person reached) than STI treatment, intervention for FSWs, and mass media campaigns but offered one of the highest rates of infections averted (Aldridge et al. 2009).

Condom distribution. The male condom has been distributed through national public health services and is available in the market. Despite claims of distribution and availability, experts noted a decline in the public distribution beginning in 2001, and the United Nations General Assembly Special Session (UNGASS) monitoring report indicated that since 2001 no obvious change in access had occurred (Valverde and Cabello 2008). Condom distribution is also routinely included in behavioral and standard interventions.

Distribution of lubricants. Early national prevention activities developed for MSM included the distribution of lubricants; however, in the four years leading up to the UNGASS monitoring report on HIV/AIDS, distribution of lubricants through public health services was not an activity that was included in the national strategy for prevention among MSM. This reversal received much criticism because access to lubricant is possible only in large cities where lubricants are sold in markets, but they have limited availability in rural or geographically distant areas (Valverde and Cabello 2008).

Behavior change messages and public education. Behavior change messages were common but have been criticized for failing to evolve in parallel with the changing HIV epidemic and failing to address new understandings of behavioral risks (Cáceres and Mendoza 2009). Although widely spread through media and school programs, educational messages have mostly been targeted toward the general audience and have largely promoted abstinence and condom use. Because messages rarely provided information regarding the increased risk associated with specific behaviors, such as multiple partners, commercial sex, or same-sex behaviors (Valverde and Cabello 2008), one can argue that MSM and other vulnerable populations were unaware that they should protect themselves or how to do so. For the younger population, HIV prevention messages are provided through the school systems; however, curricula did not include sexual diversity or rights, and a substantial proportion of students (40 percent) felt that HIV education was insufficient (Valverde and Cabello 2008).

Peer-based interventions. The National Institute of Mental Health Collaborative HIV/STD Prevention Trial Group (2009) in the United States conducted a phase III trial throughout several *barrios* in Peru from 2000 to 2002 as part of a five-country multisite study to test a community-level peer-based intervention through community popular opinion leaders (CPOLs). Using social diffusion principles, the trial tested the intervention's effectiveness in changing social norms pertaining to sexual behavior among young adult populations in Peru as well as the following groups: in China, market owners and workers; in India, male patrons of wine shops and women congregating near the shops; in the Russian Federation, dormitory students; and in Zimbabwe, those congregating in commercial areas (Cáceres, Konda, Salazar et al. 2008). The purpose of the CPOLs was to disseminate prevention messages through regular conversations among social groups, among networks, and in different venues in the *barrios*. To target heterosexually identified men, homosexually identified men, and high-risk women with multiple sex partners (*esquineros, homosexuals*, and *movidas* described by Caceres, Konda, Salazar and colleagues' [2008] research) in Peru, the team trained a total of 124 CPOLs with information on sexuality, HIV and STIs and methods for their prevention, and skill building and effective communication exercises to deliver prevention messages. They combined this training with activities to reinforce the commitment of each peer educator and keep him or her engaged. Of those invited to be a CPOL, 78 percent completed training. Success in working with CPOLs was attributed to trust established by the study team, which had been involved with the community for extended periods; credibility of working with the university that was overseeing the project; distribution of formal invitations to those eligible to be CPOLs; and frequent meetings with CPOLS to keep them engaged. Differences were seen between the three groups; homosexual men knew and felt comfortable talking to many people (including women and heterosexual men) in the *barrio*. Women, however, often were limited to reaching smaller groups of other women and men with whom they socialized, whereas heterosexual men led conversations mostly with women or with other heterosexual men and often felt more discouraged than the homosexual men when friends did not listen or mocked them during conversations. A midintervention process evaluation allowed the study team to assess CPOL training, investigate acceptability, and address any areas of concern. Overall, the intervention was acceptable to both the community and the CPOLs (Maiorana et al. 2007).

Web-based interventions. In recent years, experts have begun to encourage use of the Internet for HIV interventions, suggesting that the trend of using the Internet to meet partners has expanded to Peru and raising concerns about the role of the Internet in high-risk sexual encounters. A study of 100 HIV-positive men found that 94 percent of those who met partners through the Internet were MSM (Alva et al. 2007). In Peru, the availability of Internet access has increased with the existence of low-cost and user-friendly access provided by Internet cafés (*cabinas públicas*). They are estimated to be used by over 80 percent of Internet users and are popular for their ease of access, often open 24 hours a day and available widely across Peru, including areas of lower economic status. They often provide private areas that have been used for sexual encounters. An online survey conducted by banner ads displayed on a popular gay website found that *cabinas públicas* were the most common source for Internet access (58 percent), respondents most commonly identified as homosexual (72 percent) and the rest as bisexual, men frequently reported sex with an Internet partner in the last year (67 percent), and HIV-positive respondents sought sex partners (77 percent) and had sex with an Internet partner (67 percent) during the last year. Some participants reported sexual encounters within the *cabinas públicas* (1 percent) (Blas et al. 2006). Blas and colleagues (2007) tested the utility of banner ads displayed on a gay website in recruiting men to complete an online survey and report to health clinics for HIV testing. Ads offering health services demonstrated a higher frequency of completed surveys (5.8 percent compared with 3.4 percent) and recruited MSM who had not previously been tested for HIV; however, only 11 percent of respondents who completed the survey offering the free testing actually reported to the clinic, and among those, 6 percent had a previous diagnosis of HIV, 5 percent tested positive for HIV, and 8 percent tested positive for syphilis. A forthcoming intervention will test the effectiveness of an Internet-based intervention to conduct HIV and STI diagnosis and treatment for MSM (Curioso et al. 2007).

Mobile VCT. Vía Libre, a community-based nongovernmental organization, sought to improve access to and quality of sexual health services for MSM and TG individuals. Using mobile vans, the study employed a multidisciplinary team and frequented traditional gay venues (such as saunas and parks) and poor areas to provide comprehensive options for health service; it delivered test results within 20 minutes of collection. Participants were provided with individual case managers; condoms, lubricants, and educational materials were distributed; and those participants testing positive for HIV infection were immediately incorporated into the national highly active antiretroviral therapy (HAART) program. Investigators attributed the success of the program to immediate management of infections, online advertisement of van locations and not advertising as a gay van, visibility and availability of the van at various locations and peak times, and coordination with local authorities. One of the most important findings was the ability of the mobile unit to reach non-gay-identified individuals (Smith 2008).

Peer counseling for MSM and treatment for STIs. Peer counseling and treatment of STIs and provision of condoms to MSM (similar to interventions available for FSWs) was the common MSM-specific intervention used in the early national response.

Antiretroviral therapy. Until 2000, the national response did not encompass treatment and care, based on arguments that treatment was beyond the reach of national resources and also that treatment may lead to increased transmission. After much pressure, and later the advent of the UNGASS Declaration and the receipt of GFATM funding, treatment began to be embraced as an option for HIV programming (Cáceres and Mendoza 2009). According to UNAIDS data, 65 sites were providing ART to approximately 11,000 individuals (with a range of 9,800–12,000) by 2007, reaching about 48 percent of those in need (UNAIDS and WHO 2008), mostly in Lima and Callao (Valverde and Cabello 2008). No data are available about the number of PLWHA receiving ARVs from the private sector, where they can cost between US$1,050 annually for generic drugs and up to US$4,500 annually for first-line therapy treatments (Valverde and Cabello 2008). Deaths related to HIV ultimately peaked in the late 1990s and subsequently began to decline; the continuing decreasing trend of HIV-related deaths has been attributed to increased access to ART and improved health services (Cáceres and Mendoza 2009).

The national ART program was established in 2004, five years after HAART was initiated, providing free ART through the ministry of health and other public sources (Cáceres and Mendoza 2009). To be eligible for the HAART program, an individual must meet specific diagnostic criteria, demonstrate family support, and have a permanent residence. Many individuals benefited from the generous interpretation of these requirements, and in many cases close relatives or friends were approved at the discretion of the health care provider. Despite this flexibility, experts feel that because of stigma within families and in the health sector toward vulnerable populations such as MSM, the criteria continued to act as a barrier to treatment access. Additional barriers to accessing the HAART program included the cost of testing and the long wait for test results (Valverde and Cabello 2008). Several criticisms of the training for the

HAART program have surfaced. They include the reduced number of doctors participating even though physicians from around the country have received training. In addition, the lack of correspondence between the selection of staff to be trained and the current working staff because of the system of staff rotation within the health care facilities means the training did not encompass the interpersonal dimension for treating PLWHA and respect for the rights of PLWHA. Furthermore, poor monitoring of HAART staff is cited (Valverde and Cabello 2008). Finally, HAART placed a burden on the national health program, which was faced with structural challenges in implementing HAART that included lack of diagnostic capabilities, lack of resources to properly monitor therapy, and lack of physical resources and personnel to provide comprehensive care for the varying stages and needs of PLWHA.

HAART is used in three alternative regimens:

- The basic regimen includes provision of ARVs coupled with CD4 and viral load monitoring.
- The intermediate regimen couples the basic program with additional laboratory monitoring and imaging tests.
- The comprehensive regimen combines the treatment of opportunistic infections with the intermediate program (Aldridge et al. 2009).

Cost analysis of intervention strategies used in 2008 in Peru suggests the cost for the peer counseling and STI treatment package for MSM reached approximately US$103.00 per person, whereas intervention programs available for the general population exhibited a broad range of costs from US$0.04 per person for mass media interventions, to US$3.70 per case for STI treatment, US$40.00 per client for VCT, and US$3,792 per client for the comprehensive antiretroviral regimen (Aldridge et al. 2009). Although the peer counseling and STI treatment package for MSM was determined to be a cost-effective intervention, it falls behind peer education of FSWs and VCT in terms of strict cost-effectiveness; investigators attributed poor performance in cost-effectiveness to the analysis of the population of MSM as a single homogeneous group rather than taking into account the variations between the subpopulations. This study, however, demonstrated that providing this MSM-specific intervention program resulted in some of the highest rates of total infections averted over the course of five years and varied little over time in cost-effectiveness, unlike other interventions such as STI treatment and youth education, for which coverage varied.

Ongoing or Anticipated Interventions

Bio-behavioral interventions. A current trial (2008–11), funded by the National Institute of Mental Health and led by Cáceres and colleagues, is under way to test the effectiveness of community-level behavioral and biomedical interventions among a sample of 850 men. This study seeks to evaluate interventions to reduce high-risk behavior and decrease HIV and STI. It has four arms:

- Provision of enhanced partner therapy, in which MSM with STIs are provided with partner treatment packets that contain informational materials, prophylactic medications, and condoms for their sexual partners
- Development of Communidades Positivas, an intervention to reduce the frequency of unprotected sex with nonprimary partners by training MSM who are recognized leaders to implement a community center that provides information, support, and empowerment to MSM, their friends, and partners
- Standard care that includes traditional STI care
- A combination of enhanced partner therapy and Communidades Positivas (NIMH 2009)

Preexposure chemophylaxis. Most recently, Peru was one of the six countries included in the Preexposure Prophylaxis Initiative (iPrEx) trial that compared daily emtricitabine tenofovir disoproxil fumarate (FTC–TDF) to placebo among a random assignment of a total of 2,499 HIV-seronegative participants. Participants from Peru were recruited in Lima (N = 940) and Iquitos (N = 460). All study participants received behavioral HIV prevention measures including HIV testing, risk-reduction counseling, condoms, and management of STIs. Overall, analysis included 3,324 person-years of follow-up with a median follow-up of 1.2 years. In total, 64 infections occurred in the placebo group, and 36 infections in the experimental group, indicating a 44 percent reduction in HIV incidence (95 percent CI 15–63, $p < 0.01$) (Grant et al. 2010).

Circumcision. A similar study was conducted in 2006 in three cities of Peru as well as in Ecuador to assess willingness of MSM to participate in a trial of circumcision for the prevention of HIV acquisition. Men were enrolled in the study if they did not know their HIV status or had not received results for an HIV test in the last 12 months, totaling 2,048 enrollees with a median age of 24 years. Of those studied, 3.7 percent were circumcised, but this was more common in Lima (5.5 percent) and other large cities. Meanwhile, no significant differences were seen with respect to circumcision status when comparing HIV, syphilis infection, or sexual role. Of the participants, 54.3 percent of subjects acknowledged willingness to participate in a circumcision trial; willingness was more common (not significant) among those who tested HIV positive and had an insertive role. Possible barriers to participation included fears of surgery (45.5 percent), fears of side effects associated with surgery (47.2 percent), and fears of increased unprotected sex with partners after surgery (43.5 percent) (Guanira et al. 2007).

Conclusion

Only recently—with the encouragement of a multitude of organizations for LGBT populations, those serving PLWHA, and other civil society organizations and research institutes—has Peru begun to incorporate a human rights framework into its strategic plan and attempted to address the disproportionate prevalence of HIV infection. Peru has signed and ratified a number of international treaties and conventions, including the Universal Declaration of Human Rights; the International Covenant on Economic, Social, and Cultural Rights; the International Covenant on Civil and Political Rights; the American Convention on Human Rights, "Pact of San Jose, Costa Rica"; and the Additional Protocol to the American Convention on Human Rights in the Area of Economic, Social, and Cultural Rights, "Protocol of San Salvador"—all guaranteeing basic human rights, including the right to health. According to these laws, no professions or behaviors are illegal, such as homosexuality, injecting drug use (although sale or purchase of narcotics is illegal), or commercial sex work, and national laws protect the rights of PLWHA (Valverde and Cabello 2008). Despite these protections, discrimination, violence, and stigma targeted toward these populations run high, and many PLWHA often face great challenges in accessing or maintaining access to necessary health services (Andean Community of Nations 2003; Valverde and Cabello 2008) and many were left disappointed by government failure to protect these rights (Valverde and Cabello 2008). The 2008 review of same-sex behaviors and associated health indicators concluded that improvements in HIV services for MSM require that interventions be built on knowledge of the populations of MSM, including the size of such populations, the variety and frequencies of sexual practices and probable risk of their practices, the heterosexual relationships and bisexual practices among MSM, the prevalence of high-risk subpopulations such as those involved in sex work, and the rates and trends of HIV and STIs. Interventions should, moreover, be determined by social and behavioral investigations within populations of MSM, including knowledge, attitudes, and practices related to HIV among MSM; community mobilization and support; and legal and policy issues that affect provision and access to HIV prevention and care (Cáceres, Konda, Segura et al. 2008). These pieces have slowly come together, and continuous, informed, and coordinated efforts are necessary to meet the goal of cutting HIV transmission among MSM in Peru.

References for Brazil

Araújo, M. A., M. A. Montagner, R. M. da Silva, F. L. Lopes, and M. M. de Freitas. 2009. "Symbolic Violence Experienced by MSM in the Primary Health Services in Fortaleza, Ceará, Brazil: Negotiating Identity under Stigma." *AIDS Patient Care and STDS* 23 (8): 663–68.

Baral, S., F. Sifakis, F. Cleghorn, and C. Beyrer. 2007. "Elevated Risk for HIV Infection among Men Who Have Sex with Men in Low- and Middle-Income Countries 2000–2006: A Systematic Review." *PLoS Medicine* 4 (12): e339.

Cáceres, C.F., K. Konda, E. R. Segura, and R. Lyerla. 2008. "Epidemiology of Male Same-Sex Behaviour and Associated Sexual Health Indicators in Low- and Middle-Income Countries: 2003-2007 Estimates." *Sexually Transmitted Infections* 84 (Suppl. 1): i49–56.

Carneiro, M., F. A. Cardoso, M. Greco, E. Oliveira, J. Andrade, D. B. Greco, C. M. de Figueiredo Antunes III, and Project Horizonte team. 2003. "Determinants of Human Immunodeficiency Virus (HIV) Prevalence in Homosexual and Bisexual Men Screened for Admission to a Cohort Study of HIV Negatives in Belo Horizonte, Brazil: Project Horizonte." *Memorias do Instituto Oswaldo Cruz* 98 (3): 325–29.

CDC (Centers for Disease Control and Prevention). "The Global HIV/AIDS Pandemic, 2006." *MMWR* 55 (31): 841–44.

de Andrade, S. M., E. M. Tamaki, J. M. Vinha, M. A. Pompilio, C. W. Prieto, L. M. de Barros, L. B. de Lima, M. de Capua Chaguri, and S. A. de Lima Pompilio. 2007. "Vulnerability of Men Who Have Sex with Men in the Context of AIDS." *Cadernos de Saúde Pública* 23 (2): 479–82.

Ferreira, A. D., W. T. Caiaffa, F. I. Bastos, and S. A. Mingoti. 2006. "Profile of Male Brazilian Injecting Drug Users Who Have Sex with Men." *Cadernos de Saúde Pública* 22 (4): 849–60.

Gauri, V., C. Beyrer, and D. Vaillancourt. 2007. "From Human Rights Principles to Public Health Practice: HIV/AIDS Policy in Brazil." In *Public Health and Human Rights: Evidence Based Approaches*, ed. B. Pizer, 289–329. Baltimore, MD: Johns Hopkins University Press.

Medical News Today. 2008. "Brazilian Government Launches Initiative to Reduce HIV/AIDS among Young MSM," March 28.

Mello, M. B., A. A. Pinho, W. Tun, M. Chinaglia, A. Barbosa Jr., and J. Díaz. 2008. "Risky Sexual Behavior and HIV Seroprevalence among MSM in Campinas, SP, Brazil." Presentation at "AIDS 2008": XVII International AIDS Conference, Mexico City, August 3–8.

Ministry of Health. 2001. *AIDS: The Brazilian Experience*. São Paulo: Ministry of Health Programa Nacional de Doenças Sexual.

Périssé, A. R. S., C. M. d. Amorim, J. R. G. d. Silva, M. Schechter, and W. A. Blattner. 2006. "Relationship of Egocentric Network Characteristics and HIV Transmission among MSM in Rio de Janeiro, Brazil." Presentation at "AIDS 2006": XVI International AIDS Conference, Toronto, Canada, August 13–18.

Sampaio, M., C. Brites, R. Stall, E. S. Hudes, and N. Hearst. 2002. "Reducing AIDS Risk among Men Who Have Sex with Men in Salvador, Brazil." *AIDS and Behavior* 6 (2): 173–81.

Szwarcwald, C. L., A. Barbosa-Júnior, A. R. Pascom, and P. R. de Souza-Júnior. 2005. "Knowledge, Practices and Behaviours Related to HIV Transmission among the Brazilian Population in the 15–54 Years Age Group, 2004." *AIDS* 19 (Suppl. 4): S51–58.

Tun, W., M. de Mello, A. Pinho, M. Chinaglia, and J. Diaz. 2008. "Sexual Risk Behaviours and HIV Seroprevalence among Male Sex Workers Who Have Sex with Men and Non-Sex Workers in Campinas, Brazil." *Sexually Transmitted Infections* 84 (6): 455–57.

UNAIDS (Joint United Nations Programme on HIV/AIDS). 2008. "Epidemiological Fact Sheet on HIV and AIDS: Core Data on Epidemiology and Response—Brazil." Geneva: UNAIDS–World Health Organization Working Group on Global HIV/AIDS and Sexually Transmitted Infection Surveillance.

———. 2009. "HIV Prevention Hampered by Homophobia." January 13. http://www.unaids.org/en/Resources/PressCentre/Featurestories/2009/January/20090113MSMLATAM/.

UNAIDS (Joint United Nations Programme on HIV/AIDS) and WHO (World Health Organization). 2007. *AIDS Epidemic Update: December 2007*. Geneva: UNAIDS and WHO.

U.S. Department of State. 2009. "Background Note: Brazil." U.S. Department of State, Washington, DC. http://www.state.gov/r/pa/ei/bgn/35640.htm.

References for Peru

Aldridge, R. W., D. Iglesias, C. F. Cáceres, and J. J. Miranda. 2009. "Determining a Cost Effective Intervention Response to HIV/AIDS in Peru." *BMC Public Health* 9: 352.

Alva, I., M. Blas, P. García, R. Cabello, A. M. Kimball, and K. K. Holmes. 2007. "Riesgos y beneficios del uso de Internet entre personas viviendo con VIH/SIDA en Lima, Perú." *Revista Peruana de Medicina Experimental y Salud Pública* 24 (3): 248–53.

Andean Community of Nations. 2003. *HIV/AIDS Situation and Human Rights in the Andean Community of Nations: Monitoring of the Implementation of Obligations Stemming from the Declaration of Commitment in the Fight against HIV/AIDS*. Lima: LACCASO and Vía Libre.

Bautista, C. T., J. L. Sanchez, S. M. Montano, V. A. Laguna-Torres, J. R. Lama, J. L. Sanchez, L. Kusunoki, H. Manrique, J. Acosta, O. Montoya, et al. 2004. "Seroprevalence of and Risk Factors for HIV-1 Infection among South American Men Who Have Sex with Men." *Sexually Transmitted Infections* 80 (6): 498–504.

Blas, M. M., I. Alva, R. Cabello, P. Garcia, M. Redmon, A. Kurth, A. M. Kimball, and R. Ryan. 2006. "Response to an Internet Survey of Men Who Have Sex with Men in Peru." Poster presented at the 11th World Congress on Internet in Medicine, Toronto, Canada, October 13–20.

Blas, M. M., I. E. Alva, R. Cabello, P. J. Garcia, C. Carcamo, M. Redmon, A. M. Kimball, R. Ryan, and A. E. Kurth. 2007. "Internet as a Tool to Access High-Risk Men Who Have Sex with Men from a Resource-Constrained Setting: A Study from Peru." *Sexually Transmitted Infections* 83 (7): 567–70.

Cáceres, C. F., B. de Zalduondo, T. Hallett, C. Avila, and M. Clayton. 2010. "Combination HIV Prevention: Crafting a New Standard for the Long-Term Response to HIV." Presentation at "AIDS 2010": XVIII International AIDS Conference, Vienna, Austria, July 18–23.

Cáceres, C. F., K. A. Konda, X. Salazar, S. R. Leon, J. D. Klausner, A. G. Lescano, A. Maiorana, S. Kegeles, F. R. Jones, and T. J. Coates. 2008. "New Populations at High Risk of HIV/STIs in Low-Income, Urban Coastal Peru." *AIDS and Behavior* 12 (4): 544–51.

Cáceres, C. F., K. Konda, E. R. Segura, and R. Lyerla. 2008. "Epidemiology of Male Same-Sex Behaviour and Associated Sexual Health Indicators in Low- and Middle-Income Countries: 2003-2007 Estimates." *Sexually Transmitted Infections* 84 (Suppl. 1): i49–56.

Cáceres C. F., and W. Mendoza. 2009. "The National Response to the HIV/AIDS Epidemic in Peru: Accomplishments and Gaps—a Review." *Journal of Acquired Immune Deficiency Syndromes* 51 (Suppl. 1): S60–66.

Cáceres, C. F., W. Mendoza, K. Konda and A. Lescano. 2007. *Nuevas evidencias para las políticas y programas de salud en VIH/SIDA e infecciones de transmisión sexual en el Perú: Información disponible hasta febrero 2007*. Lima: Universidad Peruana Cayetano Heredia and Organización Panamericana de la Salud.

Clark, J. L., C. F. Cáceres, A. G. Lescano, K. A. Konda, S. R. Leon, et al. 2007. "Prevalence of Same-Sex Sexual Behavior and Associated Characteristics among Low-Income Urban Males in Peru." PLoS ONE 2 (8): e778.

Clark, J. L., K. A. Konda, C. V. Munayco, M. Pun, A. G. Lescano, S. R. Leon, J. Pajuelo, L. Suarez-Ognio, J. D. Klausner, T. J. Coates, et al. 2008. "Prevalence of HIV, Herpes Simplex Virus-2, and Syphilis in Male Sex Partners of Pregnant Women in Peru." *BMC Public Health* 8: 65.

Clark, J. L., K. A. Konda, E. R. Segura, H. J. Salvatierra, S. R. Leon, E. R. Hall, C. F. Cáceres, J. D. Klausner, and T. J. Coates. 2008. "Risk Factors for the Spread of HIV and Other Sexually Transmitted Infections among Men Who Have Sex with Men Infected with HIV in Lima, Peru." *Sexually Transmitted Infections* 84 (6): 449–54.

Curioso, W. H., M. M. Blas, B. Nodell, I. E. Alva, and A. E. Kurth. 2007. "Opportunities for Providing Web-Based Interventions to Prevent Sexually Transmitted Infections in Peru." *PLoS Med* 4 (2): e11.

Escudero Panduro, R. H., J. J. Ojeda Celi, J. M. Campos Guevara, and R. Galvan Huaman. 2000. "National Strategy of MSM Peer-Educators to Prevent STD/HIV in Peru." Presentation at the XIII International AIDS Conference, Durban, South Africa, July 9–14.

Gálvez-Buccollini, J. A., S. DeLea, P. M. Herrera, R. H. Gilman, and V. Paz-Soldan. 2009. "Sexual Behavior and Drug Consumption among Young Adults in a Shantytown in Lima, Peru." *BMC Public Health* 9: 23.

Grant, R., J. Lama, P. Anderson, V. McMahan, A. Y. Liu, L. Vargas, P. Goicochea, M. Casapía, J. V. Guanira-Carranza, M. E. Ramirez-Cardich, et al. 2010. "Preexposure Chemoprophylaxis for HIV Prevention in Men Who Have Sex with Men." *New England Journal of Medicine* 363 (27): 2587–99.

Guanira, J., J. R. Lama, P. Goicochea, P. Segura, O. Montoya, and J. Sanchez. 2007. "How Willing Are Gay Men to 'Cut Off' the Epidemic? Circumcision among MSM in the Andean Region." Presentation at the 4th IAS Conference on HIV Pathogenesis, Treatment and Prevention, Sydney, Australia, July 22–25.

Konda, K., J. L. Clark, E. R. Segura, H. J. Salvatierra, J. T. Galea, S. Leon, E. R. Hall, J. D. Klausner, C. Cáceres, and T. Coates. 2008. "Characterizing Sex Work among Male and Transgender STI Clinic Clients in Lima, Peru." Presentation at XVII International AIDS Conference, Mexico City, Mexico, August 3–8.

Konda, K. A., A. G. Lescano, E. Leontsini, P. Fernandez, J. D. Klausner, T. J. Coates, and C. F. Cáceres. 2008. "High Rates of Sex with Men among High-Risk, Heterosexually-Identified Men in Low-Income, Coastal Peru." *AIDS and Behavior* 12 (3): 483–91.

Konda, K., A. G. Lescano, C. Sandoval, J. T. Galea, T. Coates, C. Cáceres, and Group NCHSPT. 2008. "Recent Non-consensual Intercourse in Three Socially-Marginalized Populations in Low-Income, Urban, Coastal Peru." Presentation at XVII International AIDS Conference, Mexico City, Mexico, August 3–8.

Maiorana, A., S. Kegeles, P. Fernandez, X. Salazar, C. Cáceres, C. Sandoval, A. M. Rosasco, and T. Coates. 2007. "Implementation and Evaluation of an HIV/STD Intervention in Peru." *Evaluation and Program Planning* 30 (1): 82–93.

Ministerio de Salud del Perú. 2009. *Estadística: Indicadores de Salud.* Lima: Ministerio de Salud del Perú.

NIMH (National Institute of Mental Health). 2009. "Effectiveness of Community-Level Behavioral and Biomedical Interventions for Reducing HIV/STIs in Men in Peru." U.S. National Institutes of Health, Bethesda, MD. http://clinicaltrials.gov/ct2/show/NCT00670163.

Sanchez, J., J. R. Lama, L. Kusunoki, H. Manrique, P. Goicochea, A. Lucchetti, M. Rouillon, M. Pun, L. Suarez, S. Montano, J. L. Sanchez, et al. 2007. "HIV-1, Sexually Transmitted Infections, and Sexual Behavior Trends among Men Who Have Sex with Men in Lima, Peru." *Journal of Acquired Immune Deficiency Syndromes* 44 (5): 578–85.

Smith, E. S. 2008. "Using a Mobile Van to Provide Voluntary Counseling and Testing (VCT) to High-Risk and Closeted MSM." Presentation at XVII International AIDS Conference, Mexico City, Mexico, August 3–8.

Tabet, S., J. Sanchez, J. R. Lama, P. Goicochea, P. Campos, M. Rouillon, J. L. Cairo, L. Ueda, D. Watts, C. Celum, et al. 2002. "HIV, Syphilis and Heterosexual Bridging among Peruvian Men Who Have Sex with Men." *AIDS* 16 (9): 1271–77.

Ugarte Ubilluz, O., M. Arce Rodriguez, C. Acosta Saal, L. Suarez Ognio, J. L. Sebastián Mesones, and G. Rosell De Almeida. 2010. *Informe nacional sobre los progresos realizados en la aplicación del UNGASS: período: enero 2008–diciembre 2009*. Lima: Ministerio de Salud, Dirección General de Salud de las Personas.

UNAIDS (Joint United Nations Programme on HIV/AIDS) and WHO (World Health Organization). 2008. "UNAIDS/WHO Epidemiological Fact Sheets on HIV and AIDS, 2008 Update: Peru." Geneva: UNAIDS/WHO Working Group on Global HIV/AIDS and STI Surveillance.

Valverde, R., and R. Cabello. 2008. *Monitoring the Implementation of the UNGASS Declaration of Commitment: Country Report: Peru*. Lima: Organization Vía Libre.

Visser-Valfrey, M., R. Cassagnol, and M. Espinel. 2009. "UNAIDS Second Independent Evaluation 2002–2008: Country Visit to Peru, Summary Report." Presented at the 25th Meeting of the UNAIDS Programme Coordinating Board, December 8–10, Geneva.

WHO (World Health Organization), UNAIDS (Joint United Nations Programme on HIV/AIDS), and UNICEF (United Nations Children's Fund). 2009. *Towards Universal Access: Scaling Up Priority HIV/AIDS Interventions in the Health Sector: Progress Report 2009*. Geneva: WHO.

World Bank. 2009. World Development Indicators Database. http://data.worldbank .org/indicator.

CHAPTER 4

Scenario 2 Country Studies: Russian Federation and Ukraine

Russian Federation: An Expanding HIV Epidemic among MSM

Scenario: Same-sex risks are occurring within the wider context of established HIV epidemics driven by injecting drug use.

Key themes:

- The epidemic in the Russian Federation is highly concentrated among injecting drug users (IDUs), but considerable transmission occurs among men who have sex with men (MSM). Evidence indicates that the HIV epidemic is emerging among young MSM.
- Epidemiologic data on HIV infection among MSM are limited to the major urban areas, and inferences are drawn from relatively small samples.
- Despite increasing recognition of the gravity of the HIV epidemic, Russia's funding allocations to HIV prevention programs targeted to the risk groups most affected remain low.

The Russian Federation is the largest country in Eastern Europe and Central Asia, with a 2007 population of 141.4 million (U.S. Census

Bureau). The World Bank defines Russia as an upper-middle-income economy with a 2008 gross national income per capita of US$9,620 and a purchasing power parity of Int$15,630 (World Bank 2009). The first diagnosis of HIV in a Russian citizen was registered in 1987, and until 1995 the HIV epidemic grew at a very slow pace with 1,096 HIV cases reported from 160 million HIV tests during that period. However, since 1996, Russia has experienced a rapid expansion of HIV infections with HIV incidence peaking in 2001 at 60.5 per 100,000 population and remaining relatively steady through 2007 at 30.1 per 100,000 population (Federal Service for Surveillance of Consumer Rights Protection and Human Well-Being of the Russian Federation and UNAIDS 2008). Russia's epidemic has been highly concentrated among those most at risk: IDUs, their sex partners, sex workers, MSM, and vulnerable youth (Beyrer 2007; Kalichman et al. 2000). Cumulatively through 2007, among those who reported HIV risk behaviors, 82.4 percent were infected by use of nonsterile injecting equipment (Federal Service for Surveillance of Consumer Rights Protection and Human Well-Being of the Russian Federation and UNAIDS 2008). The changing social and economic conditions in post-Soviet Russia have been cited as creating the conditions necessary for the HIV epidemic: poverty and economic turmoil, increasing urbanization, mobility, crime, and rapid income growth (Moran and Jordaan 2007).

The Joint United Nations Programme on HIV/AIDS (UNAIDS) estimates that Russia accounted for approximately 66 percent of the region's newly diagnosed HIV cases in 2006 and that 1.1 percent of the country's adult population 15 to 49 years of age was living with HIV/AIDS in 2007 (UNAIDS 2008). Pronounced inconsistencies exist between UNAIDS HIV estimates and those reported by the Russian government; namely, the Russian Federal AIDS Service reports that the total number of individuals with HIV is 416,113 (less than half the UNAIDS estimate of 940,000 [560,000–1,600,000]), accounting for 0.3 percent of the total population (Federal Service for Surveillance of Consumer Rights Protection and Human Well-Being of the Russian Federation and UNAIDS 2008). However, stigma directed at people living with HIV/AIDS (PLWHA), IDUs, MSM, and sex workers is prevalent and could explain the high degree of underreporting. For example, only 43 percent of the newly reported HIV cases in 2006 had an identified route of transmission (EuroHIV 2007). A United Nations Development Programme study of PLWHA in the region identified structural barriers encountered by them and those at high risk in the areas of health care, education, and employment (UNDP 2008). Two surveys in Russia found that 70 percent of respondents felt "fear, anger or disgust towards those living with the virus" (BBC News online 2004) and that widespread ignorance and discrimination targeting PLWHA and those at high HIV risk exist among health workers and family members (Balabanova et al. 2006).

The predominant route of transmission remains injecting drug use, with 63.7 percent of new cases in 2007 (Federal Service for Surveillance of Consumer Rights Protection and Human Well-Being of the Russian Federation and UNAIDS 2008) and an estimated number of IDUs between 1.5 million and 3 million. Data from the National Scientific Narcology Centre of the Federal State Agency for Health and Social Development (2006) indicate that in 2006 the prevalence of HIV infection among registered IDUs was 11.8 percent (up from 9.3 percent in 2005). More than half (53 percent) of Russia's 89 administrative regions reported an HIV prevalence of more than 5 percent among IDUs in 2006, up from 41.6 percent in 2005 (Federal Service for Surveillance of Consumer Rights Protection and Human Well-Being of the Russian Federation and UNAIDS 2008). However, HIV prevalence estimates from second-generation surveillance efforts on IDUs vary widely by geographic region and range from 8.4 percent in Nizhny Novgorod to 64 percent in Yekaterinburg (USAID 2010).

A marked increase in the number of women infected with HIV has occurred in Russia since 2000. Among newly infected individuals, 20.6 percent were women in 2000, 38.5 percent in 2003, and 44 percent in 2007 (Federal Service for Surveillance of Consumer Rights Protection and Human Well-Being of the Russian Federation and UNAIDS 2008), indicating an increase in heterosexual transmission overall.

Data on HIV among MSM are scarce in Russia; the official HIV prevalence among MSM in 2007 was 1.1 percent, and the cumulative total of HIV cases attributable to risky behavior of MSM is 1,613 (between 1987 and 2007), even though the estimated size of the population of MSM is 2.1 million (Federal Research and Methodological Center for AIDS Prevention and Control 2005).

MSM and Transgender Typologies Used in Epidemiologic Studies in Russia

MSM in Russia live within a social context that stigmatizes and discriminates against same-sex behavior. Same-sex behavior was decriminalized in 1993 with the fall of the Soviet Union. Even though homosexuality was excluded from the list of mental health disorders in 1999, no legal protections exist for those who are discriminated against on the basis of sexual identity (Kon n.d.). A report by the Russian LGBT Network and the Moscow Helsinki Group (2007) documented incidents of discrimination and social exclusion targeting sexual minorities relating to employment and registration of noncommercial organizations. A study by Goodwin and colleagues (2003) reported that businesspeople and health professionals in the region attributed increasing rates of HIV/AIDS to a moral and social decline caused by socially marginalized groups such as MSM. Finally, MSM feel pressure to marry and keep their sexual attraction to and sexual relations with other men hidden (COC 2003).

Sexual identity of Russian MSM has not been thoroughly investigated in the literature. Information from focus group discussions and key informant interviews conducted as part of a qualitative study among MSM in Moscow, Sochi, and Kazan indicates that MSM identified as homosexual, bisexual, or heterosexual and that their identity was not directly related to their sexual practices (Kizub et al. 2009). The report did, however, demonstrate that gay-identified men are more likely to visit gay-identified venues (for example, clubs, bars, saunas, or *pleshkas* [public locations where sex work is present]), whereas less gay-identified men as well as older and ethnic minority MSM used the Internet to find male sex partners. Furthermore, the sense predominated that no organized gay community exists as it does in Western Europe or the United States. Rather, MSM in these cities socialize in fragmented groups (Kizub et al. 2009).

Data on lifetime same-sex behavior among men in Russia are lacking, except for a population-based survey of residents of St. Petersburg conducted by Amirkhanian, Kelly, and Issayev (2001), which found that 6 percent of 155 men reported a lifetime history of same-sex contacts, with none self-identifying as homosexual—most identified as bisexual. In a systematic review, Cáceres and colleagues (2008) estimated the prevalence of lifetime same-sex experience of men in Eastern Europe and Central Asia at 3 percent.

HIV Risk among MSM

UNAIDS (2009) posits that widespread stigma and discrimination targeting MSM cause official HIV surveillance data to misrepresent, by way of gross underreporting, the status of the HIV epidemic in this group. A number of studies have reported on HIV prevalence among MSM in different Russian urban areas (table 4.1).

Table 4.1 Studies Reporting HIV Prevalence among MSM in Russian Urban Areas

Source	*Year*	*HIV+*	*HIV–*	*Total N*	*HIV prevalence (%)*
Tomsk convenience sample (EuroHIV 2006)	2003	0	114	114	0.0
Yekaterinburg convenience sample (EuroHIV 2006)	2003	6	118	124	4.8
Moscow TLS (WHO Regional Office for Europe 2007)	2005	3	300	303	0.9
St. Petersburg TLS (WHO Regional Office for Europe 2007)	2005	8	209	217	3.8
Krasnoyarsk RDS (PSI Research Division 2005)	2006	2	265	267	0.8
Perm RDS (PSI Research Division 2005)	2006	5	234	239	2.2
St. Petersburg convenience sample (Sifakis et al. 2008)	2008	11	189	200	5.5
Moscow convenience sample (Sifakis et al. 2008)	2008	12	189	201	6.0
St. Petersburg network (Amirkhanian et al. 2009)	2009	2	34	36	5.6
St. Petersburg RDS (Tyusova et al. 2009)	2009	17	221	238	7.0
Total		66	1,873	1,939	3.4 (95% confidence interval: 2.6–4.2)

Source: Authors' compilation.
Note: RDS denotes respondent-driven sampling; TLS denotes time-location sampling.

Assuming that the total Russian population of MSM is 2.1 million (Federal Research and Methodological Center for AIDS Prevention and Control 2005), if the aggregate HIV prevalence estimate from table 4.1 were applied, then the expected number of HIV-positive MSM would be 73,500 (range: 56,700–90,300).

In a 2008 study in Moscow and St. Petersburg (Sifakis et al. 2008), increasing age was not associated with HIV infection, thus indicating the potential for a burgeoning epidemic among young MSM; HIV prevalence was 7.7 percent among those 18–22 years of age, 5.7 percent among those 23–25 years, 6.3 percent among those 26–28 years, and 4.1 percent among those 29 years and older. These age-disaggregated data contrast to age-specific HIV prevalence from established Western European and U.S. HIV epidemics among MSM, which show a clear increase in HIV infection with increasing age.

Bisexual MSM and Relationships with Women

Sex with women is a common occurrence reported by MSM in Russia. Because same-sex behavior is highly stigmatized, men are driven to maintain sexual relationships with women. Cáceres and colleagues (2008) estimate that lifetime report of heterosexual sex among MSM in Eastern Europe and Central Asia ranges between 44 and 53 percent, whereas the proportion of MSM who are married to women is only 7 percent. Sex with women in the prior 12 months ranged from 17.2 percent in Moscow (WHO Regional Office for Europe 2007) to 44.8 percent in Krasnoyarsk (PSI Research Division 2005) in a series of seroprevalence studies conducted on MSM in 2005–06. Kelly and colleagues (2002) recruited 434 MSM in gay-identified venues in St. Petersburg, of whom approximately 80 percent reported lifetime sex with a female and 29 percent reported bisexual behavior in the prior three months. More recently, Sifakis and colleagues (2008) reported that in St. Petersburg and Moscow in 2008, 30.2 percent of MSM engaged in sex with women and 7.3 percent were married to or cohabitating with a woman in the prior 12 months. In a 2009 study recruiting from sociocentric social networks of MSM in St. Petersburg (Amirkhanian et al. 2009), 23.7 percent of men reported sex with women in the past 12 months. Finally, in a respondent-driven sample of MSM in St. Petersburg, 19.2 percent of 180 MSM reported sex with a woman in the prior six months (Iguchi et al. 2009). These high proportions of bisexual behavior may indicate the resistance of Russian MSM to conform to western sexual roles of identity and practice during times of rapid social change or the influence of cultural pressures regarding male sexuality (Kelly et al. 2001).

Male Sex Workers

Russia's rapid social and economic transformation has resulted in rising unemployment and increasing scarcity of public health and social resources (Amirkhanian, Kelly, and Issayev 2001). Kelly and colleagues (2001) suggest that these pressures may serve as enabling factors that drive men to engage in transactional sex with other men. In a 2001 study of MSM in St. Petersburg, 22.7 percent of men reported engaging in transactional sex. These men were more likely to be younger, less educated, and unemployed than their counterparts; they also engaged in sex with women (47 percent) and high levels (45 percent) of unprotected anal intercourse in the prior three months (Kelly et al. 2001). The prevalence of transactional sex among MSM reported by other seroprevalence studies ranges between 5 percent in Tomsk (2003) and 16.5 percent in Krasnoyarsk (2006) in the year prior to study participation (Bozicevic et al. 2009). A pilot cohort study among male sex workers in Moscow reported that entry into sex work was largely through friends and partners working in the industry. Some 30 percent worked under a *seutemyorshin* (an agent for whom they worked and who handled client contacts and security), and clients were primarily met through saunas or the Internet. Approximately 86 percent of male sex workers were not originally from Moscow, 18 percent were HIV infected, and 8 percent reported injecting drug use (Baral et al. 2010). Unemployment and migration to large urban centers contribute to an increase in transactional sex among MSM and serve as a factor for further spread of HIV.

MSM and Injecting Drug Use

The preponderance of reported evidence suggests that MSM who inject illicit drugs are a relatively small proportion of MSM but at very high risk for HIV infection, especially in this context of an established IDU HIV epidemic. In seroprevalence studies in Moscow (WHO Regional Office for Europe 2007) and Perm (PSI Research Division 2005), 2 percent and 5.5 percent, respectively, of MSM reported injecting drug use. In addition, Population Services International (PSI)'s evaluation of HIV prevention programs in eight Russian regions (Kazan, Krasnoyarsk, Nizhny Novgorod, Orenburg, Pskov, St. Petersburg, Tomsk, and Vologda) reported lifetime prevalence of injecting drug use among MSM to be 3.9 percent and 4.3 percent in 2006 and 2008, respectively (Sergeyev and Gorbachev 2008). This range of estimates is corroborated by another 2008 study in Moscow and St. Petersburg, with 3.3 percent of men reporting injecting drug use behavior; however, the prevalence of HIV infection in this high-risk subset was 38.5 percent (Sifakis et al. 2008). Finally, a 2009 respondent-driven sample of MSM in St. Petersburg reported that among MSM who were IDUs, 43 percent were HIV infected (Tyusova et al. 2009). In Russia, the challenge with IDUs who are MSM is distinguishing the attributable contribution of parenteral HIV transmission among MSM; despite the relatively small numbers of this subset, MSM may acquire HIV from sharing infected injecting equipment or from increased and high-risk sexual activity driven by addiction. Furthermore, they serve as an efficient transmission subgroup, thus facilitating the spread of HIV among MSM and heterosexuals.

Interventions

Recognition of the gravity of HIV/AIDS in Russia has been increasing among Russian policy makers. Deputy Prime Minister Alexander Zhukov told an AIDS conference in 2005: "The growth of AIDS has gone beyond being a medical problem, and has become an issue of strategic, social and economic security of the country within the current demographic situation in Russia" (*Medical News Today* 2005). A federal response to the HIV/AIDS epidemic is in place, and federal funding for the response has increased more than twentyfold since 2005. In 2006–07, Rub 109 billion (US$436 million) were allocated under the National Priority Project on Health, and the subprogram AntiAIDS of the Federal Program to Prevent and Control Significant Social Diseases 2007–2010 received Rub 1.081 billion (US$43 million) (Federal Service for Surveillance of Consumer Rights Protection and Human Well-Being of the Russian Federation and UNAIDS 2008). However, these funding efforts focus primarily on treatment of AIDS rather than prevention, care, and support (USAID 2008).

The majority of harm reduction measures are supported by the Global Fund to Fight AIDS, Tuberculosis and Malaria (GFATM) and implemented through nongovernmental organizations, including the Russian Harm Reduction Network and the Global Efforts Against AIDS in Russia consortium (IHRD 2008). Under its normal funding guidelines, the GFATM would not provide support for prevention programs in Russia because of the country's high degree of economic development. However, because of Russia's inadequate funding of prevention programs for sex workers and IDUs, the GFATM extended funding for these targeted HIV prevention programs until 2011 (GFATM 2009).

The largest HIV prevention program targeting MSM in Russia is the LaSky project implemented by the PSI/Russia Center for Social Development and Information. It was launched in 1999 in Moscow and has expanded operation to 19 cities in 15 regions. LaSky activities include outreach to MSM, distribution of condoms and lubricants, counseling and social support, seminars, training and discussion panels for MSM, medical services (distribution of appointment cards for sexually transmitted infections, HIV testing, and treatment), and prevention education campaigns in media and MSM venues (http://www.lasky.ru/psi/about/). An evaluation of PSI's HIV prevention efforts for MSM reported that LaSky has been successful in promoting condom use among MSM with casual partners and transactional partners and that exposure to the HIV prevention program is associated with greater likelihood of reporting for testing for HIV or sexually transmitted infections, increased ability to negotiate condom use with different types of partners, and better information pre- and posttest counseling. Moreover, this program contributed to the increased availability of free condoms for MSM in eight Russian regions (Sergeyev and Gorbachev 2008).

Ukraine: Hidden HIV Epidemic among MSM

Scenario: Same-sex risks occur within the wider context of established HIV epidemics driven by injecting drug use.

Key themes:

- The HIV epidemic in Ukraine remains concentrated and is driven by injecting drug use; however, the extent of HIV infection among MSM is substantial.
- Sexual practices and trends indicate the potential for wider HIV spread in the general population.
- Stigma and discrimination against same-sex behavior have been widespread and institutionalized; they have, in turn, led to marked underreporting of same-sex risks and of HIV infection among MSM.

Located in Eastern Europe, Ukraine had a population of 46.3 million (U.S. Census Bureau) in 2007. The World Bank defines the country as a lower-middle-income economy with a 2008 gross national income per capita of US$3,210 and a purchasing power parity of Int$7,210 (World Bank 2009). By the end of 2007, Ukraine had 81,741 officially registered HIV cases, although the Ministry of Health of Ukraine considers that figure an underestimate because it accounts only for individuals tested in official HIV testing facilities (Ministry of Health of Ukraine 2008). In 2007 the Ukrainian AIDS Centre of the Ministry of Health revised its national estimates for HIV/AIDS using the Workbook and Spectrum methods, based on the recommendations of the UNAIDS Reference Group on Estimates, Modelling and Projections (2007). This effort produced an HIV estimate of 395,000 (range: 230,000–573,000) individuals between 15 and 49 years of age, or 1.63 percent of the adult population in Ukraine, representing the highest adult HIV prevalence in Eastern Europe and Central Asia (Kruglov et al. 2008; Ministry of Health of

Ukraine 2008; UNAIDS 2006). Even though HIV cases have been reported from all 27 regions of the country, significant geographic variability exists; 70 percent of all HIV cases have been reported in Kyiv or the southeastern provinces (that is, Dnipropetrovsk, Donetsk, Mykolayiv, and Odesa oblasts; Sevastopol; and the Autonomous Republic of Crimea) (Ministry of Health of Ukraine 2008).

The first HIV case in Ukraine was reported in 1987, and until the mid-1990s HIV was predominantly spread by sexual transmission and confined within a relatively small group of foreign students. However, an explosive epidemic among Ukrainian IDUs started in 1995, when the proportion of IDUs among all newly reported HIV infections was 68.5 percent, peaking at 83.6 percent in 1997, and since showing a decreasing trend to 40.1 percent by the end of 2007 (Ministry of Health of Ukraine 2008). The epidemic in Ukraine remains concentrated and primarily affects IDUs, sex workers, MSM, and their sexual partners; however, trends indicate the real possibility of HIV spreading in the general population. In 2007, 38.4 percent of newly reported HIV cases were attributed to sexual transmission, and of the 17,669 new HIV cases, 5,865 (33.2 percent) were among women. The contribution of indirect parenteral transmission is substantial, however, because 22 percent of HIV cases attributable to sexual transmission reported having a regular IDU sex partner in the prior 12 months (Ministry of Health of Ukraine 2008). Surveillance data on HIV among MSM are very limited and not reflected in Ukraine's official statistics because the routine HIV surveillance system does not differentiate between heterosexual and homosexual transmission. Data from sentinel surveillance activities report 158 HIV cases among MSM (or 0.13 percent of all HIV cases reported) between 1987 and 1997; in 1997, among the 17,669 newly reported HIV cases, only 43 (0.24 percent) were among MSM. These figures are a gross underestimation of HIV among MSM in Ukraine and highlight that MSM do not seek voluntary counseling and testing or do not report their behaviors because of social stigma attached to same-sex behavior.

MSM and Transgender Typologies Used in Epidemiologic Studies in Ukraine

Ukraine was the first former Soviet republic to decriminalize homosexuality (Ministry of Health of Ukraine 2008). However, the Ministry of Health of Ukraine in its 2008 United Nations General Assembly Special Session (UNGASS) on HIV/AIDS report (Ministry of Health of Ukraine 2008, 126) indicates that no "normative and legal basis . . . would protect rights of vulnerable populations, namely injecting drug users, female sex workers, men who have sex with men and others." Furthermore, the report asserts that stigma and discrimination are widespread against MSM because "MSM are generally treated as people with pathological mental deviations" (Ministry of Health of Ukraine 2008, 122). Two public opinion surveys, conducted in 2002 and 2007, showed a decreasing trend in support of equal rights for all people (42.5 percent and 34.1 percent, respectively) (Maymulakhin, Olexandr Zinchenkov, and Kravchuk 2007). In a 2004 six-city behavioral survey, 57 percent of MSM reported nondisclosure of their sexual identity to others because of fear of stigma and discrimination (Amjadeen 2005), and in 2005, approximately 57 percent of MSM reported experiencing discrimination or abuse of their rights, especially regarding employment (Gribanov et al. 2005).

In the context of widespread stigma and discrimination against MSM, sexual identity remains mostly hidden, and disclosure, especially in health and employment environments, is rare. Despite lack of extensive data on lifetime same-sex behaviors among men in Ukraine, the Ukrainian AIDS Centre has estimated the number of MSM to be 177,000–430,000 (Kruglov et al. 2008). The lower estimate was derived from triangulation of different sources of estimates (Kruglov et al. 2008). The higher estimate corroborates the estimate by Cáceres and colleagues (2008) for the prevalence of lifetime same-sex experience of men in Eastern Europe and Central Asia: approximately 3 percent of the male population. Therefore, the estimated proportion of MSM in the general population is 2.52 percent (Kruglov et al. 2008); MSM with more than one male sex partner in the prior 12 months account for 1.40 percent, and MSM with zero or one sex partner in the prior 12 months account for 0.41 percent of the total Ukrainian population (Kasianczuk et al. 2009).

HIV Risk among MSM

Seroprevalence studies among MSM recruited through respondent-driven sampling report high HIV prevalence among MSM (aggregate 10.6 percent [95 percent confidence interval 7.8–14.2]) (see table 4.2). If these prevalence estimates are applied to estimates of the population of MSM (Kruglov et al. 2008), then the expected number of HIV-positive MSM in Ukraine is between 19,470 and 47,300 (range: 14,160–60,630).

According to the UNGASS 2008 report (Ministry of Health of Ukraine 2008), in the four-city seroprevalence studies, no cases occurred among

Table 4.2 Studies Reporting HIV Prevalence among MSM in Urban Areas of Ukraine

Sources	*Location*	*Type of sample*	*Year*	*Number in sample*	*Number HIV+*	*HIV prevalence (%)*
UNAIDS and Balakiryeva 2008; Ministry of Health of Ukraine 2008	Kyiv	RDS	2007	90	4	4.40
UNAIDS and Balakiryeva 2008; Ministry of Health of Ukraine 2008	Kryviy Rig	RDS	2007	100	8	8.00
UNAIDS and Balakiryeva 2008; Ministry of Health of Ukraine 2008	Mykolayiv	RDS	2007	100	10	10.00
UNAIDS and Balakiryeva 2008; Ministry of Health of Ukraine 2008	Odessa	RDS	2007	69	16	23.20
Total				359	38	10.6 (95% confidence interval: 7.8–14.2)

Source: Authors' compilation.
Note: RDS denotes respondent-driven sampling.

MSM younger than 25 years of age. Such an indication may point to an epidemic that has been hidden from official detection and well-established in this high-risk group for some time. However, in a 2007 study of adolescents who do not have stable housing, under the United Nations Children's Fund Most At-Risk Adolescents Project, data from 10 regions indicated that 4 percent of 137 MSM (15–19 years) were HIV positive (Teltschik et al. 2008). Young MSM are very vulnerable, especially when they are socially and economically disenfranchised.

Bisexual MSM and Relationships with Women

The first estimate of bisexual behavior among MSM was recorded in 2005 from a behavioral survey among MSM in Kyiv and the Donetsk region. The survey reported that 33 percent of respondents who were MSM had an average of three female sexual partners (Substance Abuse and AIDS Prevention Foundation 2005). A survey monitoring behaviors of MSM as part of second-generation surveillance reported in 2007 that

52 percent of 359 respondents indicated lifetime sex with women, and approximately 22 percent had sex with women in the prior six months (Balakiryeva et al. 2008). Furthermore, in 2007 the Ministry of Health of Ukraine's AIDS Centre provided estimates, based on the UNAIDS Reference Group on Estimates, Modelling and Projections (2007) methods, of the number of female sexual partners of MSM in Ukraine, assuming an average of one female sexual partner per MSM. These estimates range between 177,000 and 430,000, with HIV prevalence among these women of 1.3 percent to 7.6 percent (Kruglov et al. 2008).

Male Sex Workers

Engaging in transactional sex with other males (that is, giving or receiving money or other goods in exchange for sex) is a common practice among Ukrainian MSM. In 2002, 21 percent of 227 MSM survey participants reported transactional sex with males in the prior six months (Filipov 2005). In a peer-referral convenience sample of 886 MSM in six cities conducted by the International HIV/AIDS Alliance in Ukraine in 2004, 22 percent of respondents reported transactional sex with males in the prior 12 months (Amjadeen 2005). Finally, second-generation surveillance data report that 8 percent of 359 MSM sampled through respondent-driven sampling in 2007 engaged in transactional sex with males in the one month prior to their participation in the behavioral survey (Balakiryeva et al. 2008). Thus, male sex workers are estimated to account for 0.55 percent of the total population in Ukraine (Amjadeen 2005).

MSM and Injecting Drug Use

Behavioral evidence suggests that the proportion of MSM who also inject illicit drugs is relatively small. Two reports from 2004 and 2008 (Balakiryeva et al. 2008; Centre of Social Expertise at the Institute of Sociology of the National Academy of Sciences of Ukraine 2004) indicate that 6 percent of MSM are also IDUs, which results in an estimate of that dual-risk group of 10,620–25,800, if that proportion is applied to the estimated number of MSM in Ukraine, or 0.15 percent of the total population (Balakiryeva et al. 2008). Considering that HIV prevalence among IDUs exceeded 40 percent in 2007, this subset of MSM, albeit small, is at very high risk for HIV infection. Scant corroborative evidence indicates that approximately 33 percent of MSM who are IDUs self-report being HIV infected (Centre of Social Expertise at the Institute of Sociology of the National Academy of Sciences of Ukraine 2004), whereas the majority indicate that they are bisexual and that they inject drugs occasionally but in concordance with same-sex behaviors (Amjadeen et al. 2005). Possibly, therefore, these men inject drugs to escape the social stigma of their same-sex behaviors.

Interventions

In 2004, the National Program to Ensure HIV Prevention, Support and Treatment for HIV-Infected and AIDS Patients for 2004–2008 was enacted in Ukraine, but it did not include MSM as a priority group for targeted HIV prevention. However, a 2008 update and the planned National Program for 2009 explicitly list MSM as a key target group (Ministry of Health of Ukraine 2008). Despite the strong commitment of the Ukrainian government, the country still lacks a national policy and strategy for providing HIV prevention information and educational programs that specifically target MSM (Ministry of Health of Ukraine 2008). That task has largely been carried out by civil society with funding from international donors.

The AIDS Foundation East-West, the Ukrainian Nongovernmental Organization Gay Alliance, and Noah's Ark–Red Cross Foundation, Sweden, with financial support from the Elton John AIDS Foundation, the European Union TACIS Programme, and the Swedish International Development and Cooperation Agency, implemented the MSM: HIV/STI Prevention and Support Project in Kyiv (2005–07). The project successfully advocated for the inclusion of MSM as a key group for the government's National Program to Ensure HIV Prevention, Support and Treatment for HIV-Infected and AIDS Patients. Its efforts also created a community-based network of gay-friendly social and health professionals able to provide support for HIV prevention targeted at MSM and directly engaged the community in Kyiv by distributing 44,000 condoms and 11,800 packages of lubricants.

The GFATM supported the nongovernmental International HIV/AIDS Alliance in Ukraine to conduct HIV prevention interventions among MSM. These programs were implemented by 15 subgrantee nongovernmental organizations in 12 regions (Cherkasy, Chernivtsi, Dnipropetrovsk, Donetsk, Ivano-Frankivsk, Kharkiv, Kherson, Kirovohrad, Lviv, Mykolayiv, Odesa, and Zaporizhya), the cities of Kyiv and Sevastopol, and the Autonomous Republic of Crimea. As of January 1, 2009, 19,749 MSM had been reached; in 2008, 1,446 MSM received rapid testing for HIV, and 1,521 were tested for sexually transmitted infections. Other program activities included distribution of condoms and lubricants, dissemination of educational materials, referral to services, and group and individual behavioral counseling (International HIV/AIDS Alliance in Ukraine 2008). Furthermore, the International HIV/AIDS Alliance in Ukraine supports the development of the All-Ukrainian Network of People Living with HIV/AIDS and provides technical support and capacity building for 150 nongovernmental organizations targeting at-risk groups, including MSM (International HIV/AIDS Alliance in Ukraine 2009).

The strengthening of communities across all 27 regions of the country in support of HIV prevention targeted at MSM is necessary alongside strong political will and commitment from the Ukrainian government.

References for Russian Federation

Amirkhanian, Y. A., J. A. Kelly, and D. D. Issayev. 2001. "AIDS Knowledge, Attitudes, and Behaviour in Russia: Results of a Population-Based, Random-Digit Telephone Survey in St Petersburg." *International Journal of STD and AIDS* 12 (1): 50–57.

Amirkhanian, Y. A., J. A. Kelly, J. Takacs, A. V. Kuznetsova, W. J. DiFranceisco, L. Mocsonaki, T. L. McAuliffe, R. A. Khoursine, and T. P. Toth. 2009. "HIV/STD Prevalence, Risk Behavior, and Substance Use Patterns and Predictors in Russian and Hungarian Sociocentric Social Networks of Men Who Have Sex with Men." *AIDS Education and Prevention* 21 (3): 266–79.

Balabanova, Y., R. Coker, R. A. Atun, and F. Drobniewski. 2006. "Stigma and HIV Infection in Russia." *AIDS Care* 18 (7): 846–52.

Baral, S., D. Kizub, N. F. Masenior, A. Peryskina, J. Stachowiak, M. Stibich, V. Moguilny, and C. Beyrer. 2010. "Male Sex Workers in Moscow, Russia: A Pilot Study of Demographics, Substance Use Patterns, and Prevalence of HIV-1 and Sexually Transmitted Infections." *AIDS Care* 22 (1): 112–18.

BBC News online. 2004. "Russia Campaigns against AIDS Fear." May 14. http://news.bbc.co.uk/2/hi/europe/3715599.stm.

Beyrer, C. 2007. "HIV Epidemiology Update and Transmission Factors: Risks and Risk Contexts—16th International AIDS Conference Epidemiology Plenary." *Clinical Infectious Diseases* 44 (7): 981–87.

Bozicevic, I., L. Voncina, L. Zigrovic, M. Munz, and J. V. Lazarus. 2009. "HIV Epidemics among Men Who Have Sex with Men in Central and Eastern Europe." *Sexually Transmitted Infections* 85 (5): 336–42.

Cáceres, C. F., K. Konda, E. R. Segura, and R. Lyerla. 2008. "Epidemiology of Male Same-Sex Behaviour and Associated Sexual Health Indicators in Low- and Middle-Income Countries: 2003–2007 Estimates." *Sexually Transmitted Infections* 84 (Suppl. 1): i49–56.

COC Netherlands. 2003. *Homosexuality in Eastern Europe*. Amsterdam: COC.

EuroHIV (European Centre for Epidemiological Monitoring of AIDS). 2006. *HIV/AIDS Surveillance in Europe: Mid-Year Report 2005, No. 72*. Saint-Maurice, France: Institut de Veille Sanitaire.

———. 2007. *HIV/AIDS Surveillance in Europe: End-Year Report 2006, No. 75*. Saint-Maurice, France: Institut de Veille Sanitaire.

Federal Research and Methodological Center for AIDS Prevention and Control. 2005. "A Report at the Consultation on the Universal Access to HIV Prevention, Treatment, Care and Support for the Population of the Russian Federation." Moscow, December 15–16.

Federal Service for Surveillance of Consumer Rights Protection and Human Well-Being of the Russian Federation and UNAIDS. 2008. *Country Progress Report of the Russian Federation on the Implementation of the Declaration of Commitment on HIV/AIDS. Reporting Period: January 2006–December 2007*. Moscow: Federal Service for Surveillance of Consumer Rights Protection and Human Well-Being of the Russian Federation and UNAIDS.

GFATM (Global Fund to Fight AIDS, Tuberculosis and Malaria). 2009. "Global Fund to Provide $24 Million of New Funding to Fight HIV/AIDS in Russia." Geneva, November 13.

Goodwin, R., A. Kozlova, A. Kwiatkowska, L. A. N. Luud, G. Nizharadzee, A. Realof, A. Külvetf, and A. Rämmerf. 2003. "Social Representations of HIV/AIDS in Central and Eastern Europe." *Social Science and Medicine* 56 (7): 1373–84.

Iguchi, M. Y., A. J. Ober, S. H. Berry, T. Fain, D. D. Heckathorn, P. Gorbach, R. Heimer, A. Kozlov, L. J. Ouellet, S. Shoptaw, and W. A. Zule. 2009. "Simultaneous Recruitment of Drug Users and Men Who Have Sex with Men in the United States and Russia Using Respondent-Driven Sampling: Sampling Methods and Implications." *Journal of Urban Health* 86 (1): S5–31.

IHRD (International Harm Reduction Development Program). 2008. *Harm Reduction Developments 2008: Countries with Injection-Driven HIV Epidemics.* New York: International Harm Reduction Development Program of the Open Society Institute.

Kalichman, S. C., J. A. Kelly, K. J. Sikkema, A. P. Koslov, A. Shaboltas, and J. Granskaya. 2000. "The Emerging AIDS Crisis in Russia: Review of Enabling Factors and Prevention Needs." *International Journal of STD and AIDS* 11 (2): 71–75.

Kelly, J. A., Y. A. Amirkhanian, T. L. McAuliffe, R. V. Dyatlov, J. Granskaya, O. I. Borodkina, A. A. Kukharsky, and A. P. Kozlov. 2001. "HIV Risk Behavior and Risk-Related Characteristics of Young Russian Men Who Exchange Sex for Money or Valuables from Other Men." *AIDS Education and Prevention* 13 (2): 175–88.

Kelly, J. A., Y. A. Amirkhanian, T. L. McAuliffe, J. V. Granskaya, O. I. Borodkina, R. V. Dyatlov, A. Kukharsky, and A. P. Kozlov. 2002. "HIV Risk Characteristics and Prevention Needs in a Community Sample of Bisexual Men in St. Petersburg, Russia." *AIDS Care* 14 (1): 63–76.

Kizub, D., I. Deobald, N. F. Masenior, A. Peryshkina, A. Wirtz, I. Kostetskaya, F. Sifakis, and C. Beyrer. 2009. *Advocating for HIV and STI Prevention Services and Strengthening the Advocacy Capacity of Groups Representing Men Who Have Sex with Men in the Russian Federation: Study of the Needs of Men Who Have Sex with Men with Respect to HIV and STI Prevention and Medical Care in Russia.* Moscow: AIDS infoshare.

Kon, I. S. n.d. "Homophobia as a Form of Xenophobia." In Russian. Available at http://sexology.narod.ru/info167.html.

Medical News Today. 2005. "Russia's HIV/AIDS Epidemic Poses National Security Threat, Officials Say." *Medical News Today*, April 1. http://www.medicalnews today.com/articles/22071.php (accessed April 15, 2008).

Moran, D., and J. A. Jordaan. 2007. "HIV/AIDS in Russia: Determinants of Regional Prevalence." *International Journal of Health Geographics* 6: 22.

National Scientific Narcology Centre of the Federal State Agency for Health and Social Development. 2006. "State of the Narcological Service and the Main Trends of Registered Morbidity in the Russian Federation in 2006." National Scientific Narcology Centre of the Federal State Agency for Health and Social Development, Statistical Reports, Moscow.

PSI (Population Services International) Research Division. 2005. *HIV/AIDS Study of Forms of Risky Behaviour and the Use of Medical Services by Men Having Sex with Men in Two Regions of the Russian Federation.* Moscow: PSI.

Russian LGBT Network and the Moscow Helsinki Group. 2007. "Discrimination Based on Sexual Orientation and Gender Identity in Russia." Russian LGBT Network, http://www.lgbtnet.ru/news/detail.php?ID=3453.

Sergeyev, B., and M. Gorbachev. 2008. *Russia (2008): HIV/AIDS TRaC Study of Risk, Health-Seeking Behaviors, and Their Determinants, among Men Who Have Sex with Men in Eight Regions of the Russian Federation. Second Round.* Moscow: PSI.

Sifakis, F., A. Peryskina, B. Sergeev, V. Moguilny, A. Beloglazov, N. Franck-Masenior, S. Baral, and C. Beyrer. 2008. "Rapid Assessment of HIV Infection and Associated Risk Behaviors among Men Who Have Sex with Men in Russia." Presentation at XVII International AIDS Conference, Mexico City, Mexico, August 3–8.

Tyusova, O., S. V. Verevochkin, R. Heimer, et al. 2009. "HIV in Population Groups Recruited by Respondent-Driven Sampling in St. Petersburg." Presentation at the 3rd Eastern Europe and Central Asia AIDS Conference, Moscow, October 28–30.

UNAIDS (United Nations Joint Programme on HIV/AIDS). 2008. *2008 Report on the Global AIDS Epidemic.* Geneva: UNAIDS.

———. 2009. "Hidden HIV Epidemic amongst MSM in Eastern Europe and Central Asia." UNAIDS, Press Centre, January 26.

UNDP (United Nations Development Programme). 2008. *Living with HIV in Eastern Europe and the CIS: The Human Cost of Social Exclusion*. UNDP Bratislava Regional Centre. http://europeandcis.undp.org/rhdr.aids2008/.

USAID (U.S. Agency for International Development). 2008. "HIV/AIDS Profile." USAID/Russia, Moscow. http://www.usaid.gov/our_work/global_health/aids/Countries/eande/russia_profile.pdf.

———. 2010. "HIV/AIDS Profile." USAID/Russia, Moscow. http://www.usaid.gov/our_work/global_health/aids/Countries/eande/russia_profile.pdf.

WHO (World Health Organization) Regional Office for Europe. 2007. *HIV Prevalence and Risks among Men Who Have Sex with Men in Moscow and Saint Petersburg*. Copenhagen: WHO.

World Bank. 2009. World Development Indicators Database. World Bank, Washington, DC. http://data.worldbank.org/indicator (accessed November 11, 2009).

References for Ukraine

Amjadeen, L. 2005. *Report on the Survey "Monitoring Behaviours of MSM as a Component of Second-Generation Surveillance"* [in Ukrainian]. Kyiv: International HIV/AIDS Alliance in Ukraine.

Amjadeen, L., L. Andrushchak, I. Zvershkhovska, et al. 2005. *A Review of Work with Injecting Drug Users in Ukraine in the Context of the HIV/AIDS Epidemic*. Kyiv: National Academy of Sciences of Ukraine.

Balakiryeva, O. N., T. V. Bondar, M. G. Kasyanczuk, Z. R. Kis, Y. B. Leszczynski, and S. P. Sheremet-Sheremetyev. 2008. *Report on the Survey "Monitoring Behaviours of Men Having Sex with Men as a Component of Second Generation Surveillance."* Kyiv: International HIV/AIDS Alliance in Ukraine.

Cáceres, C. F., K. Konda, E. R. Segura, and R. Lyerla. 2008. "Epidemiology of Male Same-Sex Behaviour and Associated Sexual Health Indicators in Low- and Middle-Income Countries: 2003-2007 Estimates." *Sexually Transmitted Infections* 84 (Suppl. 1): i49–56.

Centre of Social Expertise at the Institute of Sociology of the National Academy of Sciences of Ukraine. 2004. *Analytical Report: Behavioural Monitoring of MSM as a Second Generation Surveillance Component*. Kyiv: International HIV/AIDS Alliance in Ukraine.

Filipov, D. 2005. The Research of Risky Behaviour in the Context of HIV among MSM in Kyiv [in Russian]. *HIV/AIDS News* 3: 5.

Gribanov, A., Z. Kis, A. Maimulakhin, L. Chorniy, et al. 2005. *Gay Rights Are Human Rights: Report about Discrimination on the Grounds of Sexual Orientation in Ukraine*. Kyiv: Nash Mir Gay and Lesbian Center.

International HIV/AIDS Alliance in Ukraine. 2008. *Annual Report 2008*. Kyiv: International HIV/AIDS Alliance in Ukraine.

———. 2009. *Civil Society Leads National Response. Final Report: Overcoming the HIV/AIDS Epidemic in Ukraine, Funded by The Global Fund (2004–2009)*. Kyiv: International HIV/AIDS Alliance in Ukraine.

Kasianczuk, M. G., L. G. Johnston, A. V. Dovbakh, and E. B. Leszczynski. 2009. "Risk Factors Associated with Condom Use among Men Who Have Sex with Men in Ukraine." *Journal of LGBT Health Research* 5 (1–2): 51–62.

Kruglov, Y. V., Y. V. Kobyshcha, T. Salyuk, O. Varetska, A. Shakarishvili, and V. P. Saldanha. 2008. "The Most Severe HIV Epidemic in Europe: Ukraine's National HIV Prevalence Estimates for 2007." *Sexually Transmitted Infections* 84 (Suppl. 1): i37–41.

Maymulakhin, A., A. Olexandr Zinchenkov, and A. Kravchuk. 2007. *Ukrainian Homosexuals and Society: Reciprocation*. Kyiv: Nash Mir.

Ministry of Health of Ukraine. 2008. *Ukraine: National Report on Monitoring Progress towards the UNGASS Declaration of Commitment on HIV/AIDS. Reporting Period: January 2006–December 2007*. Kyiv: Ministry of Health of Ukraine.

Substance Abuse and AIDS Prevention Foundation. 2005. *Assessment of Men Who Have Sex with Men in Kiev City and Donetsk Region*. Kyiv: Substance Abuse and AIDS Prevention Foundation.

Teltschik, A., O. Balakireva, Y. Sereda, T. Bondar, and O. Sakovych. 2008. *Most At-Risk Adolescents: The Evidence Base for Strengthening the HIV Response in Ukraine*. Kyiv: UNICEF and Ukrainian Institute for Social Research after Olexander Yaremenko.

UNAIDS (Joint United Nations Programme on HIV/AIDS). 2006. *2006 Report on the Global AIDS Epidemic*. Geneva: UNAIDS.

UNAIDS Reference Group on Estimates, Modelling and Projections. 2007. "Improvements to Estimation Packages: Report of a Meeting of the UNAIDS Reference Group for Estimates, Modelling and Projections held in Glion, Switzerland, July 19–20th 2006." UNAIDS Reference Group for Estimates, Modelling and Projections, London. http://www.epidem.org/Publications/Glion2006Report.pdf.

World Bank. 2009. World Development Indicators Database. World Bank, Washington, DC. http://data.worldbank.org/indicator (accessed November 11, 2009).

CHAPTER 5

Scenario 3 Country Studies: Kenya, Malawi, and Senegal

Kenya: Developing the Evidence Base for Effective HIV Prevention among MSM

Scenario: Same-sex practices are considered in the context of expanded and mature HIV epidemics among heterosexuals.

Key themes:

- Kenya has a generalized HIV epidemic and has been a research site for the evaluation of numerous HIV prevention, treatment, and care interventions.
- Outside of South Africa, the evidence for HIV risk among men who have sex with men (MSM) in Kenya is the most well established on the African continent, and prevalence and incidence estimates have been consistently high.
- Kenya has had effective HIV prevention programs for MSM, but the coverage of these services has been limited by heightened stigma and discrimination targeting MSM.

The regional hub for trade and finance in East Africa, Kenya has a population of approximately 39 million. The country is at the upper end of low-income countries as defined by the World Bank with a gross domestic product of US$770 and a purchasing power parity of US$1,580 but has a medium ranking on the United Nations Human Development Index. The primary epidemic of HIV reached Kenya in the early 1980s with explosive growth in the early 1990s overwhelming the health care system. The traditional modes of spread dominating the HIV epidemic in Kenya have always been assumed to be high-risk heterosexual transmission and vertical transmission from mother to child. However, the last four or five years have demonstrated increased risk among other vulnerable populations including sex workers, injecting drug users (IDUs), and MSM (UNAIDS and WHO 2008).

Kenya's HIV/AIDS response is delivered under the "Three Ones" framework developed at the International Conference on AIDS and STIs in Africa, which encourages a single national AIDS coordinating authority, a single AIDS action framework to coordinate the work of partners, and a single national monitoring and evaluation system. As of 2007, Kenya had between 1.4 million and 1.8 million reproductive-age adults living with HIV, of whom approximately 68 percent were women (UNAIDS 2008). Notably, HIV incidence peaked in the late 1990s, and prevalence has also slowly been decreasing from approximately 14 percent in the mid-1990s to just over 6 percent in 2006 (UNAIDS and WHO 2008). These declines are especially apparent in urban areas and correspond with significant reductions in high-risk sexual practices among both men and women. Significant decreases in prevalence are also caused by the trend that has seen mortality secondary to HIV doubling since 1998 so that it is higher than the rate of new infections.

Kenya has adopted a significant antiretroviral therapy (ART) program that includes free treatment, but only 35 percent coverage exists among eligible HIV-positive people. According to this program's data, approximately 57,000 deaths are estimated to have been averted since 2001. This program includes a focus on prevention of mother-to-child transmission of HIV/AIDS with counseling and testing in prenatal clinics in Kenya. However, as of 2006, only about 637,000 of the 1.5 million women in need of this program were appropriately tested (NACC 2008). Moreover, of the nearly 60,000 woman found to be HIV positive, less than 40 percent received appropriate treatment. Among major issues for this ART program is that approximately 98 percent of the entire HIV budget is derived from international donors, thereby limiting national ownership and sustainability of these important initiatives.

With advances in the risk practices of the general population, increasing attention has been paid to vulnerabilities among sex workers. Female sex workers commonly work at trucking stops along the trans-Africa highway and their HIV prevalence is approximately 50 percent; they have an average of 129 different sexual partners per year. Given that up to 6 percent of women report selling sex, many are also married. Although they use condoms with casual sexual partners, they are much less likely to use condoms with their regular male partners. IDUs are also increasingly recognized as an at-risk population in Kenya (Csete et al. 2009). A 2004 United Nations Office of Drugs and Crime study found that 80 percent of IDUs in three urban centers reported sharing injection devices, with 50 percent prevalence in Mombasa (Ndetei 2004). In a World Health Organization study in Nairobi, HIV prevalence was 53 percent among IDUs with two-thirds also reporting sexual risks (Odek-Ogunde et al. 2004).

MSM and Transgender Typologies Used in Epidemiologic Studies in Kenya

Focus group discussions have revealed that MSM are from diverse age, occupational, and socioeconomic groups including both unemployed and highly educated professionals. Studies of MSM in Nairobi have revealed that many men use English-language terms of *gay*, *bisexual*, and *homosexual* to describe their sexual orientation. In Nairobi, a study of 500 MSM revealed 46 percent self-identifying as gay, 23 percent as bisexual, and 16 percent as homosexual; 12 percent self-identified in the Kiswahili term *shoga* which means gay or homosexual (Onyango-Ouma, Birungi, and Geibel 2005). *Shoga* is a term frequently used among MSM to describe themselves, but many also consider it a vulgar term, and the heterosexual population also use the term in a derogatory manner to describe MSM. *Basha* is a term often associated with men who play a masculine or insertive role during sex, whereas *shoga* have been described as predominantly receptive partners during anal intercourse. *Basha* is derived from *pasha*, which means a high-ranking official as well as being the local term for the king in packs of playing cards (Murray 2004). Although these identities do correlate with sexual positioning and thus HIV risk to some extent, these roles show significant fluidity. Moreover, few MSM self-report being transgendered, which is congruent with many studies across Africa (Onyango-Ouma, Birungi, and Geibel 2006). Qualitative evidence has also demonstrated emerging numbers of Kenyan MSM who are willing to openly advocate for their preventive health care needs (Sharma et al. 2008).

A significant proportion of Kenya's MSM likely lead closeted lifestyles, having sex with men but meeting cultural norms by marrying a woman and having children. Population-based estimates of prevalence of same-sex practices among MSM are elusive, but a few estimates have been proposed (Gouws et al. 2006). In East Africa, Cáceres and colleagues proposed that the lifetime prevalence of MSM practices is between 1 and 4 percent, which is congruent with self-reported same-sex practices among a sample of 486 men in Nairobi (Cáceres et al. 2008; Sharma et al. 2008). Same-sex practices have been posited as being more common among the coastal cities and towns than in Nairobi (NACC, World Bank, and UNAIDS 2009).

In the coastal regions of Kenya, "marriages" between men occur. Similar to female *mkungus* who provide education to girls in the duties of marriage, male *mkungus* teach young MSM. Training lasts approximately one month, at the end of which time the younger man gives the male *mkungu* special cloth and kitchen utensils as payment (Kiama 1999). In Mombasa, men who have sex only with men tend to be referred to as *shoga*, or queens, and are more likely to self-identify as gay. Men who practice only insertive anal intercourse tend to self-disclose as heterosexual and are locally referred to as *basha*, or kings (Sanders et al. 2007).

HIV Risk among MSM

MSM carry a disproportionate burden of HIV in Kenya with an average prevalence of approximately 15.2 percent (95 percent confidence interval [CI]; range 13.1–17.3), compared to an HIV prevalence among men of approximately 6.1 percent (table 5.1). Higher prevalence estimates tend to be found along the coast where a cohort has observed an overall prevalence of 22 percent (120/553) over five years of accrual with an incidence rate of 8.8 per 100 person-years (Muhaari 2009).

Estimates of the component of Kenya's HIV epidemic attributable to MSM and prison inmates are numerous. An early model estimated that MSM contributed approximately 4.5 percent of Kenya's HIV epidemic.

Table 5.1 HIV Risk among MSM in Kenya

Source	*Year*	*HIV+*	*HIV−*	*Total N*	*HIV prevalence (%)*
Angala et al. 2006	2006	83	697	780	10.6
Sanders et al. 2006, 2007; Muhaari 2009	2009	120	433	553	21.6
Total		203	1,130	1,333	15.2 (95% CI, 13.1–17.3)

Source: Authors.

More recent estimates have been higher, including 9.8 percent based on an assumption of 3 percent of men engaging in male-to-male sex (van Griensven 2007). The 2009 *Kenya HIV Prevention Response and Modes of Transmission Analysis* (NACC, World Bank, and UNAIDS 2009) estimated that 15.2 percent of incident infections are attributable to MSM. Variation based on region was significant, ranging from 6.0 percent in Nyanza to 16.4 percent in Nairobi and 20.5 percent along the coast of Kenya. The study further estimated that HIV incidence among all MSM was approximately 6.7 percent per 100 person-years and 12.6 percent per 100 person-years among incarcerated MSM.

Age-disaggregated data highlight increasing HIV prevalence associated with increasing age (odds ratio [OR] 1.1 per year, 95 percent CI 1.04–1.2). In this study, prevalence among MSM 18–24 years of age was 17.7 percent; among those 25–34, it was 26.2 percent; and among those older than 35 years, the HIV prevalence was 25.5 percent. These data suggest that many MSM are already infected by the age of 18, thus highlighting the importance of addressing the needs of young MSM (Sanders et al. 2007).

Male Sex Work

In Kenya, numerous studies have been done among male sex workers (MSWs). Available data suggest that Kenya has the most well-developed and studied network of self-identified MSWs in the region. In an initial exploratory study of MSM, 14 percent reported sex work as their primary occupation (Onyango-Ouma, Birungi, and Geibel 2005). In a sample of 285 MSM in Kenya, 74 percent reported selling sex for money or goods in the previous three months, and 40 percent of these men reported buying sex during this same time frame. Only 17 percent of the sample reported not having bought or sold sex during the preceding three months (Sanders et al. 2007). In a baseline behavioral study of 425 men who reported selling sex, levels of HIV knowledge were very low, and alcohol was associated with lower rates of condom use during transactional sex (Geibel et al. 2008; Okal et al. 2009). A follow-up study of 442 MSWs was completed after the provision of comprehensive preventive services. This study and intervention, discussed later in this chapter, demonstrated improvements across multiple domains of HIV risk status among MSWs in Mombasa (Geibel, King'ola, and Luchters 2009). A population size estimation of MSWs in Mombasa demonstrated a relatively large population of 739 men also in high need of basic preventive interventions (Geibel et al. 2007).

Bisexual MSM and Relationships with Women

Multiple studies have demonstrated high rates of active bisexuality and bisexual concurrent (BC) partnerships among MSM in Kenya. Notably, men practicing bisexuality tend to have lower rates of HIV than those practicing sex exclusively with men. Even in the female-predominant epidemics of Sub-Saharan Africa, this finding tends to be common and likely relates to sexual positioning—those who self-identify as homosexual and have only male partners tend to be the receptive partner (Lane, McIntyre, and Morin 2006; Sanders et al. 2007). In contrast, MSM who self-identify as heterosexual tend to have higher insertivity ratios, potentially explaining the lowered prevalence rates among these men.

In one study of 500 MSM in Nairobi, 23 percent self-reported as being bisexual, although 69 percent reported ever having sex with a woman, and 14 percent were either currently married or had ever been married to a woman. Of those reporting bisexual practices, 20 percent had vaginal sex with a woman in the last month, whereas 7 percent reported anal sex with a woman in the same time frame. In the more recent study by Sanders and colleagues (2007), 60 percent of 285 MSM reported having female sexual partners. Finally, a study of MSWs showed that 8 percent were currently married to a woman and another 9 percent were currently living with a woman but not married. In this study, 57 percent of 867 MSWs self-reported as being bisexual (Geibel, King'ola, and Luchters 2009).

Drug Use among MSM

Little data are available describing dual-risk Kenyan MSM who are IDUs. In the study by Sanders and colleagues (2007), only 1.4 percent of MSM reported injecting drug use, two of whom were HIV positive. Even with this small sample size, the HIV risk associated with injecting drug use nearly met statistical significance (OR 13.1, 95 percent CI 0.95–180). Given increasing reports of injecting drug use risks in the region, further evaluation of dual-risk populations of MSM in Kenya is vital (Csete et al. 2009).

Although data about injecting drug use risks among MSM are still emerging, noninjecting substance abuse, including alcohol use, has been identified as common among MSM in Kenya. In one study of MSWs, over half reported typically drinking alcohol two or more days per week. Notably, such use was associated with higher rates of unprotected anal intercourse in a multivariate model (adjusted OR [aOR] 1.63, 95 percent CI 1.05–2.54) (Geibel et al. 2008). Other reports describe the common use of *miraa* (*Catha edulis*), which is an amphetamine-like stimulant with mild to moderate capacity for dependence and is also associated with higher-risk sexual practices among MSM in Kenya (Okal et al. 2009).

Interventions

The Kenyan government has made great strides in accepting the reality that MSM are at risk in Kenya. In 1998, then Kenyan president Daniel Arap Moi told Kenya's *Daily Nation* newspaper, "Kenya has no room for homosexuals and lesbians. Homosexuality is against African norms and traditions, and even in religion it is considered a great sin" (Kiama 1999). Similarly in 1998, Maina Kahindo of the Kenyan Ministry of Health was quoted as saying that "taking into account other modes of transmission of HIV/AIDS, homosexuality is negligible and should not take up our resources and time" ("HIV and Kenya's Homosexuals" 1998). In October 2009, the Kenyan government indicated its vital need to reach out to the gay community in the form of a multicity study using respondent-driven sampling, including population size estimations and needs assessment (Wadhams 2009).

A significant body of epidemiologic and ethnographic research among MSM in Kenya exists, especially in comparison to elsewhere in Africa (Smith et al. 2009). Notably, the *Modes of Transmission Study* published by the Kenyan government highlighted that the response to MSM has received too few resources in comparison to the risk of HIV infection in this population (NACC, World Bank, and UNAIDS 2009). In 2008, in partnership with the Population Council, the Kenyan National AIDS Control Council hosted other African national AIDS control councils in discussing the health needs of MSM and prioritizing the development and implementation of effective prevention strategies (NACC and Population Council 2008). To date, the majority of work undertaken by government and research institutions has been epidemiological research in defining HIV risk and associations of risk in Kenya. However, Kenya has seen a vibrant community-led response in providing services for lesbian, gay, bisexual, and transgendered (LGBT) populations. In Kenya, at least 10 LGBT associations have emerged or are emerging in Nairobi, Mombasa, Kilifi, Nakuru, and Kisumu (Johnson 2007).

Examples of program successes for MSM include the service delivery model developed by Liverpool VCT. The MSM program at Liverpool VCT started in 2004 with a support group discussing issues of sexual identity, HIV and sexual health, condom negotiation, access to services, and disclosure. The goals of this program are to prevent spread of HIV and sexually transmitted infections among MSM and their female partners by raising awareness of the risk associated with male-to-male sex, building capacity among MSM community groups, delivering and building capacity among others to deliver MSM-sensitive voluntary counseling and testing (VCT) as well as care services at health facilities, and finally to advocate domestically, regionally, and internationally for the sexual health needs of MSM. This program has had numerous positive outcomes, including delivery of VCT to more than 3,000 MSM, development of training modules for the sensitization of health care workers to the specific needs of MSM, and distribution of 20,000 condoms and 15,000 sachets of water-based lubricant to MSM in Nairobi and Mombasa. Liverpool VCT has also trained 45 VCT and health care staff, implemented a youth sexuality counseling hotline (One2One), and collaborated with the National AIDS Control Council to ensure that MSM are included in the Kenyan National AIDS Strategic Plan (Angala et al. 2006; Liverpool VCT and Parkinson 2007).

The International Center for Reproductive Health in partnership with the Population Council also completed an evaluation of a multilevel intervention targeting MSWs in Mombasa. Starting with the opening of a drop-in center for MSM in Mombasa, the International Center for Reproductive Health then trained 40 peer educators in HIV prevention in 2007—6 of whom were trained as VCT counselors. These peer educators also received information about harm reduction in the context of alcohol and drugs. In addition, a significant effort was made to distribute condoms and water-based lubricants to sex workers. More than 100,000 condoms and 8,000 sachets of water-based lubricants were distributed. Given the significant uptake of lubricants, a further 20,000 sachets were ordered. The intervention also targeted the health sector, giving 20 service providers sensitization training and clinical training on the specific needs of MSM including anal sexually transmitted infections. This study demonstrated significant increases in the knowledge and use of condoms and lubricants. In addition, significant increases occurred in the uptake of VCT and the use of MSW-friendly clinical services. The study also demonstrated that in univariate analyses, consistent condom use among MSWs was significantly associated with exposure to peer educators, the use of MSM-friendly drop-in centers, and ever having been counseled or tested for HIV (Geibel, King'ola, and Luchters 2009).

In response to high rates of Internet use in finding male sexual partners, Gay Kenya developed and maintains a website to deliver HIV-related information, provide a safe space online for LGBT, and do advocacy (http://www.gaykenya.com/). Another group called Ishtar focuses on the needs of MSWs and partners with research organizations to complete research studies of the populations they serve. Many of these organizations are housed within the Gay and Lesbian Coalition of Kenya, which is based in Nairobi and works to effectively coordinate the many activities of active LGBT groups in Kenya (http://galck.org/).

The support from the Kenyan government, or at least lack of forceful opposition to the development of effective health care and advocacy organizations for MSM in the country, can serve as a model for its neighboring countries and the continent as a whole. The next steps include the further implementation of government-funded and evidence-based HIV interventions for MSM as well as increasing expenditures to match the evidence-based HIV risk among MSM in Kenya.

Malawi: Characterizing HIV Risk among MSM in a Generalized Epidemic

Scenario: Same-sex practices are considered in the context of expanded and mature HIV epidemics among heterosexuals.

Key themes:

- Malawi has a generalized HIV epidemic previously understood to be driven exclusively by heterosexual and vertical transmission.
- Evidence is emerging of significant HIV risk and prevalence among MSM, who report low levels of HIV-related knowledge and high levels of BC partnerships.
- Active prevention programs for MSM are currently limited to small-scale prevention programs although combination HIV prevention programs are being developed and will be implemented in 2011.

Malawi is a democratic country with a population of nearly 15 million people. It is a former British colony located in the southern region of Sub-Saharan Africa that declared independence in 1964. As of 2009, according the United Nations Human Development Index, Malawi has a ranking of low human development. The World Bank considers Malawi a low-income country, but its gross domestic product is growing by nearly 10 percent per year and is expected to keep growing through 2012. Although the economy continues to grow, poverty and famines remain major determinants of health in Malawi (World Bank 2009).

The first case of HIV in Malawi was reported in 1985, which caused the government to implement a blood-screening and education program. The National AIDS Control Program was formed in 1988 to facilitate the delivery of HIV/AIDS programs, starting with the development of a five-year AIDS plan in 1989 (NAC 2003). However, the response to

HIV was limited until 1994 with the election of President Bakili Muluzi, who recognized the importance of the HIV/AIDS epidemic and created a sense of urgency within the government to adequately respond. Active surveillance demonstrated that HIV prevalence rates in prenatal clinics had increased from 2 percent to 30 percent from 1985 to 1993, making HIV endemic in Malawi at that time (NAC 2003).

A National Strategic Framework was developed in 2000, describing a comprehensive five-year plan to mitigate the HIV epidemic, including the development of the National AIDS Commission in 2001. The government's response to the HIV epidemic increased in 2004 with the election of President Bingu Wa Mutharika who supported the development of a National AIDS Policy and appointed a Principal Secretary for HIV and AIDS housed in the government. The National AIDS Commission remains the coordinating body for the HIV/AIDS response in Malawi, delivering prevention, treatment, and care services to the general population and certain vulnerable populations.

With the support of the Global Fund to Fight AIDS, Tuberculosis and Malaria and the U.S. President's Emergency Plan for AIDS Relief, since 2003 the scale of ART has been significantly increased in Malawi (UNAIDS 2004). Specifically, Malawi had nine ART delivery sites providing treatment for approximately 3,000 people in 2003 and 377 recorded ART delivery sites supporting the needs of 198,846 people and registering 88,126 new patients per year in 2009. The latter represents approximately 65 percent of people eligible for treatment, an indicator that has demonstrated a significantly improving trend every year since 2004, when only 4.3 percent of eligible patients were receiving treatment (NAC 2010).

The most current estimates suggest a stabilization of the HIV epidemic in the general population in Malawi with approximately 930,000 people living with HIV (95 percent CI 860,000–1,000,000) and a reproductive-age prevalence rate of 11.9 percent (UNAIDS and WHO 2009). Approximately 60 percent of HIV cases in reproductive-age adults are among women. High-risk heterosexual transmission and vertical transmission remain the dominant modes of HIV spread in Malawi with an estimated 91,000 children (95 percent CI 80,000–100,000) living with HIV as of 2010 (Salter et al. 2008). Although prevalence seems to have peaked, incidence remains stable. From 1990 to 1995, the incidence rate among reproductive-age urban women was observed to be 4.2 per 100 person-years (95 percent CI 3.2–5.3) (Kumwenda et al. 2006). These data are similar to the incidence rate observed in 2004 of similarly aged women in Blantyre of 4.9 (95 percent CI 3.4–6.8) and in Lilongwe of 3.5 (95 percent CI 3.1–5.9) per 100 person-years (Kumwenda et al.

2008). Moreover, in 2006, a study of reproductive-age women in Malawi described an incidence rate of 4.5 (95 percent CI 3.0–6.1) per 100 person-years (Kumwenda et al. 2006). Thus, even in the context of comprehensive prevention targeting heterosexual and vertical transmission, HIV transmission is sustained in Malawi (Kumwenda et al. 2006).

MSM and Transgender Typologies Used in Epidemiologic Studies in Malawi

Studies have demonstrated that MSM in Malawi are from diverse socioeconomic and demographic backgrounds ranging from higher socioeconomic status with highly educated and employed professionals to those in lower socioeconomic status with lower rates of employment and income levels (Ntata, Muula, and Siziya 2008). The vast majority of MSM in Malawi have not had sexual partners from outside Malawi, only a minority has travelled to other parts of Africa, and even fewer have travelled outside the African continent. No qualitative studies of MSM have been done exploring cultural subgroups of MSM in Malawi, although these studies are planned for 2010.

HIV Risk among MSM

Malawi has a generalized HIV epidemic with an estimated prevalence of 11.5 percent among reproductive-age men. As previously described, the dominant risk factors for HIV in Malawi have been heterosexual and vertical transmission. The first seroprevalence study to assess HIV risk among MSM in Malawi was completed in 2008 and demonstrated that MSM are a high-risk group for HIV infection and human rights abuses (Baral et al. 2009). HIV prevalence was 21.4 percent, with 95.3 percent unaware of their HIV status. MSM were more likely to have received information about preventing HIV transmission with women than with men ($p < 0.05$) and were less likely to know that HIV was transmitted through anal intercourse than through vaginal intercourse ($p < 0.05$). In a multivariate model controlling for education, having had a female partner in the last six months, and number of male partners, being older than 25 ($p = 0.06$), having used the Internet to find a partner ($p = 0.07$), and not always wearing condoms with men ($p = 0.01$) were predictive for being infected with HIV. In addition, 39 percent (78/199) had experienced a human rights abuse related to their sexuality, including violence, blackmail, denial of health or housing, or rape. Univariate predictors of rights abuses included disclosing sexuality to family members ($p < 0.05$) or a health care worker ($p = 0.01$).

Male Sex Work

In the one completed study of MSM in Malawi, transactional sex was commonly reported; 62.6 percent (124/198) reporting either buying or selling sex for money or goods in the previous six months. Men were more likely to report having received money or gifts for anal intercourse in Malawi (Baral et al. 2009). Notably, having received money or goods for sex was associated with HIV, and this risk may be mediated by sexual positioning or lower rates of condom use during transactional sex.

Bisexual MSM and Relationships with Women

A study of bisexual activity and bisexual concurrency among MSM in Botswana, Malawi, and Namibia demonstrated that having any bisexual partnerships was common, but considerable heterogeneity existed by gender of partner (Beyrer et al. 2010). In terms of male sexual partners in the previous six months, the median number of partners was 2, the mean was 3.2, and some 15.2 percent of men reported 5 or more partners. About a third (34.7 percent) reported having a single regular male partner.

Among the 277 men who reported having had a female sex partner in the previous six months, the mean and median number of partners was 1.2 and 1, respectively. More than half of all men (53.7 percent) were bisexually active, ranging from a high of 63.4 percent in Malawi to a low of 43.6 percent in Botswana. Overall, some 34.1 percent of MSM were married or had a stable female partner.

Any bisexual partnerships were associated in bivariate analyses with lower education (OR 1.6, 95 percent CI 1.1–2.3), higher condom use with men and with casual male and female partners (OR 6.6, 95 percent CI 3.2–13.9), less likelihood of having ever tested for HIV (OR 1.6, 95 percent CI 1.1–2.3), less likelihood of having disclosed sexual orientation to family (OR 0.47, 95 percent CI 0.32–0.67), and greater likelihood of having received money for casual sex (OR 1.9, 95 percent CI (1.3–2.7) (table 5.2). Independent associations with bisexual partnerships included always wearing condoms with male and female sexual partners (aOR 11.7, 95 percent CI 3.9–35.5), always wearing condoms with casual male and female partners (aOR 10.2, 95 percent CI 4.7–21.9) and with regular partners (aOR 12.7, 95 percent CI 4.7–33.9), having been paid for sex (aOR 1.9, 95 percent CI 1.1–3.5), and not using water-based lubricants (aOR 2.0, 95 percent CI 1.1–3.8) (table 5.2) (Beyrer et al. 2010).

Some 16.4 percent of MSM were in BC relationships at the time of the interview (Beyrer et al. 2010). Bisexual concurrency was most common in Malawi, where 25.5 percent of all men were in such relationships, and

Table 5.2 Factors Associated with Bisexual Partnerships (Having Had Both Male and Female Sexual Partners in Preceding Six Months) among African MSM in Malawi

		Bisexually active		Univariate	Multivariate[b]
Factor	*Total[a] n (%)*	*Yes n (%)*	*No n (%)*	*OR (95% CI)*	*aOR (95% CI)*
Always wearing condoms	65/389 (16.7)	54/63 (85.7)	9/63 (14.2)	6.6 (3.2–13.9)**	11.7 (3.9–35.5)**
Always wearing condoms with casual partners	117/527 (22.2)	90/108 (83.3)	18/108 (16.6)	6.0 (3.5–10.4)**	10.2 (4.7–21.9)**
Always wearing condoms with regular partners	92/529 (17.4)	75/90 (83.3)	15/90 (16.6)	5.6 (3.1–10.0)**	12.7 (4.7–33.9)**
Receiving money for transactional sex	184/533 (34.5)	109/171 (63.7)	62/171 (36.3)	1.9 (1.3–2.7)**	1.9 (1.1–3.5)*
Taking part in transactional sex	240/532 (45.1)	134/227 (59.0)	93/227 (41.0)	1.5 (1.1–2.1)*	1.7 (0.9–2.9)
Not using water-based lubricant	210/340 (61.8)	116/202 (57.4)	86/202 (42.6)	2.0 (1.3–3.2)**	2.0 (1.1–3.8)*
Having less than secondary education	348/536 (64.9)	194/335 (57.9)	141/335 (42.1)	1.6 (1.1–2.3)**	1.3 (0.7–2.3)
Having been tested for HIV	295/530 (55.7)	150/290 (51.7)	140/290 (48.3)	1.6 (1.1–2.3)*	1.4 (0.8–2.5)
Being HIV positive	93/534 (17.4)	42/92 (45.6)	50/92 (54.3)	0.67 (0.43–1.06)	0.7 (0.3–1.4)
Being less than 24 years old	289/534 (54.1)	157/277 (56.6)	120/277 (43.3)	1.3 (0.9–1.8)	1.0 (0.5–1.8)
Being employed	251/534 (47.0)	131/245 (53.5)	114/245 (46.5)	1.0 (0.7–1.4)	0.7 (0.4–1.3)

Source: Beyrer et al. 2010.

a. Not all columns add up due to missing values.

b. For multivariate analysis, variables with a P value less than 0.05 and common confounders (education, employment, and age) were retained, but variables with significant colinearity were excluded.

* Statistically significant ($p < 0.05$); ** statistically significant ($p < 0.01$).

least common in Namibia, with only 10.3 percent of men reporting BC relationships. Men in BC relationships were much more likely to report condom use with regular male and female partners (OR = 4.6, 95 percent CI 2.8–7.7) than were men not in such relationships. Men with BC relationships were markedly less likely to have disclosed their sexual orientation to family members (OR = 0.37, 95 percent CI 0.22–0.65). Bisexual concurrency was also associated in univariate analysis with being employed (OR 1.8, 95 percent CI 1.2–2.9) and with having paid for sex with men (OR 2.0, 95 percent CI 1.2–3.2) (table 5.3). Independent associations with bisexual concurrency included always using condoms with casual sexual partners (aOR 2.7, 95 percent CI 1.6–4.5) and regular partners (aOR 4.8, 95 percent CI 2.7–8.2), having been paid (aOR 1.9, 95 percent CI 1.1–3.1) or paying for sex (aOR 1.7, 95 percent CI 1.0–2.9), having had an HIV test (aOR 1.7, 95 percent CI 1.0–2.8), and being employed (aOR 1.8, 95 percent CI 1.0–3.0) (Beyrer et al. 2010).

Drug Use among MSM

Earlier studies have demonstrated significant rates of injecting drug use among MSM in Malawi with approximately 12.2 percent (18/147) reporting injecting illegal drugs in the previous six months (Baral et al. 2009). No other qualitative or quantitative data describe the risks associated with injecting drug use in Malawi, but these data demonstrate that it may constitute a previously understudied risk of HIV transmission in Malawi.

Interventions

In the context of the generalized epidemics of Sub-Saharan Africa, the HIV response has focused on the prevention and treatment of HIV infections in the general population of children and reproductive-age adults. With the scale-up of ART, HIV incidence and prevalence rates in the general population have peaked in certain places, whereas in others, surveillance data characterize an epidemic in decline. Concurrently, as presented here, evidence is emerging of the disproportionate burden of HIV risk in most at-risk populations, including MSM, sex workers, and people who use drugs.

In contrast to the general population, data describing effective HIV interventions for these populations are scarce, as is evidence of such interventions being brought to scale and resulting in decreased HIV prevalence or incidence rates. Moreover, consensual same-sex practices between men are criminalized in Malawi, and these laws have been increasingly enforced, resulting in numerous arrests, such as the highly profiled 2010 arrests, trial, conviction, and eventual pardon of Tiwonge Chimbalanga and Steven Monjeza ("Malawi: 'Marriage Trial' Threatens Rights" 2010).

Table 5.3 Factors Associated with Bisexual Concurrency (Active Regular Relationships with Both a Man and a Woman at Study Interview) among African MSM in Malawi, 2008

		Bisexually concurrent		*Univariate*	*Multivariate*[b]
Factor	*Total*[a] *n (%)*	*Yes n (%)*	*No n (%)*	*OR (95% CI)*	*aOR (95% CI)*
Always wearing condoms	65/389 (16.7)	20/64 (31.3)	44/64 (68.7)	1.7 (1.0–3.1)	1.6 (0.9–3.1)
Always wearing condoms with casual partners	117/527 (22.2)	32/115 (27.8)	83/115 (72.2)	2.5 (1.5–4.0)**	2.7 (1.6–4.5)**
Always wearing condoms with regular partners	92/529 (17.4)	35/91 (38.5)	56/91 (61.5)	4.6 (2.8–7.7)	4.8 (2.7–8.2)**
Receiving money for transactional sex	184/533 (34.5)	41/180 (22.8)	139/180 (77.2)	2.0 (1.2–3.1)**	1.9 (1.1–3.1)**
Paying money for transactional sex	151/534 (28.3)	35/148 (23.6)	113/148 (76.4)	2.0 (1.2–3.2)**	1.7 (1.0–2.9)*
Taking part in transactional sex	240/532 (45.1)	48/235 (20.4)	187/235 (79.5)	1.7 (1.1–2.7)	1.6 (0.9–2.6)
Having been tested for HIV	295/530 (55.7)	36/288 (12.5)	252/288 (87.5)	1.8 (1.1–2.9)	1.7 (1.0–2.8)*
Being HIV positive	93/534 (17.4)	15/93 (16.1)	78/93 (83.8)	0.96 (0.5–1.8)	0.6 (0.3–1.3)
Being employed	251/534 (47.0)	52/247 (21.1)	195/247 (78.9)	1.8 (1.2–2.9)	1.8 (1.0–3.0)*
Being less than 24 years old	289/534 (54.1)	43/283 (15.2)	240/283 (84.8)	0.8 (0.5–1.3)	1.0 (0.6–1.8)

Source: Beyrer et al. 2010.

a. Not all columns add up due to missing values.

b. For multivariate analysis, variables with a P value less than 0.05 and common confounders (education, employment, and age) were retained, but variables with significant colinearity were excluded.

* Statistically significant ($p < 0.05$); ** statistically significant ($p < 0.01$).

Criminalization, stigma, and lack of targeted HIV prevention programs exacerbate HIV risk among MSM in Malawi by limiting the provision and uptake of evidence-based HIV prevention programs. Given this context, no evaluation has been done of HIV prevention services targeting MSM in Malawi. However, some services are currently being delivered by a community group situated in Lilongwe and Blantyre, including the provision of condoms and water-based lubricants as well as risk reduction counseling. A pilot comprehensive HIV prevention program is planned to launch in 2010 that will generate useful data to better understand the effectiveness of targeted and comprehensive interventions for MSM in Malawi. This program is innovative because it aims to be the first to characterize and pilot combination HIV prevention interventions for MSM in Malawi. It will provide novel insight into the recruitment and retention of a high-risk and criminalized population in the context of a generalized HIV epidemic in Africa. Anecdotal reports indicate that the implementation of this project has faced many barriers that range from the paucity of regional data describing effective HIV prevention interventions for MSM to the issue of homosexuality being highlighted on a daily basis by domestic Malawian and international media.

Senegal: An HIV Epidemic among MSM That Is Not Linked to That of the General Population

Scenario: MSM, IDUs, and heterosexual transmissions all contribute to the HIV epidemic.

Key themes:

- Senegal has experienced a limited HIV epidemic in the general population secondary to early adoption of evidence-based HIV prevention and treatment strategies.
- Consistent evidence shows a significant disproportionate burden of HIV risk and infection among MSM in Senegal compared to the general population.[a]
- Recent arrests of MSM and targeted stigma have limited provision and uptake of previously effective HIV prevention, treatment, and care services.

a. Following the algorithm and based on available data, Senegal would also be assigned to scenario 4 but is somewhat of an outlier in the category, as there exist some uncertainties in risks and prevalence of HIV for female sex workers, IDU, and MSM, which make characterization difficult. In this case, and there are doubtless others; more refined epidemiologic studies will likely be required to characterize these dynamics epidemics among MSM and others at risk.

Senegal remains one of the most stable democracies in Africa with a population of nearly 13 million people. It is just on the cusp between being a low-income and lower-middle-income country with a gross national income per capita of US$970 but is considered to have a low Human Development Index by the United Nations Development Programme (Drain et al. 2004). Notably, Senegal is a religious country that is approximately 93 percent Muslim and 5 percent Christian and thus has extremely high rates of circumcision (USAID 2009).

Six initial cases of AIDS were reported in Senegal in 1986. Subsequently, a national AIDS program was developed by 1987 that included a screening system for HIV antibodies in the blood supply (Thior et al. 1997). Politicians in Senegal were progressive in discussing and developing domestic policy to promote sexual and reproductive health among the general population. Moreover, the government was a major driving force behind the declaration on AIDS made by the heads of state members of the Organization of African Unity in June 1992 (Pisani et al. 1999). This initial declaration focused on the need to launch government-led comprehensive and evidence-based responses to HIV across Africa involving multiple stakeholders including political, religious, and community leadership. To fund the implementation of this declaration, the Senegalese government invested nearly US$20 million between 1992 and 1996, including a major focus on condom availability and use. Other early initiatives focused on stakeholder conferences including people living with HIV/AIDS, community-based organizations, media, and key parliamentarians to complete needs assessments for each of these stakeholders and promote open lines of communication (Pisani et al. 1999).

Given the important role of religion in Senegal, Muslim and Christian leaders were involved in the HIV/AIDS response at an early stage (UNAIDS 2009). Exemplifying this movement was a conference in 1995 of 260 senior Islamic leaders where consensus was reached on the need to support AIDS prevention efforts. Christian church leaders followed suit in 1996 with a conference including all Senegalese bishops that reached a similar consensus. This dialogue between scientists, community leaders, and religious leaders facilitated the willingness of the religious leaders to have discussions about HIV/AIDS in mosques and churches throughout Senegal. In mosques, these discussions included the promotion of condom use between married couples, whereas Christian church leaders were willing to refer constituents to places where they could receive these services (Pisani et al. 1999).

The community response in Senegal has also been vibrant from the beginning of the epidemic. In 1995, 200 community-based AIDS-support organizations and more than 400 other community-based organizations represented over half a million members supporting AIDS-related activities, including a variety of awareness-raising campaigns. An umbrella organization representing 100 of these groups was soon formed with the mission of representing the needs of and developing capacity among member organizations (Pisani et al. 1999).

Female sex work has been legal in Senegal since 1969, although sex workers are required to register with the government and have regular health checks. Early in the HIV/AIDS epidemic, the high risk faced by sex workers for acquisition and transmission of HIV became clear (Piot and Laga 1988; Thior et al. 1997). During the regular health checks mandated by the government, education campaigns focusing on HIV transmission were implemented, condoms were distributed, and their use was promoted. Furthermore, 30 groups for sex workers were developed with the goal of implementing community-led preventive health education and programming for their members. These groups were also charged with providing outreach to unregistered female sex workers (FSWs). Finally, programs were developed addressing the needs of the clients of sex workers to educate them about the risks of HIV and to promote the use of condoms during transactional sex (Pisani et al. 1999).

Other key interventions highlighting the Senegalese government's comprehensive response in the mid-1990s were the integration of sexual health education programs in primary and secondary school curricula. In addition, Senegal developed one of the first surveillance and treatment programs for syndromic sexually transmitted infections (STIs) in Africa. Finally, educating care providers on the need to encourage and educate their clients on the necessity of HIV disclosure and partner notification was a focus (Pisani et al. 1999).

Although these significant early prevention efforts have likely played a major role in attenuating the HIV epidemic in Senegal, biological determinants have also played a role in mitigating the epidemic in Senegal. Specifically, rates of HIV-2 tended to be higher in Senegal compared to HIV-1. HIV-1 is between five and nine times more infectious then HIV-2, and vertical transmission is 15–20 times more likely with HIV-1 than with HIV-2 (Saar et al. 1998). Finally, HIV-1 is significantly more likely to result in lowered CD4 counts and AIDS than is HIV-2 (Saar et al. 1998). In addition, given that more than 95 percent of the male population is circumcised, this factor likely afforded some protection for men from acquiring HIV from FSWs (Krieger et al. 2005).

In 2007, Senegal spent US$8.5 million of national funds, up from US$5.8 million in 2006 (UNAIDS and WHO 2008). In 2007, Senegal was estimated to have an HIV prevalence of 1 percent among reproductive-age adults, up from 0.4 percent in 2001. During this time frame, the estimated ratio of HIV among women to men decreased from 1.55 in 2001 to 1.46 in 2007 with absolute values of 9,000 men and 14,000 women infected in 2001 compared to 26,000 men and 38,000 women in 2007. Fortunately, relatively few children are infected; the most recent estimates in 2007 are 3,100 across the country, compared with 1,200 in 2001 (UNAIDS 2008). In 2007, 68 sites were providing ART in Senegal, serving 6,700 people, which is just over half the 12,000 estimated to be in need of such treatment (UNAIDS and WHO 2008).

Although Senegal's HIV epidemic is expanding and now is at the borderline of meeting the criteria for a generalized epidemic, it is still considered an HIV prevention success story among Sub-Saharan African countries. The epidemic dynamics in Senegal are different from those in other scenario 3 countries such as Kenya and Malawi where heterosexual transmission among reproductive-age adults who do not report additional risk factors such as transactional sex, injecting drug use, or same-sex practices accounts for the majority of infections. In Senegal, the epidemic is much more concentrated among populations of MSM and among FSWs. In addition, new anecdotal evidence reports injecting drug use in Senegal. The HIV epidemic among MSM is the most severe, with the highest HIV prevalence rates reported for any risk group in the country. The national Senegalese AIDS strategy for 2007–11 identifies MSM as a key target population for prevention, and the Senegalese Ministry of Health is implementing programs to reach them. Senegalese LGBT organizations are partners in prevention programs run by ENDA (Environnement et Développement du Tiers Monde)-Santé (Johnson 2007). In December 2008, the International Conference on AIDS and STIs in Africa was held in Dakar. There, Senegalese government officials publicly pledged their support to reducing HIV among sexual minorities (IAS and SAA 2009).

The willingness of the Ministry of Health to address HIV among MSM appears to have led to a political backlash. Within weeks of the conference, police arrested nine male HIV prevention workers in Dakar on suspicion of engaging in homosexual conduct. Article 319.3 of the Senegalese penal code states that "whoever commits an improper or unnatural act with a person of the same sex" will be punished by imprisonment of between one and five years and a fine of CFAF 100,000 to 1,500,000 (US$200–US$3,000). In January 2009, these men were sentenced to eight years in prison and a CFAF 500,000 fine. The arrest and sentencing were widely publicized locally and garnered international attention ("Senegal: Growing Intolerance towards Gay Men" 2009; "Senegal: Nine Gay Men Arrested, Convicted and Given Harsh Sentences" 2009).

MSM and Transgender Typologies Used in Epidemiologic Studies in Senegal

As in other parts of Africa, in Senegal some MSM are openly gay whereas others are more closeted (Teunis 2001). Gay men in Senegal tend to self-identify in Wolof as *gor jigeen*, meaning literally "man-woman," or in French as *homosexuels*. *Gor jigeen* is also used by the general population as a derogatory term to describe MSM. Although these men sometimes have effeminate characteristics, they often do not show these traits in open society for justified fear of violence. In broad terms, two relatively distinct groups exist: *gor jigeen ibbis* (or *oubis*), meaning *open*, and *yoos* (or *yauss*), meaning *fallen women* (or a term for bad women, including sex workers). *Ibbis* tend to use feminine pronouns when describing each other and also tend to be the receptive partner during anal intercourse. *Yoos* tend to self-identify as heterosexual, not as *gor jigeen*, and tend to be the insertive partner during anal intercourse. Moreover, these men generally have bisexual concurrent partnerships with girlfriends or wives while having sex or relationships with men (Niang et al. 2002, 2003).

In heterosexual relationships, a man commonly gives a gift to a woman before sex. Similarly, in relationships between *yoos* and *ibbis*, the *yoos* tend to give a gift to the *ibbis* before sex. This relationship is considered distinct from transactional sex, especially because *ibbis* tend to be wealthier than many *yoos*. In other countries, more fluidity between the various subgroups of MSM tends to exist, but an early ethnographic study found that these identities were surprisingly fixed in Senegal. However, sexual practices among men with these identities are less fixed, and some *ibbis* reported being the insertive partner and *yoos* reported enjoying being the receptive partner (Teunis 2001).

HIV Risk among MSM

One of the earliest published studies of HIV prevalence among MSM in Africa was completed in Senegal and published in 2005 (table 5.4). In it, 463 MSM accrued using snowball sampling from Dakar and four other

Table 5.4 HIV Risk among MSM in Senegal

Source	*Year*	*HIV+*	*HIV–*	*Total N*	*HIV prevalence (%)*
Wade et al. 2005	2005	100	363	463	21.5
Moreau et al. 2007	2007	88	175	263	33.5
Wade et al. 2008	2008	110	391	501	21.8
Total		298	929	1,227	24.3 (95% CI 19.4–29.2)

Source: Authors.

urban communities demonstrated an HIV prevalence of 21.5 percent (95 percent CI 17.7–25.3). STI prevalences among MSM were 4.8 percent (95 percent CI 3.0–7.2), 22.3 (95 percent CI 18.5–26.4), 4.1 percent (95 percent CI 2.4–6.4), and 5.4 percent (95 percent CI 3.5–8.0) for active syphilis, herpes simplex virus 2 (HSV-2), chlamydia, and gonorrhea, respectively (Wade et al. 2005). Men in this study reported high rates of risky sexual behavior in the month prior to the interview, including unprotected receptive anal intercourse (20 percent), unprotected insertive anal intercourse with a male partner (24 percent), and unprotected intercourse with a female partner (18 percent). Determinants of HIV infection in this study were being older, having a higher number of lifetime male partners, and being a waiter. Notably, evidence also existed of increased risk in the capital city of Dakar, because MSM living in Dakar were more than three times more likely to be infected with HIV (OR 3.33, 95 percent CI 1.07–3.43). A 2007 follow-up study after the implementation of prevention programs of 501 MSM demonstrated an HIV prevalence of 21.8 percent (95 percent CI 18.3–25.7), which was essentially unchanged from the previous survey (Wade et al. 2008). Using these data and assuming that 3 percent of men engage in male-to-male sex, then in Senegal one could estimate 19.7 percent of the HIV epidemic would be attributed to MSM (van Griensven 2007).

Senegal is one of the only countries in Africa to have molecular epidemiological data of circulating strains among MSM (Ndiaye et al. 2009). These molecular analyses were performed on the HIV-positive samples from the 2005 study by Wade and colleagues. Some key differences were seen in the circulating strains among MSM compared to those in the general population, including a significantly higher proportion of the potentially more virulent clade C HIV among MSM as compared to sex workers (40 percent compared with less than 5 percent). However, each of the variants described among MSM has been previously demonstrated to circulate among the general population and FSWs in Senegal, highlighting that the epidemic among MSM is not separate from that of the general population (Ndiaye et al. 2009).

Male Sex Work

As previously mentioned, the tradition in Senegal of men giving women money or gifts before sex applies to sex between men where one partner gives money or gifts to another for sex. No accepted definition exists of what constitutes transactional sex compared to male sex work or whether, in the Senegalese context, these two populations can be distinguished. This situation is relevant because preliminary data suggest that many of the same men both buy and sell sex from and to men at different times. Transactional sex, as defined by anal intercourse in exchange for money or gifts with a casual partner, seems to be commonly reported in studies of MSM, but relatively little is known about how often they sell sex, their health needs, and their history of rights abrogations. In one study in Senegal, two-thirds of the participants reported receiving money and 9 percent reported exchanging money for their most recent sexual encounter with another man (Niang et al. 2002).

In the 2005 study evaluating HIV prevalence, 78 of 463 MSM reported that their first sexual encounter with another man was paid. Notably, a trend was seen toward higher HIV prevalence in men reporting receiving money for their first sexual encounter (28.2 percent compared with 19.9 percent, $p = 0.1$). In the preceding 12 months, 20 percent of men reported receiving money for sex. Among those reporting inconsistent use of condoms during transactional sex, 32.2 percent were HIV positive compared to 17.6 percent HIV positive among those reporting consistent condom use during transactional sex ($p < 0.05$) (Wade et al. 2005).

Bisexual MSM and Relationships with Women

Active bisexuality has been reported as being common among MSM in Senegal, although less is known about the prevalence of BC partnerships. Of 463 MSM interviewed in a study in Senegal, 94.1 percent reported ever having sexual activity with women, and approximately 10 percent reported ever having been married to a woman (Wade et al. 2005). The mean number of lifetime female partners was four (interquartile range 2–9); 74.1 percent had at least one female partner in the preceding year, of whom more than 30 percent reported more than three female partners. Finally, in this study, 18 percent of men reported having at least one unprotected sexual encounter with a woman, although this figure decreased to 12 percent ($p < 0.01$) in the follow-up study completed in 2007 (Wade et al. 2005, 2008).

In another Senegalese study, 88 percent of 250 MSM reported having sex with a woman, of whom 20 percent reported anal sex, 21 percent reported giving money for sex with women, and 13 percent reported receiving money for sex with women. Finally, only 37 percent of men reporting bisexual practices reported using a condom the last time that they had sex with a woman (Niang et al. 2002).

Drug Use among MSM

Little is known about additional risks of injecting drug use or risk associated with noninjecting drug use among MSM in Senegal. As in other parts of Africa, a trend exists toward increased HIV risk with alcohol consumption. In the 2005 study (Wade et al.), 17 percent reported consuming alcohol in the last week and had an HIV prevalence of 27.8 percent, compared to 20.1 percent among those who did not consume alcohol in the last week ($p = 0.013$).

Interventions

A 2001 study conducted in Dakar by the Population Council found that many MSM had been victims of verbal and physical abuse based on their sexual orientation and that most felt keeping their same-sex behavior and relationships secret was important to avoid violence and discrimination (Niang et al. 2002). MSM were particularly resistant to the idea of revealing anal symptoms at clinics and hospitals, and some avoided the health care system altogether because of the risk of exposing their homosexuality. Some men reported that health center staff had treated them with scorn or ignored them completely and did not respect their confidentiality. At the same time, respondents expressed a preference for treatment at public hospitals and dispensaries if they were affordable and treated clients with confidentiality and respect (Moreau et al. 2007). In response, the Horizons Program initiated a series of interventions, including peer education, media interventions, and increased HIV/STI services.

The peer education component included recruiting and training 40 MSM to serve as leaders and peer educators tasked with improving knowledge about HIV prevention, increasing condom use, and increasing uptake of preventive services among MSM. The peer educators were selected based on their capacity as social influence leaders, including ability to mobilize other MSM, excellent communication skills, and understanding of and agreement with the aims of the project. In return, the peer educators received a small stipend for their work. Peer educators worked within networks using one-on-one meetings, community discussions, and focus group discussions. They distributed condoms, disseminated information about where to access condoms, and provided referrals to MSM-friendly health care providers (Moreau et al. 2007).

The media component evaluated an intervention targeting the media to decrease stigma aimed at MSM. A series of key informant interviews and focus group discussions were completed with 20 leaders of different media groups exploring the feasibility of a media communication consensus-building workshop. A two-day seminar was completed with 29 journalists from 20 media groups to discuss public health–based approaches to reducing vulnerability among MSM. A media content analysis was completed of coverage of issues involving MSM in Senegal that demonstrated significant stigma and discrimination, and participants formulated a set of recommendations. A pre- and postseminar evaluation of the participants was performed, demonstrating significant increases in knowledge, attitudes, and perceptions of journalists toward MSM and intentions to change reporting practices. Media content analyses completed after the intervention demonstrated encouraging results and a more favorable attitude toward the promotion of social justice for MSM in Senegal. This study highlighted the possibility of using the media as a powerful tool to help improve social contexts among MSM (Diouf et al. 2004).

The final component of these interventions included a health sector intervention to improve access to comprehensive health services for MSM. The Ministry of Health, in collaboration with Family Health International, trained a network of health providers to be sensitized to the needs of MSM as well as to have a better understanding of the specific clinical needs of these men. The education components focused on improved provision of VCT, syndromic surveillance and treatment of STIs, and referral for ART. The previously described peer educators were made aware of these specific providers and disseminated this information to other members of the community (Moreau et al. 2007).

These interventions were evaluated using various means. Results demonstrated a significantly increased awareness of the existence of STIs and HIV/AIDS, reaching 99 percent by the end of the study ($p < 0.01$). Moreover, understanding of the role of condoms in preventing HIV and STI transmission increased, as did HIV testing rates. However, no significant increase occurred in the consistent use of condoms or water-based lubricants during anal intercourse. Although the MSM-friendly health services were significantly appreciated, the uptake among non-gay-identified MSM was relatively low (Moreau et al. 2007).

Another intervention targeting MSM was the World Bank–sponsored Multi-Country HIV/AIDS Program, which was active in Burkina Faso, The Gambia, and Senegal. Through an assessment of existing gaps and by developing the funding mechanisms to meet these needs, the Multi-Country HIV/AIDS Program was able to increase access to HIV/AIDS prevention, care, support, and treatment programs for MSM and male sex workers, as well as other high-risk groups (Niang et al. 2004).

A further evaluation of HIV risk among MSM in 2007 demonstrated that HIV prevalence remained high; however, reductions in high-risk practices among MSM were observed. Specifically, MSM reporting at least one incident of unprotected insertive anal intercourse during the last month with a male partner decreased from 24 percent to 9 percent ($p < 0.01$), as did the rates of unprotected receptive anal intercourse from 20 percent to 10 percent ($p < 0.01$). Finally, unprotected sex with female sexual partners decreased from 18 percent to 12 percent ($p < 0.01$). Estimates of incidence are likely needed to assess the efficacy of these interventions and decreased risk status among MSM (Wade et al. 2008).

References for Kenya

Angala, P., A. Parkinson, N. Kilonzo, A. Natecho, and M. Taegtmeye. 2006. "Men Who Have Sex with Men (MSM) as Presented in VCT Data in Kenya." Presentation at "AIDS 2006": XVI International AIDS Conference, Toronto, Canada, August 13–18.

Cáceres, C. F., K. Konda, E. R. Segura, and R. Lyerla. 2008. "Epidemiology of Male Same-Sex Behaviour and Associated Sexual Health Indicators in Low- and Middle-Income Countries: 2003-2007 Estimates." *Sexually Transmitted Infections* 84 (Suppl. 1): i49–56.

Csete, J., A. Gathumbi, D. Wolfe, and J. Cohen. 2009. "Lives to Save: PEPFAR, HIV, and Injecting Drug Use in Africa." *Lancet* 373 (9680): 2006–7.

Geibel, S., N. King'ola, and S. Luchters. 2009. "Impact of Male Sex Worker Peer Education on Condom Use in Mombasa, Kenya." Presentation at the 5th IAS Conference on HIV Pathogenesis, Treatment and Prevention, Cape Town, South Africa, July 19–22.

Geibel, S., S. Luchters, N. King'ola, E. Esu-Williams, A. Rinyiru, and W. Tun. 2008. "Factors Associated with Self-Reported Unprotected Anal Sex among Male Sex Workers in Mombasa, Kenya." *Sexually Transmitted Diseases* 35 (8): 746–52.

Geibel, S., E. M. van der Elst, N. King'ola, S. Luchters, A. Davies, E. M. Getambu, N. Peshu, S. M. Graham, R. S. McClelland, and E. J. Sanders. 2007. "'Are You on the Market?': A Capture-Recapture Enumeration of Men Who Sell Sex to Men in and around Mombasa, Kenya." *AIDS* 21 (10): 1349–54.

Gouws, E., P. J. White, J. Stover, and T. Brown. 2006. "Short Term Estimates of Adult HIV Incidence by Mode of Transmission: Kenya and Thailand as Examples." *Sexually Transmitted Infections* 82 (Suppl. 3): iii51–55.

"HIV and Kenya's Homosexuals." 1998. *African Health* 20 (6): 48.

Johnson, C. A. 2007. *Off the Map: How HIV/AIDS Programming Is Failing Same-Sex Practicing People in Africa.* New York: International Gay and Lesbian Human Rights Commission.

Kiama, W. 1999. "Where Are Kenya's Homosexuals?" *AIDS Analysis Africa* 9 (5): 9–10.

Lane, T., J. McIntyre, and S. Morin. 2006. "High-Risk Sex among Black MSM in South Africa: Results from the Gauteng MSM Survey." Presentation at "AIDS 2006": XVI International AIDS Conference, Toronto, Canada, August 13–18.

Liverpool VCT and A. Parkinson. 2007. *Reducing HIV and STI Transmission among Men Who Have Sex with Men in Kenya.* Nairobi: Liverpool VCT.

Muhaari, A. 2009. "High HIV-1 Incidence in Men Who Have Sex with Men in Mombasa, Kenya." Presented at the MSM Satellite Meeting of the 4th Southern African AIDS Conference, Durban, South Africa, March 31–April 3.

Murray, S. O. 2004. "Africa: Sub-Saharan, Pre-Independence." In *glbtq: An Encyclopedia of Gay, Lesbian, Bisexual, Transgender, and Queer Culture,* ed. C. J. Summers. Chicago, IL: glbtq, Inc. http://www.glbtq.com/social-sciences/africa_pre.html.

NACC (National AIDS Control Council, Office of the President, Kenya). 2008. *UNGASS 2008 Country Report for Kenya.* Nairobi: NACC.

NACC (National AIDS Control Council, Office of the President, Kenya) and Population Council. 2008. *The Overlooked Epidemic: Addressing HIV Prevention and Treatment among Men Who Have Sex with Men in Sub-Saharan Africa; Report of a Consultation, Nairobi, Kenya, 14–15 May 2008.* Nairobi: Population Council.

NACC (National AIDS Control Council, Office of the President, Kenya), World Bank, and UNAIDS (Joint United Nations Programme for HIV/AIDS). 2009. *Kenya HIV Prevention Response and Modes of Transmission Analysis.* Nairobi: NACC.

Ndetei, D. 2004. *Study on the Assessment of the Linkages between Drug Abuse, Injecting Drug Abuse and HIV/AIDS in Kenya: A Rapid Situation Assessment.* Nairobi: United Nations Office on Drugs and Crime.

Odek-Ogunde, M., F. A. Okoth, W. Lore, and F. R. Owiti. 2004. "Seroprevalence of HIV, HBC and HCV in Injecting Drug Users in Nairobi, Kenya: World Health Organization Drug Injecting Study Phase II Findings." Presentation at the 15th International Conference on AIDS, Bangkok, Thailand, July 11–16.

Okal, J., S. Luchters, S. Geibel, M. F. Chersich, D. Lango, and M. Temmerman. 2009. "Social Context, Sexual Risk Perceptions and Stigma: HIV Vulnerability among Male Sex Workers in Mombasa, Kenya." *Culture, Health, and Sexuality* 11 (8): 811–26.

Onyango-Ouma, W., H. Birungi, and S. Geibel. 2005. *Understanding the HIV/STI Risks and Prevention Needs of Men Who Have Sex with Men in Nairobi, Kenya.* Horizons Final Report. Washington, DC: Population Council.

———. 2006. "Understanding the HIV/STI Prevention Needs of Men Who Have Sex with Men in Kenya." Horizons Research Summary. Washington, DC: Population Council.

Sanders, E. J., S. M. Graham, H. S. Okuku, E. M. van der Elst, A. Muhaari, A. Davies, N. Peshu, M. Price, R. S. McClelland, and A. D. Smith. 2007. "HIV-1 Infection in High Risk Men Who Have Sex with Men in Mombasa, Kenya." *AIDS* 21 (18): 2513–20.

Sanders, E. J., S. Graham, E. M. van der Elst, M. Mwangome, T. Mumba, and S. Mutimba. 2006. "Establishing a High Risk HIV-Negative Cohort in Kilifi, Kenya." Presentation at AIDS Vaccine 2006 Conference, Amsterdam, August 29–September 1.

Sharma, A., E. Bukusi, P. Gorbach, C. R. Cohen, C. Muga, Z. Kwena, and K. K. Holmes. 2008. "Sexual Identity and Risk of HIV/STI among Men Who Have Sex with Men in Nairobi." *Sexually Transmitted Diseases* 35 (4): 352–54.

Smith, A. D., P. Tapsoba, N. Peshu, E. J. Sanders, and H. W. Jaffe. 2009. "Men Who Have Sex with Men and HIV/AIDS in Sub-Saharan Africa." *Lancet* 374 (9687): 416–22.

UNAIDS (United Nations Joint Programme on HIV/AIDS). 2008. *2008 Report on the Global AIDS Epidemic.* Geneva: UNAIDS.

UNAIDS (United Nations Joint Programme on HIV/AIDS) and WHO (World Health Organization). 2008. *Sub-Saharan Africa: AIDS Epidemic Update Regional Summary.* Geneva: UNAIDS and WHO.

van Griensven, F. 2007. "Men Who Have Sex with Men and Their HIV Epidemics in Africa." *AIDS* 21 (10): 1361–62.

Wadhams, N. 2009. "In Fight against AIDS, Kenya Confronts Gay Taboo." Time.com/Nairobi, November 7.

References for Malawi

Baral, S., G. Trapence, F. Motimedi, E. Umar, S. Iipinge, F. Dausab, and C. Beyrer. 2009. "HIV Prevalence, Risks for HIV Infection, and Human Rights among Men Who Have Sex with Men (MSM) in Malawi, Namibia, and Botswana." *PLoS One* 4 (3): e4997.

Beyrer, C., G. Trapence, F. Motimedi, E. Umar, S. Iipinge, F. Dausab, and S. Baral. 2010. "Bisexual Concurrency, Bisexual Partnerships, and HIV among Southern African Men Who Have Sex with Men (MSM)." *Sexually Transmitted Infections* 86: 323–27.

Kumwenda, N., I. Hoffman, M. Chirenje, C. Kelly, A. Coletti, A. Ristow, F. Martinson, J. Brown, D. Chilongozi, B. Richardson, et al. 2006. "HIV Incidence among Women of Reproductive Age in Malawi and Zimbabwe." *Sexually Transmitted Diseases* 33 (11): 646–51.

Kumwenda, N., J. Kumwenda, G. Kafulafula, B. Makanani, F. Taulo, C. Nkhoma, and T. Taha. 2008. "HIV-1 Incidence among Women of Reproductive Age in Malawi." *International Journal of STD and AIDS* 19 (5): 339–41.

"Malawi: 'Marriage Trial' Threatens Rights." 2010. *Human Rights Watch*, New York, NY, April 1. http://www.hrw.org/en/news/2010/04/01/malawi-marriage-trial-threatens-rights.

NAC (National AIDS Commission). 2003. "Estimating National HIV Prevalence in Malawi from Sentinel Surveillance Data: Technical Report." Lilongwe, Malawi: Ministry of Health.

———. 2010. *Malawi HIV and AIDS Monitoring and Evaluation Report 2008–2009: UNGASS Country Progress Report; Reporting Period: January 2008–December 2009*. Lilongwe, Malawi: Office of the President and Cabinet of the Republic of Malawi.

Ntata, P. R., A. S. Muula, and S. Siziya. 2008. "Socio-demographic Characteristics and Sexual Health Related Attitudes and Practices of Men Having Sex with Men in Central and Southern Malawi." *Tanzania Journal of Health Research* 10 (3): 124–30.

Salter, M. L., V. F. Go, D. D. Celentano, M. Diener-West, C. M. Nkhoma, N. Kumwenda, and T. Taha. 2008. "The Role of Men in Women's Acceptance of an Intravaginal Gel in a Randomized Clinical Trial in Blantyre, Malawi: A Qualitative and Quantitative Analysis." *AIDS Care* 20 (7): 853–62.

UNAIDS (Joint United Nations Programme on HIV/AIDS). 2004. *2004 Report on the Global AIDS Epidemic: 4th Global Report*. Geneva: UNAIDS.

UNAIDS (Joint United Nations Programme on HIV/AIDS) and WHO (World Health Organization). 2009. *AIDS Epidemic Update: December 2009*. Geneva: UNAIDS and WHO.

World Bank. 2009. "Gross National Income Per Capita 2008, Atlas Method and PPP." World Development Indicators database, World Bank, October 7.

References for Senegal

Diouf, D., A. Moreau, C. Castle, G. Engelberg, and P. Tapsoba. 2004. "Working with the Media to Reduce Stigma and Discrimination towards MSM in Senegal." Presentation at the XV International AIDS Conference, Bangkok, Thailand, July 14–16.

Drain, P. K., J. S. Smith, J. P. Hughes, D. T. Halperin, and K. K. Holmes. 2004. "Correlates of National HIV Seroprevalence: An Ecologic Analysis of 122 Developing Countries." *Journal of Acquired Immune Deficiency Syndromes* 35 (4): 407–20.

IAS (International AIDS Society) and SAA (Society for AIDS in Africa). 2009. "Public Health Leaders Call on Government of Senegal to Release 9 Men Imprisoned for Eight Years Based on Their Sexual Orientation." Joint Statement, IAS, Geneva, Switzerland, and SAA, Abuja, Nigeria, January 12.

Johnson, C. 2007. *Off the Map: How HIV/AIDS Programming Is Failing Same-Sex Practicing People in Africa*. New York: International Gay and Lesbian Human Rights Commission.

Krieger, J. N., R. C. Bailey, J. Opeya, B. Ayieko, F. Opiyo, K. Agot, C. Parker, J. O. Ndinya-Achola, G. A. Magoha, and S. Moses. 2005. "Adult Male Circumcision: Results of a Standardized Procedure in Kisumu District, Kenya." *BJU International* 96 (7): 1109–13.

Moreau, A., P. Tapsoba, A. Ly, C. Niang, and A. K. Diop. 2007. "Implementing STI/HIV Prevention and Care Interventions for Men Who Have Sex with Men in Dakar, Senegal." Horizons Research Summary. Washington, DC: Population Council.

Ndiaye, H. D., C. T. Kane, N. Vidal, F. R. Niama, P. A. Niang-Diallo, T. Dièye, A. Gaye-Diallo, A. S. Wade, M. Peeters, and S. Mboup. 2009. "Surprisingly High Prevalence of Subtype C and Specific HIV-1 Subtype/CRF Distribution in Men Having Sex with Men in Senegal." *Journal of Acquired Immune Deficiency Syndromes* 52 (2): 249–52.

Niang, C., M. Diagne, Y. Niang, A. Moreau, D. Gomis, M. Diouf, K. Seck, A. S. Wade, P. Tapsoba, and C. Castle. 2002. *Meeting the Sexual Health Needs of Men Who Have Sex with Men in Senegal*. Washington, DC: Population Council.

Niang, C., A. Moreau, K. Kostermans, H. Binswanger, C. Compaore, M. Diagne, et al. 2004. "Men Who Have Sex with Men in Burkina Faso, Senegal, and The Gambia: The Multi-Country HIV/AIDS Program Approach." Presentation at the XV International AIDS Conference, Bangkok, Thailand, July 14–16.

Niang, C., P. Tapsoba, E. Weiss, M. Diagne, Y. Niang, A. Moreau, D. Gomis, A. S. Wade, K. Seck, and C. Castle. 2003. "'It's Raining Stones': Stigma, Violence and HIV Vulnerability among Men Who Have Sex with Men in Dakar, Senegal." *Culture, Health and Sexuality* 5 (6): 499–512.

Piot, P., and M. Laga. 1988. "Prostitutes: A High Risk Group for HIV Infection?" *Sozial- und Präventivmedizin* 33 (7): 336–39.

Pisani, E., M. Caraël, I. Ndoye, N. Meda, S. M'boup, A. S. Wade, S. Ndiaye, C. Niang, F. Sarr, and I. Diop. 1999. *Acting Early to Prevent AIDS: The Case of Senegal*. Geneva: UNAIDS.

Sarr, A. D., D. J. Hamel, I. Thior, E. Kokkotou, J. L. Sankalé, R. G. Marlink, E. M. Coll-Seck, M. E. Essex, T. Siby, I. NDoye, et al. 1998. "HIV-1 and HIV-2 Dual Infection: Lack of HIV-2 Provirus Correlates with Low CD4+ Lymphocyte Counts." *AIDS* 12 (2): 131–37.

"Senegal: Growing Intolerance towards Gay Men." 2009. *HIV/AIDS Policy and Law Review* 14 (1): 31.

"Senegal: Nine Gay Men Arrested, Convicted and Given Harsh Sentences." 2009. *HIV/AIDS Policy and Law Review* 14 (1): 49–50.

Teunis, N. 2001. "Same-Sex Sexuality in Africa: A Case Study from Senegal." *AIDS and Behavior* 5 (2): 173–82.

Thior, I., G. Diouf, I. K. Diaw, A. D. Sarr, C. C. Hsieh, I. Ndoye, S. Mboup, L. Chen, M. Essex, R. Marlink, et al. 1997. "Sexually Transmitted Diseases and Risk of HIV Infection in Men Attending a Sexually Transmitted Diseases Clinic in Dakar, Senegal." *African Journal of Reproductive Health* 1 (2): 26–35.

UNAIDS (Joint United Nations Programme on HIV/AIDS). 2008. *Sub-Saharan Africa: AIDS Epidemic Update; Regional Summary*. Geneva: UNAIDS.

———. 2009. "Leadership in Senegal's AIDS Response." UNAIDS, Press Centre, feature story, April 9.

UNAIDS (United Nations Joint Programme on HIV/AIDS) and WHO (World Health Organization). 2008. "UNAIDS/WHO Epidemiological Fact Sheet on HIV and AIDS, 2008 Update: Senegal." Geneva: UNAIDS/WHO Working Group on Global HIV/AIDS and STI Surveillance.

USAID (U.S. Agency for International Development). 2009. "Supporting Senegal's Fight against HIV/AIDS since 1987." USAID/Senegal, Dakar.

van Griensven, F. 2007. "Men Who Have Sex with Men and Their HIV Epidemics in Africa." *AIDS* 21 (10): 1361–62.

Wade, A. S., C. T. Kane, P. A. Diallo, A. K. Diop, K. Gueye, S. Mboup, I. Ndoye, and E. Lagarde. 2005. "HIV Infection and Sexually Transmitted Infections among Men Who Have Sex with Men in Senegal." *AIDS* 19 (18): 2133–40.

Wade, A. S., J. Larmarange, A. K. Diop, O. Diop, K. Gueye, A. Marra, A. Sene, C. Ene, S. Ba, P. Niang Diallo, et al. 2008. "Reduction of Risk Behaviors among MSM in Senegal after Targeted Prevention Interventions." Presentation at "AIDS 2008": XVII International AIDS Conference, Mexico City, August 3–8.

CHAPTER 6

Scenario 4 Country Studies: India and Thailand

India: Complex Taxonomies of MSM with Multifaceted Epidemics of HIV

Scenario: Men who have sex with men (MSM), injecting drug users (IDUs), and heterosexual transmissions all contribute to the HIV epidemic.

Key themes:

- India has multiple concurrent HIV epidemics with differing dynamics based on geography and diversity of risks.
- Commonalities of these different Indian HIV epidemics are that they are concentrated among key risk groups including MSM, sex workers, and IDUs.
- MSM and transgendered (TG) populations in India have a complex taxonomy with varying HIV risk practices and consequent HIV risk.
- Although coverage is limited in some settings, effective HIV interventions have been developed and implemented for MSM in India with a focus on combined behavioral and structural approaches.

Since the 1990s, India has been making sustained development progress on a scale, size, and pace that is unprecedented in its history. A low-income country with mass poverty at the time of its independence in 1947, India now has a diminishing pool of very poor people and is poised to cross the threshold to join the ranks of the world's middle-income countries with a 2008 gross national income per capita of US$1,070.

Estimates of the HIV epidemic in India over the last decade have fluctuated significantly. As of 2004, the National AIDS Control Organisation (NACO) estimated more than 5 million reproductive-age adults were infected with HIV in India, representing a prevalence of less than 1 percent. Given India's large population, even a minor difference in prevalence estimations results in significant differences in the absolute estimations of burden of disease. The Joint United Nations Programme on HIV/AIDS has postulated that NACO's figure overestimated the actual number of people living with HIV secondary to sampling of high-risk subsets of the population and then generalizing the disease burden to the general population (Steinbrook 2007). More recent estimates suggest that India has approximately 2.3 million people living with HIV with a disproportionate burden of disease in the southern states of Andhra Pradesh, Karnataka, Maharashtra, and Tamil Nadu and the northeastern states of Manipur and Nagaland (NACO 2008; NIHFW and NACO 2007). Although this estimate is approximately half of earlier estimates of absolute infections, it still represents the third-most infections in any country globally. These data points suggest that the HIV epidemic has stabilized or declined among heterosexual populations in the southern states, presumably as a result of intensive intervention and treatment efforts and improved epidemiologic surveillance mechanisms (Arora et al. 2008). Of new infections, 85 percent have been assumed to be secondary to heterosexual transmission, but much of heterosexual transmission is likely secondary to male partners of female sex workers (FSWs) (Kumar et al. 2006). These data suggest that declining prevalence does not reflect all risk populations, and recent and consistent data suggest the HIV epidemic continues to concentrate among particular populations in India (Chandrasekaran et al. 2006).

Female sex work is common in many of the southern states, with 11 percent of adult urban men reportedly often paying for sex—although nearly 30 percent reported ever having paid for sex. A complex typology of FSWs exists in India, including one that defines sex workers by geography of work, such as brothel-based, street-based, home-based, lodge-based, *dhaba* (a local restaurant)-based, and highway-based FSWs.

Numerous other populations of sex workers exist. For example, indirect-primary sex workers solicit clients at their places of work, which are venues where facilitating sex work is the primary purpose (massage parlors, bars); indirect-secondary sex workers generally solicit clients at their places of work but are in non-sex-work-related industries (agriculture, construction); and phone-based sex workers primarily solicit clients through telephones (Buzdugan, Halli, and Cowan 2009). Notably, the evidence base for the health effects—including effects on HIV and sexually transmitted infections (STIs)—of sex trafficking in India is modest but growing (Silverman et al. 2006, 2007). In a series of important papers about women and girls trafficked between Nepal and India, Silverman and colleagues (2007) have studied the HIV and STI associations with trafficking in this extensive prostitution context. In a 2007 *JAMA* paper (Silverman et al. 2007), they reported that girls trafficked into sex work before reaching 15 years of age were at markedly higher risk for HIV infection than those trafficked at 18 years or older, with an adjusted odds ratio (aOR) of 3.7 (95 percent confidence interval [CI] = 1.32–10.34). These youngest trafficking victims, albeit a small sample (N = 33) had over a 60 percent prevalence of HIV infection. Having been trafficked to Mumbai, rather than other destinations in India, was associated with a markedly higher aOR for HIV infection, as was longer duration of forced prostitution, suggesting structural factors likely play key roles in the risks for HIV among these girls and women.

Risk practices among the general population of women in India tend to be low, given social norms in much of India. More than 90 percent of women report having a single sexual partner and marriage by 25 years of age, suggesting that their primary risk for infection is mediated by marriage. In addition, more than 90 percent of HIV-positive women reported being married and in a monogamous relationship, reinforcing the concept that HIV risk is mediated by marriage. In India, many seropositive women reportedly find out about their HIV status when pregnant as a result of prenatal care (Solomon et al. 2003). Within marriage, rates of reported intimate partner violence have been high, which is associated with higher rates of extramarital high-risk sexual practices among abusive men, thus further increasing risk status among married women. These complex modes of transmission are generally not accounted for when discussing heterosexual transmission between couples. Differentiating the role of transmission of HIV secondary to same-sex practices among men is equally difficult. The majority of MSM in

India do not openly self-disclose their sexual practices or self-identify as being gay or homosexual, thereby making assessment of their relative contribution to the epidemic difficult with traditional surveillance mechanisms. As such, the HIV prevention response in India over the past two decades has focused on heterosexual transmission and prevention of transmission from mother to child (NACO 2005).

Taxonomy of MSM in India

The taxonomy of different subpopulations in India is likely the most complex and well developed globally (Asthana and Oostvogels 2001). Sexualities are fluid, and developing and assigning rigid definitions of subpopulations of MSM is somewhat artificial although it serves the purpose of facilitating an understanding of the public health needs of these men. *Hijras* are biological or anatomical males who reject their masculine identity and self-identify either as a woman or as a third gender: "not-man," "between man and woman," or "neither man nor woman." Some *hijras* are born as hermaphrodites or intersex people, but this situation is likely rare compared to male-to-female TG persons or TG women (Pisal 2006). *Hijras* are often inaccurately described as eunuchs, which is a term used to describe men who were castrated by accident, coercion, or punishment, generally leaving the penis intact. In contrast, many *hijras* voluntarily remove all of their external male genitalia, including both the scrotum and the penis. In Tamil Nadu, *hijras* are called *aravanis*, which is a term developed by *hijra* communities to replace the derogatory term *Ali* (Chakrapani 2005).

Hijra communities have multiple subpopulations, including those who have undergone *salvation* or *nirvana*. These *nirvan* or *nirvan kothi*s have undergone surgical removal of all their male genitalia and are thus incapable of insertive anal intercourse. TG women who have not had sexual reassignment surgery are called *ackwa* or *ackwa kothi*. Some *ackwa* are in training for community rites of passage until they are ready to achieve *nirvana* with sexual reassignment surgery. *Zenanas* are *hijras* who may dress as men or women but who have some effeminate characteristics. This population has the greatest overlap with *kothi* populations, highlighting the fluidity of Indian sexualities. *Hijras* tend to be the receptive partner when having sex with men, thus potentiating their risk for HIV and STIs. Notably, not all *hijras* assess their sexual practices as being homosexual because they consider the receptive partner to play the female role and the insertive partner to assume the male role irrespective of their gender at birth. Although active bisexuality among *hijras* is rare, some *hijras* are married and may have children before joining the *hijra* community (Asthana and Oostvogels 2001).

Kothis describe a wide continuum of sexualities but are generally men who display effeminate characteristics. Many of these men are predominantly the receptive partner for anal and oral intercourse, which increases their risk of acquiring HIV infection compared to predominantly insertive MSM. However, given the diversity among *kothis*, some, called *khada kothis*, in northern India, for example, practice insertive anal intercourse. Many *kothis* have bisexual concurrent partnerships and are often married to women. The continuum of sexualities in India means significant overlap occurs between *hijra* and *kothi* populations, and many *hijras* self-identify as *kothis*. The distinction is that *hijras* almost exclusively dress as women and are more likely to have undergone sexual reassignment surgery than are *kothis*. *Kothis* are more likely to be in active bisexual partnerships or to practice bisexual concurrency than are *hijras*, who tend to leave their families when they join the *hijra* community (Pisal 2006).

Panthi is a term generally used by *kothis* and *hijras* to refer to MSM who practice exclusively insertive or penetrative sex and rarely display any female characteristics. *Panthi* has also been used to describe heterosexual men who do not have sex with *hijras* or *kothis*, so not all *panthis* are necessarily MSM. *Panthis* are nearly always married to women, though some *hijras* or *kothis* consider themselves married to a *panthi* even if the *panthi* is married to a woman (Chakrapani 2005).

Finally, some MSM are referred to as *double-deckers* or *DD*. This term describes sexual practices more than identity because these men may be *kothis* or more rarely *hijras* or *panthis*. Some double-deckers have subtle effeminate characteristics, but most tend to be actively bisexual and often marry women.

Although these sexualities are diverse, open display of homosexual identities remains relatively uncommon, secondary to societal norms as well as the criminalization of these practices under the Indian penal code as a legacy of British colonial rule (Asthana and Oostvogels 2001; Herget 2006). Section 377 of the Indian Penal Code was overturned in July 2009, but a long time will be needed for societal norms to change and for structural barriers to evidence-based prevention, treatment, and care services to be mitigated. Exclusion from health services, stigma, discrimination, and police-mediated violence remain common human rights violations making MSM difficult to study (Chakrapani et al. 2007; Chandrasekaran et al. 2006; Safren et al. 2006).

HIV Risk among MSM

Although research among MSM in India is challenging, the last decade has seen a significant increase in the evidence base describing HIV risk in this population. A recent systematic review identified 48 manuscripts exploring risk status among MSM in India; 12 manuscripts focused exclusively on health risks faced by MSM (Setia et al. 2008). The prevalence of same-sex practices in India remains unknown, in part because of the limitations of current strategies for population size estimations, including demographic health surveys. Moreover, given the different social dynamics and epidemic patterns of south and north India, one estimate will likely not be generalizable for the whole country. However, some studies have found prevalence rates of same-sex practices ranging from 3 percent to 12 percent when accruing male participants from a variety of settings, including a hospital or rural district. Current data describing HIV prevalence among MSM are derived from government-managed passive and active surveillance mechanisms, targeted research studies, and programmatic evaluations.

Surveillance mechanisms rely on self-reported sexual practices and thus tend to underestimate the true prevalence of same-sex practices, especially in the context of heightened stigma and discrimination. In addition, in 2007, only 40 of 1,134 national surveillance sites were devoted to MSM, thus limiting the generalizability of these data (NACO 2008). However, surveillance has demonstrated that in contrast to the general population, HIV prevalence among MSM is increasing. The current estimate is 7.6 percent—with significant disparities across the country, including estimates of 17 percent in the southern states of Andhra Pradesh and Karnataka (NACO 2008).

Setia and colleagues' (2008) systematic review of the literature on MSM in India demonstrated a pooled estimate of HIV prevalence of 16.5 percent (95 percent CI 11–22 percent) and 55 percent (95 percent CI 40–71 percent) in TG individuals. The first known study dates to 1989 and demonstrated disproportionate burden of hepatitis B as well as several STIs, including syphilis and gonorrhea. More recent studies demonstrated low levels of condom use. Moreover, when condoms were used, often no access to safe lubricants was available, thereby mitigating the benefit of the condom. In a study from Mumbai published in 2006, the HIV prevalence among MSM was 11 percent (Hernandez et al. 2006). Condom rates in this study were low, with 90 percent of these men reporting never having used a condom. In a study of MSM from Chennai, approximately 7 percent were infected, and only 50 percent had ever been tested for HIV. Low perceived risk of HIV infection was an important driver for the lack of testing among MSM in Chennai. In addition, 85 percent of men reported having been harassed by police and did not feel comfortable seeking testing services in government hospitals, which represented the main regional provider of HIV services (Chakrapani et al. 2007). Research completed in Pune (in the southern state of Maharashtra) among all men found that 7 percent reported same-sex practices. Among these MSM, the HIV prevalence was 19 percent with 6 percent being seropositive for syphilis antibodies. This study also demonstrated that genital ulcerative diseases (GUDs) were associated with HIV infection among MSM (odds ratio [OR] = 1.86, 95 percent CI 1.23–2.81). In a study from Mumbai, prevalence was found to be much higher among TG women than among MSM; specifically, the HIV prevalence was 68 percent among TG women and 17 percent among MSM. Again, GUDs were found to be associated among MSM with HIV infection, herpes simplex virus 2 (OR = 9.0, 95 percent CI 2.2–36.9), and syphilis (OR = 6.0, 95 percent CI 1.5–24.0). In addition, having had receptive anal sex more than five times in six months was highly associated with HIV infection (OR = 4.3, 95 percent CI = 1.2–15.0) (Setia et al. 2006). Similarly, among TG individuals, GUDs were significant markers of HIV risk with herpes simplex virus 2 (OR 6.7, 95 percent CI = 1.1–40.4) and syphilis (OR = 9.8, 95 percent CI = 1.5–63.9). As with other studies among MSM, condom use rates were low; 59 percent of MSM and 54 percent of TG individuals reported never or rarely using condoms during anal sex (Setia et al. 2008). A qualitative study completed in Chennai has since demonstrated that condoms were not used because of decreased pleasure, assumed low risk of male sexual partners, or difficulties with condom negotiation, especially during transactional sex (Chakrapani et al. 2007). A large study of 4,597 MSM in the southern states of Andhra Pradesh, Karnataka, Maharashtra, and Tamil Nadu described a population at high risk with low HIV testing rates ranging from 13 percent (Andhra Pradesh) to 56 percent (Maharashtra); the rates in Tamil Nadu and Karnataka were 43 percent and 36 percent, respectively (Brahmam et al. 2008). Of those who reported having been tested for HIV, approximately 20 percent reported having done so voluntarily.

Male Sex Work

As data are continually emerging describing the development of communities of MSM, so too are data describing risk status of male sex workers

(MSWs) and prevalence of transactional sex in India (Lahiri and Kar 2007). Prevalence of sex work or transactional sex varies significantly, with estimates ranging from 11 percent of MSM to 96 percent of TG persons in Mumbai (Hernandez et al. 2006; Setia et al. 2006; Shinde et al. 2009). Several studies have demonstrated that self-defined MSWs and MSM practicing transactional sex is fairly common in India although it is higher in certain subpopulations of MSM including *hijras* and TG populations. In a study of 6,661 MSM in Andhra Pradesh, 1,776 (26.7 percent) reported ever selling sex, 1,098 reported often practicing transactional sex, and nearly 700 reported infrequent practice of transactional sex. Risk status in this population was high with 146/1,000 (estimated range = 116–179) expected to acquire HIV annually and expected to transmit HIV annually to 55 men or women who do not sell sex. MSWs were 6.7 times more likely (95 percent CI 4.9–9.2) to acquire HIV than FSWs and 2.5 times more likely (95 percent CI 2.0–3.2) to transmit infection than their female counterparts. Notably, risk was higher among non-sex-worker MSM than among FSWs in this study (Dandona et al. 2006).

A study evaluating correlates of transactional sex among 200 men was completed in Tamil Nadu. It compared MSWs to MSM who did not engage in transactional sex and found that men who sell sex had a significantly higher mean number of male partners in the past month (31 compared with 4), were more likely to use condoms, and were more likely to report having been harassed (Asthana and Oostvogels 2001). Also important, of these men, 32.5 percent reported never having been tested for HIV. In a study of 4,597 MSM from the southern states of India, many were included based on a definition of having exchanged money or goods for sex with another man. HIV prevalence ranged from 7 percent to 21 percent (Brahmam et al. 2008).

Bisexual MSM and Relationships with Women

As described in the section on taxonomies of MSM in India, bisexuality is common among many of these subpopulations. Specifically, studies demonstrate that between 30 percent and 60 percent of Indian MSM are married (Go et al. 2004; Gupta et al. 2006). No consistent finding of HIV risk based on bisexuality has been made; in some studies, risk has been higher among actively bisexual men, and in some cases, it has been lower (Brahmam et al. 2008; Hernandez et al. 2006; Setia et al. 2008). Preliminary results suggest that being married is associated with higher risk of HIV infection—a recent study from Mumbai demonstrated that MSM who were married had an aOR of being infected with HIV of 2.7

(95 percent CI 1.6-4.8) (Kumta et al. 2010). In addition, studies have shown that compared to unmarried MSM, married men report lower rates of condom use, higher rates of anal sex, and greater numbers of sexual partners—both male and female (Chakrapani et al. 2007; Dandona et al. 2005; Verma and Collumbien 2004). Condom use rates with female sexual partners or wives tend to be quite low, which potentiates risk for acquiring HIV infection for these women (Dandona et al. 2006; Newman et al. 2008). For example, in one study of 821 MSM in Mumbai, 53 percent reported never using a condom with their female partners because of availability, low risk perception, or reduced pleasure (Kumta et al. 2010)

Drug Use among MSM

India has an estimated 3 million opiate users, of whom approximately 164,820 to 1.1 million inject drugs (Arora et al. 2008; UNODC 2009). Although epidemics of HIV among MSM seem to be concentrated in the southern states, the northeastern states of India (including Manipur and Nagaland) have the highest reported rates of drug use secondary to proximity of this region to the Golden Triangle and the long land borders with Myanmar, a major heroin exporter (Beyrer et al. 2000). Given this large population of IDUs, a relatively large population of dual-risk IDUs and MSM likely exists, especially given the reports of increasing injecting drug use in the southern states. The *National Behavioural Surveillance Survey (BSS) 2006* (NACO 2006b) included behavioral assessments of 2,638 MSM in 10 sites across the country. Drug use rates among MSM were reported to be highest in the northern states compared to the southern states, with 60.4 percent of MSM reporting ever injecting drugs in Delhi and 21.1 percent in Bangalore, compared to 2.2 percent in Chennai. In Delhi, recent drug use was common, with 30.4 percent reported injecting illicit drugs in the last year compared to no respondents in Chennai or Kolkata reporting this practice. Similarly, 9.1 percent of MSM in Goa and Gujarat reported injecting drugs in the last 12 months compared to again no MSM reporting this practice in the southern state of Andhra Pradesh. Notably, injecting drugs has become more common in Delhi and Mumbai since the 2001 *BSS* was completed. Fortunately, rates are lower in the south, including Chennai and Kolkata, and the proportion of MSM reporting ever trying a drug has decreased significantly from a similar *BSS* completed in 2001. Across all states, 32.4 percent of MSM in Uttar Pradesh reported ever using a drug, compared to only 0.4 percent in Andhra Pradesh.

Interventions

India's NACO was established in 1990 and coordinates the HIV response in India. The early NACO prevention programs targeted specific key populations including FSWs, migrants, truck drivers, and IDUs. At that time, the relative contribution of men to the HIV epidemic was focused on extramarital concurrent sexual partnerships with FSWs as well as being at risk for parenteral transmission through injecting drugs with little attention focused on the role of transmission secondary to men having sex with men (Setia et al. 2008). Consequently, few HIV prevention interventions targeted MSM in India throughout much of the first two decades of the response, although a current objective of NACO's third National AIDS Control Programme is to increase access to HIV prevention and care services among MSM (NACO 2006a). As such, NACO has developed a resource pack for HIV prevention services for MSM and *hijra* communities in India (National AIDS Control Programme 2006). The need for these programs has been well established and discussed throughout this report—they have the highest HIV prevalence rates of any population in India, low rates of HIV testing, low rates of consistent condom use or the use of lubricants, low rates of knowledge about antiretroviral treatment, high rates of transactional sex and formal sex work, and high rates of bisexual concurrency. Contextualizing all of this risk are the recently repealed laws criminalizing same-sex practices as well as prevalent reports of stigma, discrimination, and exclusion from health services.

Although international partners have launched large-scale initiatives coordinated by NACO, the majority of initiatives addressing the needs of MSM have been community based and supported by such organizations as the Naz Foundation International and the Humsafar Trust. Other key international nongovernmental organizations (NGOs) have been OxFam and the International HIV/AIDS Alliance. A major initiative launched in India has been the Avahan India AIDS Initiative (Avahan), which is an HIV prevention program for most at-risk populations. Avahan was implemented in the six Indian states that account for 80 percent of the infections in India: the four southern states of Andhra Pradesh, Karnataka, Maharashtra, and Tamil Nadu, and the two northeastern states of Manipur and Nagaland. The two most at-risk populations addressed in the first five years of the program were FSWs and high-risk MSM, with a goal of reaching 217,000 sex workers and 80,000 MSM. This program has been scaled up quickly, and within five years 67 percent of MSM ever contacted had used STI treatment services at least once, and 75 percent of MSM had received the comprehensive package of services focused on drop-in centers, condom distribution, and peer educators (Avahan 2008).

Structural drivers of risk, including exclusion from health services and stigma and discrimination, have been addressed though these initiatives that are generally launched by community-based organizations (Passano 2006). For example, the need to intervene to improve the delivery of health services for MSM through health sector interventions, including the development of clinical guidelines for the management of MSM and TG patients, has been recognized. The key objective of a handbook for STI/HIV and sexual health care providers was to increase their knowledge and enhance their skills on the specific health needs of sexual minorities as a way of improving the quality of services available to these populations in India (Chakrapani 2005). The media have also been recognized as a key resource available for advocacy, and Dev Anand of the Gelaya Trust provides support to groups in developing media advocacy and communication plans. One key victory for improving the health and realizing the rights of MSM in India was the repeal of the law criminalizing these practices (Bondyopadhyay 2008). This action took many years of dedicated advocacy before the law was overturned in 2009, although as previously stated, social attitudes will take many years to change as will the decrease in levels of stigma. A key component will be community systems strengthening and support for domestic community-based organizations supporting the needs of populations of MSM. In 2009, the Global Fund to Fight AIDS, Tuberculosis and Malaria has recognized this need by awarding a large-scale regional program supporting capacity building for MSM in South Asia as part of Round 9. One of the primary recipients was the Naz Foundation International in India. As these programs are brought to scale, one hopes the epidemic of HIV among MSM in India will be curbed and follow the same decreasing trajectory of HIV in other key populations in India.

Thailand: High HIV Prevalence and Incidence among Gay Men, other MSM, and Transgenders (*Katoey*)

Scenario: MSM, IDUs, and heterosexual transmissions all contribute to the HIV epidemic.

Key themes:

- Thailand has a generalized HIV epidemic that has been marked by a number of waves among different populations with linked risk factors throughout the last 25 years.

- Currently, the overall HIV epidemic in Thailand appears to be stable with significant prevalence attributed to MSM, IDUs, and sex workers.
- Recent HIV incidence data highlight an explosive epidemic among MSM including MSWs and TG populations, and the overall epidemic trajectory in Thailand appears to be increasing, driven by the MSM component.
- Thailand has implemented numerous innovative HIV interventions for MSM, but high incidence rates highlight the need to increase coverage, quality, and uptake of these services.

Thailand has justly been heralded for a number of achievements in HIV prevention, treatment, and care (Ainsworth, Beyrer, and Soucat 2003). The country was among the first Asian states to develop a national plan for HIV/AIDS, to establish a national AIDS commission chaired by a prime minister, to establish a national HIV sentinel surveillance system, and to develop and implement the "100 percent condom campaign," a structural intervention in the national sex industry that became a regional model. As antiretroviral treatment became available, Thailand was the first Asian country to commit to universal access to antiretrovirals. Thailand has also been a key international partner in HIV research, including being the first—and still only—developing country to conduct two efficacy trials of HIV vaccines. Despite these remarkable successes, the Thai response has also been marked by the long-standing exclusion of MSM (Celentano 2005). MSM were not included in the national HIV surveillance system (with the exception of MSWs in some sentinel sites, including Bangkok), until 2007, delaying understanding of the dynamics of the Thai epidemic and limiting the public sector response.

The Thai HIV epidemic has been marked by phases of spread—the very first wave described by Weniger and colleagues (1991) was among MSM and MSWs in 1985–88. In 1988–89, an explosive epidemic was detected among IDUs, initially in Bangkok but within a few months throughout the country (Weniger et al. 1991). Asia's most severe heterosexual epidemic followed shortly thereafter, driven by high rates of commercial sex worker patronage by young Thai men across the country (Nelson et al. 1996). By 1992–93, Thailand had a generalized epidemic of HIV-1, and the spread from men to female sex partners was well established. Evidence from a range of studies suggests that the Thai epidemic peaked in 1995–96, and HIV rates among most populations in the sentinel surveillance declined steadily thereafter. IDUs have been a marked exception, with high and sustained HIV rates across sentinel rounds. MSM, because they were not included until the 2007–11 National Plan, cannot be readily studied through the sentinel system (NAPaA Committee 2007). Nevertheless, data from cohort studies, from several other studies of military recruits and drug users, and from the work of van Griensven and colleagues in Bangkok, Chiang Mai, Pattaya, and Phuket, demonstrate a severe and expanding epidemic of HIV among MSM across the country (Beyrer et al. 2005; Guadamuz et al. 2009; van Griensven et al. 2005). HIV rates in Bangkok MSM evaluated through venue time sampling increased from an estimated 17.3 percent in 2003 to 28.3 percent in 2005 and to 30.7 percent in 2007, the highest in the region (van Griensven et al. 2009). The overall increase in prevalence from 2003 to 2007 was significant for trend ($p < 0.001$). Among young MSM (15–22 years of age), the estimated incidence rose from 4.1 percent in 2003 to 6.4 percent in 2005 to an extraordinarily high rate of 7.7 percent in 2007 ($p > 0.02$ for trend) (van Griensven et al. 2009). These incidence measures are among the few data sets available among MSM in low- and middle-income countries and demonstrate both the power of well-done research and the intensity of the force of the spread of HIV among these young men as soon as sexual debut with other men has occurred; median age of anal sexual debut across the sample rounds was 17 and did not change. This age was slightly older than the median age of sexual debut among all young Thai men, reported to be 16.5 years from military recruit studies (Nelson et al. 1996).

MSM and Transgender Typologies Used in Epidemiologic Studies in Thailand

Thai sexual behavior and gender identity have been extensively studied, and multiple investigations have linked behaviors and identities to HIV risks and vulnerabilities. Thai culture has a long-standing traditional third gender category: *katoey*, who are TG biological males who take on female identities and roles and speak the female-gendered dialect of Thai (Jackson and Cook 1999). With the advent of modern sexual reassignment surgery, which is widely available in Thailand, some *katoey* have chosen gender reassignment and become TG women. Male partners of *katoey* were traditionally not seen as homosexual but were considered *puchai* (that is, men), as long as they maintained masculine behavior and appearance. In a study among 2,005 Thai men admitted for drug detoxification in northern Thailand, 3.8 percent reported lifetime history of sex with another male; 84.8 percent of these MSM had only ever had a *katoey* sex partner; and only 10.6 percent of drug-using MSM reported ever having had sex with a male-identified man (Beyrer et al. 2005).

Contemporary Thai culture has seen the emergence of openly gay men who are male identified and no longer fit the *katoey/puchai* paradigm. The social research construct MSM is itself increasingly used by Thai men to self-describe their identity. Bisexuality is also a common identity, and the Thai term *seua bi* (literally, "bi flesh") refers to men who enjoy sex with both men and women. MSWs, a considerable population in some commercial sex areas (principally Bangkok, Chiang Mai, Pattaya, Phuket, and virtual online domains), may be heterosexually identified, bisexual, homosexual, or *katoey*, although the majority (62.9 percent) in a three-city study in 2005 reported heterosexual orientation (CDC 2006). Exchange or transactional sex is a feature of Thai culture broadly, and caution must be used in defining men who report having had exchange sex as sex workers (van Griensven et al. 2009).

A U.S. Centers for Disease Control and Prevention–Ministry of Public Health collaboration has used three categories for Thai MSM: MSM, MSWs, and TG individuals. This paradigm has the advantage of simplicity and makes the key distinction of separating out sex workers, who have differing risks and service needs, from other MSM. It has least specificity for MSM, because this category includes homosexually identified men, hidden MSM, and bisexual men in a single broad group.

Differential Risks of HIV among Thai MSM Populations

The 2005 *Morbidity and Mortality Weekly Report* (*MMWR*) data on three categories of MSM—MSM, MSW, and TG individuals—identified differential HIV risks and rates across sampling sites (table 6.1). These populations were venue time sampled with sites in Bangkok, Chiang Mai, and Phuket, which are major MSM and commercial sex centers (CDC 2006).

Table 6.1 HIV Rates among Categories of Thai MSM, in Bangkok, Chiang Mai, and Phuket, 2005

		HIV+ (%)			
Subgroup	*N*	*Bangkok*	*Chiang Mai*	*Phuket*	*Variance by site*
MSM	821	28.3	15.3	5.5	$p < 0.001$
MSWs	754	18.9	11.4	11.5	..
TG individuals	474	11.5	17.6	11.9	..

Source: Adapted from CDC 2006.
Note: .. = not significant.

Risks for HIV infection also varied across subgroups of MSM in this study. For MSM, residing in Bangkok or Chiang Mai, older age, drug use, and nondisclosure of past HIV tests were independently associated with HIV infection. Among MSWs, park or street recruitment and self-reported GUDs were independent associations, whereas sex with a woman in the past three months was inversely associated with HIV. Among TG individuals, older age, street or park recruitment, and lower educational level were associated with HIV infection. These differing risks argue for targeted prevention and outreach programs for these different groups.

A significant concern in both the *MMWR* study and the 2009 report by van Griensven and colleagues was the lack of awareness of current HIV status among Thai MSM (Adam 2009; van Griensven et al. 2009). In the 2005 data from among a total of 340 HIV-positive men, 274 (80.6 percent) reported they were not HIV infected. The U.S. Centers for Disease Control and Prevention group recommended encouragement of much more frequent HIV testing among all groups of MSM to address this concern.

Several encouraging trends in reported risk behaviors were seen among all MSM in the 2009 study. Having ever had an HIV test increased from 43.8 percent of men in 2003 to 52.3 percent of men in 2007 ($p = 0.04$ for trend), a modest increase. Reported anal intercourse decreased from 97.9 percent of men in 2003 to 87.5 percent of men in 2007 ($p < 0.001$ for trend); having had one or more casual partners in the past three months declined from 65.3 percent in 2003 to 38.5 percent in 2007 ($p < 0.001$ for trend). Unfortunately, the proportion of men reporting always using condoms with other men did not change and was at about two-thirds (64 percent) across all three survey rounds (van Griensven et al. 2009). Reports of ever having sex with a woman were also stable from 2003 to 2007 and were reported by about one-third (37 percent) of all MSM.

Drug Use among MSM

Most studies of MSM in Thailand have found relatively low reported rates of active injecting drug use. Drug use was associated with HIV infection in the *MMWR* report only in MSM, and this use was largely a history of smoked methamphetamine rather than injecting drug use (CDC 2006). Rates of noninjected drug use, mostly methamphetamine, were high across the populations, however, and were reported by 38.5 percent of MSWs, 24.1 percent of TG individuals, and 15.5 percent of MSM in

2005. Trend analysis in the paper by van Griensven and colleagues (2009) showed a marked and statistically significant increase in reported drug use (amphetamine-like substances, amphetamine-type stimulants, and benzodiazepines) in the past three months, from 3.6 percent of MSM in 2003 to 17.5 percent in 2005 and 20.8 percent in 2007 ($p < 0.001$ for trend). Drug use during last sex, another measure of risk used in this study, also increased significantly and was reported by 5.5 percent of MSM in 2007 (van Griensven et al. 2009).

One large study of drug users explored behaviors of both IDUs and non-IDUs among MSM presenting for voluntary drug treatment in northern Thailand (Beyrer et al. 2005). This study of 1,752 sexually experienced drug-using men found that 3.8 percent reported a lifetime history of sex with another male; the great majority of their partners were TG *katoey*. Comparing drug-using MSM to drug-using men who reported a lifetime history of only female sexual partners, drug-using MSM had higher HIV rates (OR 2.32, 95 percent CI 1.36–3.96) and were younger ($p < 0.0001$), were more likely to be Thai ($p < 0.0001$), were better educated ($p < 0.0001$), had more lifetime sex partners ($p < 0.0001$), had more female partners ($p < 0.002$), were more likely to have injected than other drug-using men ($p < 0.0001$), and were more likely to have hepatitis C infection (OR 2.59, 95 percent CI 1.55–4.34). As with the Bangkok study, most non-IDUs in this population were methamphetamine (amphetamine-type stimulant) smokers.

The proportion of drug users with a lifetime history as MSM (3.8 percent) is in accord with recent estimates of behavior of MSM in Southeast Asia. Adam and colleagues (2009) found an estimate of 3.5 percent to 4.5 percent of Southeast Asian men reported same-sex relations in the previous year.

MSWs and Migration

One particularly understudied subset of MSM in Thailand is migrant MSWs. In northern Thailand, a recent report was that 48.6 percent of 181 MSWs working in commercial sex venues were non-Thai migrants, the majority ethnic Shan from Myanmar (64.7 percent of non-Thais) (Guadamuz et al. 2009). HIV rates and risks were significantly higher among the Thai than the migrant MSWs (11.8 percent compared with 3.4 percent; $p < 0.001$), but this difference is likely to reflect the relatively high turnover rate of migrant MSWs. Ethnic migrants from Myanmar were very poorly educated; 34.1 percent had no formal schooling in their lifetimes. Sexual identities varied markedly between Thai and non-Thai MSWs in this sample. Non-Thai men were overwhelmingly heterosexual in orientation (84.7 percent) with only 3.5 percent identifying as gay and 5.9 percent bisexual. Thai MSWs were much more heterogeneous, with 22.7 percent reporting being gay, 11.4 percent bisexual, 3.4 percent TG, and 53.4 percent heterosexual. Migrant men will likely require culturally and linguistically targeted interventions to reduce their risks while selling sex in Thailand.

Interventions

Despite the early evidence of HIV infection among MSM in Thailand, few interventions were taken to scale in the early years of HIV spread in the country. The Thai 100 percent condom campaign did target MSWs working at known male sex venues (gay bars, brothels, saunas, and clubs) from 1992 onward (Kunawararak et al. 1995), and NGOs were active in Chiang Mai and Bangkok during this same period at gay bars and clubs where MSWs worked.

In 2003, Thai policy toward gay venues changed abruptly with the "Law and Order Campaign." This punitive and legalistic policy approach of crack-downs on gay bars, clubs, and saunas featured highly public sauna raids, public humiliation, and public nudity of detained clients and workers, including sale of humiliating images to the Thai press. Most dangerous from a public health perspective was the equation of condom availability at gay venues with the "promotion of homosexuality." This policy was a complete reversal of the Thai 100 percent condom campaign, which had recognized that although sex work was illegal, condoms in sex venues were a public health good. Although homosexuality was not illegal, the 2003 "Law and Order Campaign" nevertheless punished gay venue management for providing condoms and lubricant. These prevention tools rapidly disappeared from gay venues (Beyrer 2007).

The period from 2003 to 2007 was marked by rapid spread of HIV among MSM in Thailand. From 2007 forward, HIV prevention policy has shifted toward inclusion of MSM in the National Plan (NAPaA Committee 2007) in response to rising HIV rates among MSM and advocacy on the part of increasingly organized MSM and lesbian, gay, bisexual, and transgender networks. This shift has also included implementation of a range of prevention and treatment programs for MSM, MSWs, and TG individuals. A range of stakeholders have played important roles in these HIV prevention, treatment, and care and support activities. In the NGO sector these groups have included the Rainbow Sky Association; Rainbow

Sky Regional Offices including Bangkok Rainbow; the lesbian, gay, bisexual, and transgender rights group Anjaree; the Thai Network of People Living with HIV/AIDS; and the Thai Drug User Network, which has had a primary focus on providing harm reduction services and human rights for drug users. International NGOs with programming for MSM have included Family Health International, Médecins Sans Frontières, the Ford Foundation, and the Rockefeller Foundation. In addition to government entities, including the Ministry of Public Health, Thai organizations such as the Thai Red Cross Program on AIDS, and the bilateral U.S. Centers for Disease Control and Prevention–Thai Ministry of Public Health collaboration on HIV/AIDS have played key roles in the response.

In the 10th National HIV Plan (for years 2007–11), preventive intervention activities targeted to MSM accounted for a modest 1.3 percent of the total proposed budget. Some 16.1 percent of the overall budget is for prevention for all populations. Treatment and care for MSM were included in the national health insurance scheme for antiretroviral drugs, but MSM-targeted treatment programs were not included (USAID Health Policy Initiative 2006).

Despite a wide array of prevention programs from the NGO, government, and bilateral sectors, remarkably few data are available on the efficacy of HIV prevention programs for MSM in Thailand. The epidemiology suggests that HIV incidence densities have been very high but may have begun leveling off in 2007. This trend will need to be evaluated when the 2008 and 2009 sentinel surveillance data are available. If real, it would suggest prevention activities may be affecting transmission rates among MSM. The data from 2003–07 suggest that HIV prevention efforts were not succeeding in achieving reductions in rates.

Novel HIV Preventive Interventions for MSM in Thailand

A large multicountry trial is currently under way for preexposure prophylaxis with Truvada among HIV-uninfected MSM in several countries that includes a trial site in Chiang Mai led by Dr. Suwat Chariyalertsuk of Chiang Mai University. The Chiang Mai site was targeted to enroll some 200 MSM in a daily Truvada compared to placebo regimen. The results have demonstrated efficacy of the trial (Grant et al. 2010). At least one additional randomized controlled trial of oral chemoprophylaxis with Truvada will likely be required before this intervention is accepted for use in programs, but it does represent a potentially powerful biomedical prevention tool for MSM and other at-risk individuals.

References for India

Arora, P., R. Kumar, M. Bhattacharya, N. Nagelkerke, and P. Jha. 2008. "Trends in HIV Incidence in India from 2000 to 2007." *Lancet* 372 (9635): 289–90.

Asthana, S., and R. Oostvogels. 2001. "The Social Construction of Male 'Homosexuality' in India: Implications for HIV Transmission and Prevention." *Social Science and Medicine* 52 (5): 707–21.

Avahan. 2008. *Avahan—the India AIDS Initiative: The Business of HIV Prevention at Scale.* New Delhi: The Bill and Melinda Gates Foundation.

Beyrer, C., M. H. Razak, K. Lisam, J. Chen, W. Lui, and X-F. Yu. 2000. "Overland Heroin Trafficking Routes and HIV-1 Spread in South and South-East Asia." *AIDS* 14 (1): 75–83.

Bondyopadhyay, A. 2008. "Human Rights, Sexuality and the Indian Legal System." International Lesbian and Gay Law Association, Delhi.

Brahmam, G., V. Kodavalla, H. Rajkumar, H. K. Rachakulla, S. Kallam, S. P. Myakala, R. S. Paranjape, M. D. Gupte, L. Ramakrishnan, A. Kohli, et al. 2008. "Sexual Practices, HIV and Sexually Transmitted Infections among Self-Identified Men Who Have Sex with Men in Four High HIV Prevalence States of India." *AIDS* 22 (Suppl. 5): S45–57.

Buzdugan, R., S. S. Halli, and F. M. Cowan. 2009. "The Female Sex Work Typology in India in the Context of HIV/AIDS." *Tropical Medicine and International Health* 14 (6): 673–87.

Chakrapani, V. 2005. *Understanding Men Who Have Sex with Men (MSM) and Hijras & Providing HIV/STI Risk Reduction Information. Handbook for STI/HIV and Sexual Health Care Providers.* Mumbai: Indian Network for People Living with HIV/AIDS.

Chakrapani, V., P. A. Newman, M. Shunmugam, A. McLuckie, and F. Melwin. 2007. "Structural Violence against Kothi-Identified Men Who Have Sex with Men in Chennai, India: A Qualitative Investigation." *AIDS Education and Prevention* 19 (4): 346–64.

Chandrasekaran, P., G. Dallabetta, V. Loo, S. Rao, H. Gayle, and A. Alexander. 2006. "Containing HIV/AIDS in India: The Unfinished Agenda." *Lancet Infectious Diseases* 6 (8): 508–21.

Dandona, L., R. Dandona, J. P. Gutierrez, G. A. Kumar, S. McPherson, and S. M. Bertozzi. 2005. "Sex Behaviour of Men Who Have Sex with Men and Risk of HIV in Andhra Pradesh, India." *AIDS* 19 (6): 611–19.

Dandona, L., R. Dandona, G. A. Kumar, J. P. Gutierrez, S. McPherson, and S. M. Bertozzi. 2006. "How Much Attention Is Needed towards Men Who Sell Sex to Men for HIV Prevention in India?" *BMC Public Health* 6: 31.

Go, V. F., A. K. Srikrishnan, S. Sivaram, G. K. Murugavel, N. Galai, S. C. Johnson, T. Sripaipan, S. Solomon, and D. D. Celentano. 2004. "High HIV Prevalence and Risk Behaviors in Men Who Have Sex with Men in Chennai, India." *Journal of Acquired Immune Deficiency Syndromes* 35 (3): 314–19.

Gupta, A., S. Mehta, S. V. Godbole, S. Sahay, L. Walshe, S. J. Reynolds, M. Ghate, R. R. Gangakhedkar, A. D. Divekar, A. R. Risbud, et al. 2006. "Same-Sex Behavior and High Rates of HIV among Men Attending Sexually Transmitted Infection Clinics in Pune, India (1993–2002)." *Journal of Acquired Immune Deficiency Syndromes* 43 (4): 483–90.

Herget, G. 2006. "India: UNAIDS Claims Law Criminalizing Homosexuality Hinders HIV Prevention." *HIV/AIDS Policy and Law Review* 11 (1): 35–36.

Hernandez, A., C. Lindan, M. Mathur, M. Ekstrand, P. Madhivanan, E. S. Stein, S. Gregorich, S. Kundu, A. Gogate, and J. R. Jerajani. 2006. "Sexual Behavior among Men Who Have Sex with Women, Men, and Hijras in Mumbai, India—Multiple Sexual Risks." *AIDS and Behavior* 10 (4 Suppl.): S5–16.

Kumar, R., P. Jha, P. Arora, P. Mony, P. Bhatia, P. Millson, N. Dhingra, M. Bhattacharya, R. S. Remis, and N. Nagelkerke for the International Studies of HIV/AIDS Investigators. 2006. "Trends in HIV-1 in Young Adults in South India from 2000 to 2004: A Prevalence Study." *Lancet* 367 (9517): 1164–72.

Kumta, S., M. Lurie, S. Weitzen, H. Jerajani, A. Gogate, A. Row Kavi, V. Anand, H. Makadon, and K. H. Mayer. 2010. "Bisexuality, Sexual Risk Taking, and HIV Prevalence among Men Who Have Sex with Men Accessing Voluntary Counseling and Testing Services in Mumbai, India." *Journal of Acquired Immune Deficiency Syndromes* 53 (2): 227–33.

Lahiri, A., and S. Kar. 2007. *Dancing Boys: Traditional Prostitution of Young Males in India*. Kolkata, India: People Like Us (PLUS).

NACO (National AIDS Control Organisation). 2005. *An Overview of the Spread and Prevalence of HIV/AIDS in India*. New Delhi: NACO.

———. 2006a. *National AIDS Control Programme Phase III (2006–2011): Strategy and Implementation Plan*. New Delhi: NACO.

———. 2006b. *National Behavioural Surveillance Survey (BSS) 2006: Men Who Have Sex with Men (MSM) and Injecting Drug Users (IDUs)*. New Delhi: National AIDS Control Organisation, Ministry of Health and Family Welfare, Government of India.

———. 2008. *HIV Sentinel Surveillance and HIV Estimation in India 2007: A Technical Brief.* New Delhi: NACO.

National AIDS Control Programme. 2006. "Resource Pack for Interventions with MSM and Hijras." New Delhi: National AIDS Control Programme, Ministry of Health and Family Welfare.

Newman, P. A., V. Chakrapani, C. Cook, M. Shunmugam, and L. Kakinami. 2008. "Correlates of Paid Sex among Men Who Have Sex with Men in Chennai, India." *Sexually Transmitted Infections* 84 (6): 434–38.

NIHFW (National Institute of Health and Family Welfare) and NACO (National AIDS Control Organisation). 2007. *Annual HIV Sentinel Surveillance Country Report 2006*. New Delhi: NIHFW and NACO.

Passano, P. 2006. "The MSM Initiative." Mumbai: Population Services International, India.

Pisal, H. 2006. "Culture and Health of *Hijras* in India: A Study of a Marginalized Community in Pune and Mumbai." Report submitted to the faculty of the Swiss Tropical Institute, University of Basel, Switzerland.

Safren, S., C. Martin, S. Menon, J. Greer, S. Solomon, M. J. Mimiaga, and K. H. Mayer. 2006. "A Survey of MSM HIV Prevention Outreach Workers in Chennai, India." *AIDS Education and Prevention* 18 (4): 323–32.

Setia, M., P. Brassard, H. Jerajani, S. Bharat, A. Gogate, S. Kumta, A. Row Kavi, V. Anand, and J. F. Boivin. 2008. "Men Who Have Sex with Men in India: A Systematic Review of the Literature." *Journal of LGBT Health Research* 4 (2–3): 51–70.

Setia, M., C. Lindan, H. Jerajani, S. Kumta, M. Ekstrand, M. Mathur, A. Gogate, A. Row Kavi, V. Anand, and J. D. Klausner. 2006. "Men Who Have Sex with Men and Transgenders in Mumbai, India: An Emerging Risk Group for STIs and HIV." *Indian Journal of Dermatology, Venereology and Leprology* 72 (6): 425–31.

Shinde, S., M. Setia, A. Row Kavi, V. Anand, and H. Jerajani. 2009. "Male Sex Workers: Are We Ignoring a Risk Group in Mumbai, India?" *Indian Journal of Dermatology, Venereology and Leprology* 75 (1): 41–46.

Silverman, J. G., M. R. Decker, J. Gupta, A. Maheshwari, V. Patel, and A. Raj. 2006. "HIV Prevalence and Predictors among Rescued Sex-Trafficked Women and Girls in Mumbai, India." *Journal of Acquired Immune Deficiency Syndromes* 43 (5): 588–93.

Silverman, J. G., M. R. Decker, J. Gupta, A. Maheshwari, B. M. Willis, and A. Raj. 2007. "HIV Prevalence and Predictors of Infection in Sex-Trafficked Nepalese Girls and Women." *JAMA* 298 (5): 536–42.

Solomon, S., J. Buck, S. K. Chaguturu, A. K. Ganesh, N. Kumarasamy. 2003. "Stopping HIV before It Begins: Issues Faced by Women in India." *Nature Immunology* 4: 719–21.

Steinbrook, R. 2007. "HIV in India—a Complex Epidemic." *New England Journal of Medicine* 356 (11): 1089–1093.

UNODC (United Nations Office on Drugs and Crime). 2009. *World Drug Report 2009*. Vienna: UNODC.

Verma, R., and M. Collumbien. 2004. "Homosexual Activity among Rural Indian Men: Implications for HIV Interventions." *AIDS* 18 (13): 1845–47.

References for Thailand

Adam, P. C. G., J. B. F. de Wit, I. Toskin, B. M. Mathers, M. Nashkhoev, I. Zablotska, R. Lyerla, and D. Rugg. 2009. "Estimating Levels of HIV Testing, HIV Prevention Coverage, HIV Knowledge, and Condom Use among Men Who Have Sex with Men (MSM) in Low-Income and Middle-Income Countries." *Journal of Acquired Immune Deficiency Syndromes* 52 (Suppl. 2): S143–51.

Ainsworth, M., C. Beyrer, and A. Soucat. 2003. "AIDS and Public Policy: The Lessons and Challenges of 'Success' in Thailand." *Health Policy* 64 (1): 13–37.

Beyrer, C. 2007. "STD Prevention in Vulnerable Populations: Human Rights Issues and Ways to Move Forward." Presentation at the 17th International Society for STD Research Conference, Seattle, WA, July 29–August 1.

Beyrer, C., T. Sripaipan, S. Tovanabutra, J. Jittiwutikarn, V. Suriyanon, T. Vongchak, N. Srirak, S. Kawichai, M. H. Razak, and D. D. Celentano. 2005. "High HIV, Hepatitis C and Sexual Risks among Drug-Using Men Who Have Sex with Men in Northern Thailand." *AIDS* 19 (14): 1535–40.

CDC (U.S. Centers for Disease Control and Prevention). 2006. "HIV Prevalence among Populations of Men Who Have Sex with Men—Thailand, 2003 and 2005." *Morbidity and Mortality Weekly Report* 55 (31): 844–48.

Celentano, D. D. 2005. "Why Has the Thai HIV Epidemic in Men Who Have Sex with Men Been So Silent?" *AIDS* 19 (16): 1931.

Grant, R., J. Lama, P. Anderson, V. McMahan, A. Y. Liu, L. Vargas, P. Goicochea, M. Casapía, J. V. Guanira-Carranza, M. E. Ramirez-Cardich, et al. 2010. "Preexposure Chemoprophylaxis for HIV Prevention in Men Who Have Sex with Men." *New England Journal of Medicine* 363 (27): 2587–99.

Guadamuz, T. E., W. Wimonsate, A. Varangrat, P. Phanuphak, R. Jommaroeng, P. A. Mock, J. W. Tappero, and F. van Griensven. 2009. "Correlates of Forced Sex among Populations of Men Who Have Sex with Men in Thailand." *Archives of Sexual Behavior*.

Jackson, P. A., and N. M. Cook, eds. 1999. *Genders and Sexualities in Modern Thailand*. Chiang Mai, Thailand: Silkworm Books.

Kunawararak, P., C. Beyrer, C. Natpratan, W. Feng, D. D. Celentano, M. de Boer, K. E. Nelson, and C. Khamboonruang. 1995. "The Epidemiology of HIV and Syphilis among Male Commercial Sex Workers in Northern Thailand." *AIDS* 9 (5): 517–21.

NAPaA Committee (National HIV and AIDS Prevention and Alleviation Committee). 2007. *National Plan for Strategic and Integrated HIV and AIDS*

Prevention and Alleviation (2007–2011). Nonthaburi, Thailand: The National Committee for HIV and AIDS Prevention and Alleviation Drafting Working Group on the National Plan for Strategic and Integrated HIV and AIDS Prevention and Alleviation 2007–2011.

Nelson, K. E., D. D. Celentano, S. Eiumtrakol, D. R. Hoover, C. Beyrer, S. Suprasert, S. Kuntolbutra, and C. Khamboonruang. 1996. "Changes in Sexual Behavior and a Decline in HIV Infection among Young Men in Thailand." *New England Journal of Medicine* 335 (5): 297–303.

USAID (U.S. Agency for International Development) Health Policy Initiative. 2006. "HIV Expenditure on MSM Programming in the Asia-Pacific Region." Background paper produced for the International Consultation on Male Sexual Health and HIV in Asia and the Pacific titled "Risks and Responsibilities," New Delhi, India, September 22–26. Washington, DC: USAID Health Policy Initiative, Task Order 1, Constella Futures.

van Griensven, F., S. Thanprasertsuk, R. Jommaroeng, G. Mansergh, S. Naorat, R. A. Jenkins, K. Ungchusak, P. Phanuphak, J. W. Tappero, and Bangkok MSM Study Group. 2005. "Evidence of a Previously Undocumented Epidemic of HIV Infection among Men Who Have Sex with Men in Bangkok, Thailand." *AIDS* 19 (5): 521–26.

van Griensven, F., A. Varangrat, W. Wimonsate, S. Tanpradech, K. Kladsawad, T. Chemnasiri, O. Suksripanich, P. Phanuphak, P. Mock, K. Kanggarnrua, et al. 2009. "Trends in HIV Prevalence, Estimated HIV Incidence, and Risk Behavior among Men Who Have Sex with Men in Bangkok, Thailand, 2003–2007." *Journal of Acquired Immune Deficiency Syndromes* 53 (2): 234–39.

Weniger, B. G., K. Limpakarnjanarat, K. Ungchusak, S. Thanprasertsuk, K. Choopanya, S. Vanichseni, T. Uneklabh, P. Thongcharoen, and C. Wasi. 1991. "The Epidemiology of HIV Infection and AIDS in Thailand." *AIDS* 5 (Suppl. 2): S71–85.

CHAPTER 7

Middle East and North Africa

Key themes:

- HIV epidemics in the Middle East and North Africa (MENA) have been limited in the general population; fewer than 400,000 people are estimated to be living with HIV in the region.
- Although surveillance and research have been limited, the primary drivers of HIV infection in the region appear to be sexual and parenteral (injecting drug use) transmission.
- Emerging evidence indicates a disproportionate burden of HIV in the region among key vulnerable populations including men who have sex with men (MSM).
- In some MENA countries, evidence also shows an increased investment in HIV prevention programs for MSM, yet coverage remains limited.

MENA is a geographically defined set of countries including both high-income, well-developed nations and low- and middle-income countries with lower ratings on the United Nations (UN) Human Development Index (Shawky, Soliman, and Sawires 2009). The data on HIV in this large and diverse region are limited. The studies that have been done and the surveillance data that have been made public suggest that HIV spread in these nations tends to be quite limited. In most, the HIV epidemic stage can be defined as low-level epidemics or very low HIV prevalence in the general population. Data on high-risk populations, including MSM, are even more limited (Abu-Raddad et al. 2010). In 2007, the region had an estimated 40,000 incident HIV infections, bringing the total number of people living with HIV in this region to about 380,000 (Shawky, Soliman, Kassak et al. 2009). Most HIV infections in the region occur in men and in urban contexts, with the exception of Sudan, which has been found to have higher rates among women and in rural areas, similar to other parts of southern and eastern Africa. The two primary drivers of HIV infection in the MENA region appear to be parenteral transmission through the shared use of injection equipment among drug users and sexual transmission (Soliman et al. 2010). Limited data are available for most at-risk populations, and the prevalence data that do exist tend to be derived from surveillance data rather than specific research studies addressing these populations. Passive surveillance mechanisms for HIV reporting tend to underestimate the role of specific high-risk practices, such as same-sex practices, in driving HIV acquisition and transmission because of fear of disclosure of these practices to interviewers. Populations of MSM at high risk for HIV transmission because of high-risk sexual practices, low levels of condom use, and low levels of HIV knowledge have been observed in several MENA countries.

Data are available from six low- and middle-income MENA countries: the Arab Republic of Egypt, Lebanon, Morocco, Pakistan, Sudan, and Tunisia. These data include prevalence data characterizing the burden of disease of HIV among MSM in the MENA region and explore risk factors for HIV infection among these men. Some formative studies have evaluated populations of MSM in other countries, including Afghanistan, but these data remain preliminary and are not reviewed here. A thorough review of HIV/AIDS in the MENA region has recently been published that includes descriptions of epidemic patterns in all MENA countries as defined by the World Bank (Abu-Raddad et al. 2010). Although an increasing amount of data describe HIV risks among MSM in the MENA low- and middle-income countries, little exploration of the social and structural drivers of HIV risk included in the biobehavioral studies has been completed to date. Given documented human rights violations of MSM in many of these settings, exploring the relationship between rights violations and HIV risk among MSM is an important future direction for research.

Egypt

Egypt is a lower-middle-income country and is classified in the medium range according to the UN Human Development Index. The HIV epidemic has been limited in Egypt. Approximately 9,200 people are estimated to be living with HIV of a population of more than 80 million, and fewer than 500 people are estimated to need antiretroviral therapy, 313 of whom currently receive treatment. However, growing risk status of HIV among MSM in Egypt has increasingly been recognized (El-Rahman 2004; El-Sayyed, Kabbash, and El-Gueniedy 2008; Kabbash et al. 2007; Symington 2008). Relatively small studies had been completed until a large HIV/AIDS Bio-Behavioral Surveillance Survey was completed in 2006 by the Ministry of Health and Family Health International (FHI 2007) that included most at-risk populations, focusing on MSM, sex workers, and injecting drug users (Egypt National AIDS Program 2010; Soliman et al. 2008). The study included 267 MSM with an overall HIV prevalence of 6.2 percent. Bisexual activity was common; 56.2 percent reported ever having had sex with a woman, and 5.2 percent reported bisexual concurrency in being married to a woman (Soliman et al. 2008). Commercial or transactional sex was also common in this population with nearly half the sample (42 percent, n = 120) reporting this practice. Importantly, condom use rates were low during sex with men: 9.2 percent of MSM reported using a condom with their last male partner during transactional sex, and 12.7 percent reported condom use during nontransactional sex. In a baseline assessment of HIV programming, 79 percent of MSM knew that condoms were the most effective way of preventing transmission of HIV and sexually transmitted infections (STIs), but only 28 percent reported using condoms with their last male partners. Surveillance has also demonstrated that drug use is fairly common among MSM, with 10.9 percent reporting injecting drugs in the last month. Capture-recapture size estimations completed in high-prevalence settings in Egypt demonstrated that 16.9 percent of all men seeking voluntary counseling and testing services were MSM (Egypt National AIDS Program 2010). Enumeration methods were used in 79 areas of Cairo in 2009 and demonstrated that 30.9 percent of male clients in voluntary counseling and testing centers were MSM (n = 914/2,960) (Egypt National AIDS Program 2010). The 2010 United Nations General Assembly Special Session (UNGASS) report for Egypt noted that the country may be experiencing a concentrated epidemic among MSM (Egypt National AIDS Program 2010). Notably, as found in the Bio-Behavioral Surveillance Survey, high-risk sexual practices between men are common, and levels of sexual health-related knowledge are suboptimal.

The Egyptian government has developed and implemented early responses aiming to decrease risk among MSM including distribution of 8,805 condoms and lubricant sachets to 779 MSM since the middle of 2009 (Egypt National AIDS Program 2010). Although providing some prevention programming is a major development, these data highlight that the interventions have yet to be brought to scale. The Egyptian government has endorsed addressing the continuum of risk factors for HIV infection among MSM, ranging from individual level to structural or societal determinants of HIV risk. The programs include developing community-based outreach services and providing referrals to medical, legal, and mental health service providers.

Lebanon

Lebanon is an upper-middle-income country with a population of just over 4 million. As in Egypt, the HIV epidemic has been estimated to be quite limited with a total of approximately 3,000 people living with HIV, representing a modest increase from 2,200 in 2001 (UNAIDS and WHO 2008). In Lebanon, an integrated bio-behavioral survey termed "Mishwar" was attempted in 2007–08 using respondent-driven sampling to assess risk among most at-risk populations including MSM (DeJong et al. 2009; Helem 2009). Formative research indicated significant social networks of MSM in the Greater Beirut area as well as two community-based organizations focused on addressing the needs of MSM. However, given significant levels of fear and distrust in the community, accrual of MSM into this study was not successful, and only 37 MSM were recruited of a planned 620. Specifically, fear was associated with visiting the offices of the community-based organizations because MSM would be associated with the activities of this organization. The limited data available highlighted a high-risk population. Less than 50 percent of MSM reported using a condom with their last male partner, and 30 percent of MSM had been tested for HIV in the last 12 months and were aware of their status. Earlier assessments not including HIV testing have been more successful in accruing MSM, including a rapid assessment by the International HIV/AIDS Alliance in partnership with the local organization Helem. These assessments have confirmed a prevalence of risk practices with limited levels of knowledge among MSM in Lebanon. Some services have been initiated for MSM, including the funding of an STI clinic managed by a community-based organization and mobile-van outreach services that have served 464 MSM (National AIDS Control Program–Lebanon 2010). In addition, some formative mapping programs have assessed MSM-friendly clinical health services.

Morocco

Morocco is a lower-middle-income country, with a gross domestic product of US$1,667 per inhabitant in 2004 dollars. Similar to other countries in MENA, Morocco has a limited HIV epidemic with approximately 20,000 people living with HIV in the country and 1,000 deaths attributable to AIDS yearly (UNAIDS and WHO 2009a). Surveillance estimates have indicated an HIV prevalence of approximately 4.4 percent among MSM, compared to a background general population prevalence of 0.1 percent (Yatine 2009). Prevention programs for MSM have been increasing in scale with the UNGASS 2010 report indicating that 23,374 MSM were reached with preventive services in 2009, representing an increase from 11,967 in 2005 (Royaume du Maroc 2010). Moreover, 9 percent of all people tested for HIV in Morocco from 2008 to 2009 were MSM. Notably, all funding supporting MSM services is derived internationally; US$687,301 of US$24,707,204 total funding spent was on targeted preventive services, or 2.7 percent of the total HIV-related budget (Royaume du Maroc 2010). No peer-reviewed published literature was found describing the epidemiology of HIV among MSM or any description of programs being provided for MSM, but reports from the field have indicated that both the government and several community-based organizations are providing services (CCMM 2006; Royaume du Maroc 2010).

Pakistan

Pakistan is a low-income and populous country with more than 150 million people. Given Pakistan's history, including the country in the MENA region is debatable. Similar to many MENA countries, Pakistan has a limited HIV epidemic in the general population with approximately 0.1 percent of reproductive-age adults infected. The Joint United Nations Programme on HIV/AIDS estimates that between 70,000 and 150,000 people are infected with HIV, although Pakistan's National AIDS Control Program has identified only 3,000 cases of HIV (National AIDS Control Program–Pakistan 2010; UNAIDS and WHO 2009b).

Given identified concentrated epidemics among injecting drug users, sex workers, and MSM, Pakistan has a concentrated epidemic (Mayhew et al. 2009; Rajabali et al. 2008). Pakistan has an estimated 500,000 people who use drugs, mostly opium and heroin smokers, of whom 60,000 are estimated to inject (Strathdee et al. 2003). In urban centers such as Karachi, high rates of HIV infection have been identified. In Pakistan, researchers have used peer ethnography to characterize sexual identities among male and transgendered sex workers (Collumbien et al. 2009). These analyses have also been used to design quantitative studies evaluating HIV risk status and to inform HIV prevention strategies for these MSM (Hawkes et al. 2009). Specifically, Pakistan has multiple populations of MSM, including third-gender populations such as *hijras* and zenanas. *Hijra* is a self-identified term that translates roughly as not man and not woman, but a third gender. *Hijras* tend to cross-dress publicly and privately and are a part of a social, religious, and cultural community. Ritual castration is common among them, but not all *hijras* are castrated. Sex with men is common. Zenanas tend to be males who feminize their behaviors to attract more male-identified sexual partners and tend to be the receptive partner during intercourse. Although marriage among *hijras* is uncommon, zenanas may also be married to women. In a bio-behavioral survey completed in Karachi and Lahore, HIV prevalence of these groups varied significantly by city (NACP MoH, FHI, and DfID 2005). In Karachi, the HIV prevalence was 1.5 percent (3/197) among *hijras* and 4 percent (n = 17/401) among self-identified male sex workers (MSWs). Rates were lower in Lahore, however, with 0.5 percent (n = 1/191) prevalence among *hijras* and 0 percent (n = 0/387) among MSWs. Self-reported STI symptoms were common, with 38 percent of MSWs reporting these clinical symptoms in the previous year and 30 percent of *hijras* reporting the same across both cities. Of importance, less than 40 percent of *hijras* or MSWs sought care for these symptoms (NACP MoH, FHI, and DfID 2005). This point is especially relevant given that more than 90 percent of these MSWs and *hijras* report unprotected anal intercourse, and only a small proportion reported regular use of condoms with male partners. In addition, less than 1 percent of either *hijras* or MSWs reported the use of water-based lubricants during anal intercourse although approximately 70 percent to 80 percent reported the use of other lubricants. Syphilis rates were very high in these two populations, with 35.6 percent (n = 144/399) of MSWs infected and 60.2 percent (n = 118/196) of *hijras* infected in Karachi and 5.7 percent (n = 22/387) and 11.5 percent (n = 22/192), respectively, infected in Lahore.

Information is limited on HIV prevention programming that has been launched in response to these data. Moreover, data on structural or social drivers of HIV risk among MSM in Pakistan are scarce (Khan 2009).

Sudan

Sudan is a low-income country with a low ranking on the UN Human Development Index. The first AIDS case in Sudan was reported in 1986, and up to 2004, 17,000 cases of HIV have been reported (Lino 2010; SNAP 2010). A few formative studies have been completed in Sudan with a focus on accrual in Khartoum, which is Sudan's most populous city and its commercial center. One study was completed among men who practice exclusively receptive anal intercourse and excluded bisexual MSM and those reporting insertive anal intercourse. This study accrued 384 MSM who were registered as MSM with the Society Security Police department registry of MSM (Elrashied 2006a). The voluntarism of this study cannot be ascertained from published reports. Snowball sampling was used to accrue further MSM for a total of 713 MSM (Elrashied 2006b). Nearly all study participants were Muslims born in Sudan, and more than 90 percent were literate with relatively high levels of education. Levels of HIV-related knowledge were inadequate in this population, with 55.3 percent (n = 380/687) reporting that anal sex was protective for HIV; only 20.2 percent (n = 139/687) of the men had ever been tested for HIV. Some 14 percent (n = 83/603) of the men had ever used a condom, but only 7.7 percent of those who used condoms did so to protect against HIV acquisition or transmission. Bisexuality was common, with 71.2 percent ever having sex with a female, of whom 71.1 percent had 1 to 5 female partners in the previous six months and 16.7 percent had 6 to 10 female partners in this time frame. Moreover, 22.9 percent (n = 163/712) reported being married. Furthermore, 71.2 percent of the men reported transactional sex in the previous six months, and only 58.5 percent of them reported using a condom with their last partner. Alcohol use was prevalent among MSM; nearly 80 percent reported drinking in the previous month. Besides alcohol, approximately one-quarter of the sample had used some form of illicit drugs, and the majority of these men (96.6 percent) had used drugs within the preceding month. Of MSM who used drugs, 5.2 percent (n = 9/172) reported injecting heroin, whereas the majority (162/172) reported smoking Cannabis. In total, 9.3 percent of the men were HIV positive. These data were consistent with a study of insertive MSM from

Khartoum state where HIV prevalence was found to be 7.8 percent among a sample of predominantly Muslim men with high levels of transactional sex and bisexual practices (Elrashied 2008).

Tunisia

The HIV epidemic in Tunisia has been limited, with approximately 1,499 HIV cases registered from 1985 to 2008 and 490 deaths secondary to AIDS (UNAIDS and WHO 2009c). As of 2008, 1,009 individuals were living with HIV, equating to a prevalence of 0.09 percent. With a low general population prevalence of less than 0.1 percent, an estimated 4.9 percent of MSM in Tunisia are infected with HIV, and approximately 1.1 percent is also positive for hepatitis C virus (DDSB 2010). Active surveillance was completed among 1,778 MSM in Tunisia in 2008, and high-risk HIV practices were found to be common (Hsairi 2007). Specifically, more than 90 percent reported having multiple male partners in the previous six months, and nearly 75 percent of the sample reported unprotected anal intercourse during this time frame. Bisexual practices were also prevalent, with 69 percent of the sample reporting having sex with women. Furthermore, 92.2 percent of the sample reported having at least one unprotected same-sex partner and one unprotected female sexual partner in the previous six months. Although access to condoms was observed as being moderately high, condom use was inadequate with less than 20 percent reporting always using condoms with male partners and about 50 percent having used condoms during transactional sex. Only 15.6 percent reported using lubricants during sex with men, but whether these were water-based or petroleum-based lubricants was not reported. Drug use was prevalent, with 14.7 percent of MSM reported injecting illicit drugs in the last year; 35.6 percent reported using Cannabis during this time frame (Hsairi 2007; UNAIDS and WHO 2009c). In addition, 35.9 percent reported having had symptoms consistent with an STI, although 49.4 percent of participants reported not having consulted a doctor for their symptoms. Only 34 percent of the men studied had reported having ever had an HIV test.

References

Abu-Raddad, L. J., F. A. Akala, I. Semini, G. Riedner, D. Wilson, and O. Tawil. 2010. *Characterizing the HIV/AIDS Epidemic in the Middle East and North Africa: Time for Strategic Action*. Washington, DC: World Bank.

CCMM (Country Coordinating Mechanism Morocco). 2006. *Sixth Call for Proposals of the Global Fund to Fight Aids, Tuberculosis and Malaria: Proposal of the CCM for Morocco: HIV/AIDS and Tuberculosis Components*. Rabat: Kingdom of Morocco.

Collumbien, M., A. A. Qureshi, S. H. Mayhew, N. Rizvi, A. Rabbani, B. Rolfe, R. K. Verma, H. Rehman, Naveed-i-Rahat. 2009. "Understanding the Context of Male and Transgender Sex Work Using Peer Ethnography." *Sexually Transmitted Infections* 85 (Suppl. 2): ii3–7.

DDSB (République Tunisienne, Ministère de la Santé Publique, Direction des Soins de Santé de Base). 2010. *Rapport de Situation National à l'Intention de l'UNGASS 2010: Janvier 2008–décembre 2009*. Tunis: DDSB and ONUSIDA.

DeJong, J., Z. Mahfoud, D. Khoury, F. Barbir, and R. A. Afifi. 2009. "Ethical Considerations in HIV/AIDS Biobehavioral Surveys That Use Respondent-Driven Sampling: Illustrations from Lebanon." *American Journal of Public Health* 99 (9): 1562–67.

Egypt National AIDS Program. 2010. *UNGASS Country Progress Report: Arab Republic of Egypt, January 2008–December 2009*. Cairo: Egypt National AIDS Program.

El-Rahman, A. 2004. "Risky Behaviors for HIV/AIDS Infection among a Sample of Homosexuals in Cairo City, Egypt." Presentation at the XV International Conference on AIDS, Bangkok, Thailand, July 11–16.

Elrashied, S. M. 2006a. "Generating Strategic Information and Assessing HIV/AIDS Knowledge, Attitude and Behaviour and Practices as Well as Prevalence of HIV1 among MSM in Khartoum State, 2005." A draft report submitted to the Sudan National AIDS Control Programme, Together Against AIDS Organization (TAG), Khartoum, Sudan.

———. 2006b. "Prevalence, Knowledge and Related Risky Sexual Behaviours of HIV/AIDS among Receptive Men Who Have Sex with Men (MSM) in Khartoum State, Sudan, 2005." Presentation at "AIDS 2006": XVI International AIDS Conference, Toronto, Canada, August 13–18.

———. 2008. "HIV Sero-Prevalence and Related Risky Sexual Behaviours among Insertive Men Having Sex with Men (IMSM) in Khartoum State, Sudan, 2007." Presentation at "AIDS 2008": XVII International AIDS Conference, Mexico City, Mexico, August 3–8.

El-Sayyed, N., I. A. Kabbash, and M. El-Gueniedy. 2008. "Risk Behaviours for HIV/AIDS Infection among Men Who Have Sex with Men in Cairo, Egypt." *Eastern Mediterranean Health Journal* 14 (4): 905–15.

FHI (Family Health International). 2007. *Egypt Final Report April 1999–September 2007 for USAID's Implementing AIDS Prevention and Care (IMPACT) Project*. Arlington, VA: FHI.

Hawkes, S., M. Collumbien, L. Platt, N. Lalji, N. Rizvi, A. Andreasen, J. Chow, R. Muzaffar, H. ur-Rehman, N. Siddiqui, et al. 2009. "HIV and Other Sexually Transmitted Infections among Men, Transgenders and Women Selling Sex in Two Cities in Pakistan: A Cross-Sectional Prevalence Survey." *Sexually Transmitted Infections* 85 (Suppl. 2): ii8–16.

Helem. 2009. *"Mishwar": An Integrated Bio-Behavioural Surveillance Study among Four Vulnerable Groups in Lebanon: Men Who Have Sex with Men, Commercial Sex Workers, and Injection Drug Users*. Beirut: Helem.

Hsairi, M. A. 2007. "Synthèse de l'enquête sérocomportementale auprès des hommes ayant des rapports sexuels avec des hommes en Tunisie." PowerPoint presentation, Tunis, Tunisia.

Kabbash, I. A., N. M. El-Sayed, A. N. Al-Nawawy, I. K. Shady, and M. S. Abou Zeid. 2007. "Condom Use among Males (15–49 Years) in Lower Egypt: Knowledge, Attitudes and Patterns of Use." *Eastern Mediterranean Health Journal* 13 (6): 1405–16.

Khan, F. H. 2009. "HIV and Homosexuality in Pakistan." *Lancet Infectious Diseases* 9 (4): 204–205.

Lino, E. 2010. *HIV/AIDS Situation in Southern Sudan*. Khartoum: Ministry of Health, Sudan.

Mayhew, S., M. Collumbien, A. Qureshi, L. Platt, N. Rafiq, A. Faisel, N. Lalji, and S. Hawkes. 2009. "Protecting the Unprotected: Mixed-Method Research on Drug Use, Sex Work and Rights in Pakistan's Fight against HIV/AIDS." *Sexually Transmitted Infections* 85 (Suppl. 2): ii31–ii6.

NACP MoH (National AIDS Control Program, Ministry of Health, Government of Pakistan), FHI (Family Health International), and DfID (Department for International Development). 2005. *National Study of Reproductive Tract and Sexually Transmitted Infections: Survey of High-Risk Groups in Lahore and Karachi, 2005*. Karachi, Pakistan: Ministry of Health, DfID, and FHI.

National AIDS Control Program, Lebanese Republic Ministry of Public Health. 2010. *UNGASS Country Progress Report: Lebanon, March 2010*. Beirut: Lebanese Republic Ministry of Public Health.

National AIDS Control Program, Ministry of Health, Government of Pakistan. 2010. *UNGASS Pakistan Report: Progress Report on the Declaration of Commitment on HIV/AIDS for the United Nations General Assembly Special Session on HIV/AIDS*. Islamabad: Ministry of Health.

Rajabali, A., S. Khan, H. J. Warraich, M. R. Khanani, and S. H. Ali. 2008. "HIV and Homosexuality in Pakistan." *Lancet Infectious Diseases* 8 (8): 511–15.

Royaume du Maroc. 2010. *Mise en oeuvre de la declaration d'engagement sur le VIH/SIDA: Rapport national 2010; Période considérée: Janvier 2008–décembre 2009*. Rabat: Royaume du Maroc.

Shawky, S., C. Soliman, K. M. Kassak, D. Oraby, D. El-Khoury, and I. Kabore. 2009. "HIV Surveillance and Epidemic Profile in the Middle East and North Africa." *Journal of Acquired Immune Deficiency Syndromes* 51 (Suppl. 3): S83–95.

Shawky, S., C. Soliman, and S. Sawires. 2009. "Gender and HIV in the Middle East and North Africa: Lessons for Low Prevalence Scenarios." *Journal of Acquired Immune Deficiency Syndromes* 51 (Suppl. 3): S73–74.

Soliman, C., Z. El Taher, A. Abed El Sattar, S. Shawky, B. Feyisetan, D. Oraby, S. Elkamhawi, D. Khaled, E. Salah, and N. El Sayed. 2008. "Key Findings of Bio-BSS among High Risk Groups in the Middle East, Egypt Case Study." Presentation at the XVII International AIDS Conference, Mexico City, August 3–8.

Soliman, C., I. A. Rahman, S. Shawky, T. Bahaa, S. Elkamhawi, A. A. El Sattar, D. Oraby, D. Khaled, B. Feyisetan, E. Salah, et al. 2010. "HIV Prevalence and Risk Behaviors of Male Injection Drug Users in Cairo, Egypt." *AIDS* 24 (Suppl. 2): S33–38.

Strathdee, S. A., T. Zafar, H. Brahmbhatt, A. Baksh, and S. ul Hassan. 2003. "Rise in Needle Sharing among Injection Drug Users in Pakistan during the Afghanistan War." *Drug and Alcohol Dependence* 71 (1): 17–24.

SNAP (Sudan National AIDS Control Programme). 2010. *United Nations General Assembly Special Session on HIV/AIDS (UNGASS) Report 2008–2009: North Sudan*. Khartoum: Federal Ministry of Health.

Symington, A. 2008. "Egypt: Court Convicts Men for 'Debauchery.'" *HIV AIDS Policy and Law Review* 13 (1): 63–64.

UNAIDS (United Nations Joint Programme for HIV/AIDS) and World Health Organization (WHO). 2008. "UNAIDS/WHO Epidemiological Fact Sheet on HIV and AIDS, Lebanon 2008 Update: Core Data on Epidemiology and Response." Geneva: UNAIDS and WHO.

———. 2009a. "Morocco: Epidemiologic Country Profile on HIV/AIDS." WHO Global Atlas, Epidemiological Fact Sheet Country Profiles, 2008 Update.

———. 2009b. "Pakistan: Epidemiologic Country Profile on HIV/AIDS." WHO Global Atlas, Epidemiological Fact Sheet Country Profiles, 2008 Update.

———. 2009c. "Tunisia: Epidemiologic Country Profile on HIV/AIDS." WHO Global Atlas, Epidemiological Fact Sheet Country Profiles, 2008 Update.

Yatine, Y. 2009. "Prévenir l'infection à VIH auprès des HSH dans le contexte Arabo-musulman: Expérience de l'ALCS Maroc." PowerPoint presentation by Coordinateur National des actions prévention HSH ALCS MAROC in Copenhagen.

PART II

Combination HIV Prevention Interventions

CHAPTER 8

Combination HIV Prevention Interventions for MSM

An Umbrella Review of the Evidence and Recommendations

Key themes:

- A broad strategy for evaluating data must be implemented in effective HIV prevention strategies for marginalized populations, including men who have sex with men (MSM).
- Several effective behavioral HIV prevention strategies are targeting increasing condom use during anal sex for MSM, but studies consistently demonstrate that the benefits are subject to decay with episodic interventions.
- Emerging biomedical HIV prevention strategies for MSM include oral and rectal antiviral chemoprophylaxis that aim to decrease HIV acquisition and transmission risks.
- Although research evidence supporting structural interventions is limited, significant programmatic experience and causal inference highlight the need for these interventions to target structural change at the levels of communities, populations, and governments by attempting to modify social, political, and environmental factors.

Although increasing data highlight risk among MSM in low- and middle-income settings, the data set describing best practices for prevention, treatment, and care for this at-risk population remains limited. In response, several processes were under way in 2009–10 along with the creation of some key documents. These include a recommended package of comprehensive HIV preventive services for MSM in Asia, published by the United Nations Development Programme (UNDP)'s Asia Pacific Coalition on Male Sexual Health, and an ongoing process of global guideline development for prevention and management of HIV and sexually transmitted infection (STI) in clinical settings for MSM being conducted by the World Health Organization (WHO) (UNDP et al. 2009). This book has endeavored to harmonize the approaches used here with both the UNDP and WHO efforts through regular communication with both groups to ensure congruence across their approaches. These approaches are not duplicative, however, because this chapter includes consideration of community-level interventions and includes antiretroviral (ARV) treatment and access to that treatment in its consideration of preventive packages. This approach is supported by the emerging literature on the transmission effect of undiagnosed and untreated HIV infections in networks of risk and by encouraging data from Donnell and others (2010) on the potent role of ARV therapy (ART) in transmission in discordant couples. An unknown but presumably substantial number of MSM in all settings are in discordant-couple relationships, so the authors and their community and scientific partners agreed that these effects should be investigated among MSM.

The process used in this chapter relied on a series of systematic reviews of the literature in combination with a global consultation for implementation science data and community best practices. Preliminary results have indicated that the different methods of reviewing evidence used by the WHO, UNDP's Asia Pacific Coalition on Male Sexual Health, and this book have consistent themes. One of those themes is that responding to multiple levels of HIV risk among MSM requires combination HIV prevention interventions (CHPIs) that are applied on multiple levels and through multiple modes to maximize potential effectiveness (Piot et al. 2008). The analogy to HIV treatment is poignant—application of a single antiviral agent is not beneficial and, indeed, it may be harmful because of the development of resistant strains (Coates, Richter, and Cáceres 2008). The implementation of a single mode of HIV prevention will similarly not provide effective control of the HIV epidemic at a population level and has the potential to increase risk at the individual level secondary to treatment optimism (Merson, Padian et al. 2008). Biomedical interventions are analogous to harm reduction interventions in that they aim to decrease transmission and acquisition risk of HIV rather than to decrease the prevalence of the behavior itself. To date, condoms and lubricants are the best-evidenced biomedical HIV prevention tools; other biomedical strategies have so far failed to demonstrate efficacy, especially among MSM, or have not been evaluated in these men (Kaldor, Guy, and Wilson 2008; Vermund, Allen, and Karim 2009). An exception is ART, which has recently been demonstrated to have potent HIV prevention impacts (greater than 92 percent efficacy) among discordant couples (Donnell et al. 2010). No biological basis exists for assuming the preventive effects of ART will be less for male same-sex discordant couples than heterosexual ones because the effects of ART on viral load have been repeatedly shown to be independent of route of acquisition. Nevertheless, the behavioral aspects of this biomedical preventive intervention among MSM require urgent study. Given reports of treatment optimism associated with certain biomedical strategies, coupling these strategies with behavioral interventions that aim to decrease the high-risk practices themselves with increased condom use is key (Reisner, Mimiaga, Case et al. 2009). Structural-level risk interventions among MSM have rarely been appropriately evaluated, in part because of the complexity of the study designs required to characterize efficacy and effectiveness of these interventions and in part because of logistical and cost considerations. Structural interventions also target social change in the general population, creating as a secondary outcome improved access of MSM to appropriate health services. Notably, CHPIs do not represent comprehensive health care programming for MSM; rather, this package focuses on those interventions known or theorized to decrease risk of HIV acquisition or transmission. HIV prevention is complex, and if successful strategies are to be designed and implemented, the research and implementation agenda needs to address this complexity and receive appropriate resources (Piot et al. 2008).

Methods

The Highest Attainable STandard of Evidence (HASTE) system was developed and used to evaluate evidence based on three distinct categories given equal weight: efficacy data, implementation science data, and plausibility.

Assessing the Quality of Evidence

Within the realm of clinical medicine, evidence-based medicine is now considered the basis on which to define standards of clinical care. Defining packages of clinical services has been predicated on systematic reviews of individually randomized double-blinded placebo-controlled trials of medications or services for patients with varying clinical conditions. The Grading of Recommendations Assessment, Development and Evaluation (GRADE) system has been widely endorsed as the most effective method with which to grade the current state of evidence for a variety of clinical interventions (Coates, Richter, and Cáceres 2008; Merson et al. 2008). GRADE was designed for individual-level clinical interventions where the traditional hierarchy of evidence is applied. Specifically, the highest-quality evidence is derived from randomized double-blinded placebo-controlled trials, followed by unblinded randomized controlled trials, prospective cohort studies, case-control studies, clinical case series, and finally consensus among experts. Additional weight is given to appropriately executed systematic reviews and meta-analyses of studies with little heterogeneity among participants, methods, and results. To further standardize the presentation of evidence in clinical interventions and meta-analyses, criteria including CONSORT and QUOROM were developed that have facilitated the grading of evidence (Kaldor, Guy, and Wilson 2008; Vermund, Allen, and Karim 2009). Given the nature of individual-level clinical interventions, GRADE has facilitated the development of clinical practice guidelines and other clinical practice tools to promote the practice of evidence-based medicine (Donnell et al. 2010). The GRADE system is also relevant because it integrates the potential for a separation between quality of evidence and strength of recommendations based on extenuating circumstances such as cost-efficacy, risk-benefit, and contextual factors (Reisner, Mimiaga, Case et al. 2009).

Although the use of GRADE is generally accepted in clinical medicine, no widely accepted standard exists for grading public health interventions, although a series of different algorithms and hierarchies of evidence have been proposed (Begg et al. 1996; Clarke 2000; Guyatt et al. 2008; UNAIDS 2009). The International Agency for Research on Cancer, the United States Preventive Task Force, the newly revived Canadian Task Force on Preventive Health Care, and the National Institute for Health and Clinical Excellence in the United Kingdom, among others, use varying algorithms for evaluating public health interventions. (McQueen 2002; Petticrew and Roberts 2003; Rychetnik et al. 2000; Stroup et al. 2000). Although Sir Bradford Hill's (1965) criteria for causality—including strength of the relationship, dose-response, temporality, experimental evidence, analogy, and biologic plausibility—still apply to public health interventions, demonstrating efficacy using traditional evaluation strategies is more difficult (Ansari, Tsertsvadze, and Moher 2009). One reason is that public health interventions tend to be context-specific and are generally multifaceted. Moreover, primary prevention strategies targeting populations at risk may be subject to the prevention paradox first described by the seminal epidemiologist Dr. Geoffrey Rose (Rose 1985; Briss et al. 2000). The prevention paradox describes a situation where an effective population-level public health intervention may provide only little benefit at the individual level while being significant at the population level.

Responding to this possibility, the current work developed a novel system of evaluating evidence for HIV interventions that targets decreasing HIV risk specifically among most-at-risk populations. This chapter proposes the use of the term the *Highest Attainable STandard of Evidence*. HASTE was initially used to define a package of services for preventing HIV infection among MSM in low- and middle-income countries (LMICs). A derivative of the GRADE approach targeting public health interventions has been proposed by investigators from the World Health Organization (Begg et al. 1996). Although GRADE was initially designed as a clinical decision making support tool, it can serve as the basis for which to evaluate the quality of public health interventions. The system proposed by Tang, Choi, and Beaglehole (2008) focuses on three main causality criteria: strong association, consistency of results, and biologic plausibility. However, Tang and colleagues' system was developed for evaluating health promotion interventions in the context of chronic disease prevention strategies. When stigma affecting most-at-risk populations is compounded with the difficulties and limitations of randomized controlled trials evaluating public health interventions with biological endpoints, the evidence base for any HIV intervention supporting these vulnerable populations is limited. Thus, although this chapter initially intended to use the GRADE methodology to evaluate individual interventions, it became clear that the system required modification to include the assessments of what were termed the highest attainable standards of evidence. This "highest attainable standard of evidence" deliberately echoes the language of human rights conventions on the right to health, which accept that what can realistically be *attained* in resource-constrained environments can still serve as life-saving aspirational goals.

The HASTE system proposed here is specific to HIV interventions among most-at-risk populations and focuses on three main characteristics with equal importance—efficacy data, implementation science data, and biological and public health plausibility—although it may be adaptable to other public health areas and disciplines. The inclusion of a review of efficacy data is a common denominator across all systems evaluating levels of evidence. However, the response to preventing HIV infection has differed from most other clinical conditions in that the implementation of these preventive measures is generally managed by civil society and not-for-profit nongovernmental institutions rather than health care facilities. Notably, with increasing evidence of effective biomedical interventions to prevent HIV infection, including circumcision and topical and oral chemoprophylaxis, this balance may eventually change. Although peer-reviewed data from these implementers is often unobtainable, these interventions constitute a predominant majority of HIV prevention services in LMICs. Thus, this chapter considered capturing of these implementation science data crucial in informing the optimal package of services for MSM.

Hill's criteria for causality remain the most relevant set of determinants of whether a risk factor causes disease or an intervention causes prevention or mitigation of a disease. One of these criteria is plausibility, and this chapter considered this criterion vital, as others have previously done (Begg et al. 1996). However, in considering public health plausibility of an intervention, this chapter assessed whether a preventive intervention with limited demonstrated efficacy in preventing HIV as a biological endpoint was within the causal pathway of another intervention that does have demonstrable effectiveness in preventing HIV infection.

HASTE includes four grades of evidence, depending on the amount of peer-reviewed and implementation data available, as well as the plausibility of these interventions (table 8.1):

- Strong (Grade 1)
- Conditional (Grade 2)
- Insufficient (Grade 3)
- Inappropriate (Grade 4)

Grade 1, or strong, recommendations are given when available data indicate the desirable effect of an intervention clearly outweighs the potential risks or data indicate the intervention addresses a known causal risk factor of HIV risk among most-at-risk populations. Grade 2, or conditional, recommendations are given when an intervention has potential efficacy, but further research is required. Conditional recommendations may be given when only one or a few studies have evaluated a particular

Table 8.1 Four HASTE Levels of Evidence for Public Health Interventions

HASTE level	*Strength of recommendation*	*Explanation*
Grade 1	Strong	• Efficacy is consistent. • Intervention is biologically plausible. • Implementation data are available.
Grade 2a	Probable	• Efficacy data are limited. • Intervention is biologically plausible.
Grade 2b	Possible	• Efficacy is inconsistent. • Intervention is biologically plausible. • Consensus exists from implementation science data.
Grade 2c	Pending	• Definitive trials are ongoing. • Intervention is biologically plausible.
Grade 3	Insufficient	• Data are inconsistent. • Plausibility is undefined.
Grade 4	Inappropriate	• Consistent data demonstrate lack of efficacy. • Consensus exists from implementation data of inappropriate intervention.

Source: Stefan Baral, Chris Beyrer, and Andrea Wirtz.

intervention, but a strong association was shown. Alternatively, efficacy data may be limited but with strong plausibility in the context of strong consensus and experience from implementation or programmatic research that this particular intervention constitutes an important component of comprehensive HIV interventions for most-at-risk populations. In either of these scenarios, the intervention would be defined as Grade 2a, or probable. If data on efficacy are inconsistent, but the intervention is biologically plausible and a consensus exists from reviews of implementation science, then it would be called Grade 2b, or possible. A grade of possible can be given if the intervention in question has limited data but has public health plausibility in being a component of a causal pathway of another intervention of demonstrated value. Grade 2c, or pending, recommendations are given when definitive trials among most-at-risk populations are ongoing. Grade 3, or insufficient, is applied when evidence for the efficacy of a particular intervention is inconsistent, the causal pathway is unclear or not well defined, and consensus from community experience about a particular intervention is limited. Grade 4, or inappropriate, is given when no evidence of efficacy or effectiveness of an intervention exists, where risks outweigh potential benefits, or where consensus exists from implementation data that the intervention is inappropriate.

Validation and External Review

The previously mentioned global consultation meeting served as an interim validation and review of the recommendations suggested in the package of services. A separate process for ensuring the appropriateness of the review included peer review by HIV/AIDS prevention experts not connected with the study. The external reviewers included both (a) academic experts in HIV/AIDS epidemiology and targeted interventions for MSM and (b) experts in implementation of interventions for MSM in both high- and low-income settings.

Findings

The package of HIV interventions for MSM in LMICs must be multimodal to address the multiple levels of HIV risk.

Targeting Individual-Level Risk

Evidence is emerging for biomedical strategies such as oral and topical antiviral chemoprophylaxis, but lessons from behavioral interventions are vital to ensure adherence to these preventive strategies.

Barrier protection and water- and silicone-based lubricants. A significant body of literature highlights the efficacy of barrier devices in protecting from HIV infection in both penile-vaginal as well as penile-anal sex (Coates, Richter, and Cáceres 2008; Weller and Davis-Beaty 2002). The Multicenter AIDS Cohort Study (MACS) and the Collaborative HIV Seroincidence Study have provided convincing data that condom use lies at the core of CHPI (Buchbinder et al. 2005; Vittinghoff et al. 1999). Following 2,189 MSM in multiple sites across the United States for a total of 2,633 person-years and 60 recorded seroconversions, the research team was able to generate per contact risks of sexual contact among MSM. The highest risk was from unprotected receptive anal intercourse at 0.82 percent (95 percent confidence interval [CI] 0.24–2.76) per coital act when the partner was known to be HIV positive and 0.27 percent (95 percent CI 0.06–0.49) when partners of unknown HIV status were included. Unprotected insertive anal intercourse with HIV-positive and status-unknown partners was associated with a per coital transmission risk of 0.06 percent (95 percent CI 0.02–0.19), which is approximately six times higher than the HIV transmission per coital act for penile-vaginal sex (Wawer et al. 2005). Unprotected oral intercourse was associated with a low rate of HIV transmission, which is congruent with the observations that although saliva contains antibodies to HIV, live virus is not sustained. Consistently using condoms was associated with much lower per contact rates of risk for receptive intercourse with HIV-positive and unknown-serostatus partners (0.18 percent, 95 percent CI 0.10–0.28) (Vittinghoff et al. 1999). Researchers stipulated that based on specific histories of the seroconversions associated with protected sex, infections were secondary to condom failure, including breakage and slippage.

Ensuring that MSM have access to appropriate condoms remains at the core of any prevention program for MSM. Providing condoms is necessary, but community-driven evidence has highlighted the need to also effectively distribute condoms in a way to ensure that MSM have access to these condoms when needed. No experimental studies were found comparing distribution systems for condoms, but community-driven experience strongly suggests that providing free condoms in settings ranging from bathhouses to service centers for MSM has advantages over making condoms available for purchase in stores. This community-driven evidence and plausibility for the effective provision of condoms, the efficacy data around the use of condoms in preventing HIV, and the fact that all available experimental data are consistent with the need for effective distribution of condoms and lubricants result in a Grade 1, or strong, recommendation for including this intervention in CHPIs.

Although condoms remain a cornerstone of HIV prevention for MSM, significant issues have been associated with their use, including breakage, slippage, and lack of effective condom negotiation by receptive partners (Silverman and Gross 1997). User determinants associated with condom failure among MSM include longer penile length and larger penile circumference, self-identification as black or minority ethnic, use of petroleum-based lubricants, and lack of additional lubricant during anal intercourse (Golombok, Harding, and Sheldon 2001). Moreover, some lessons on the application value of lubricants can be gleaned from studies of vaginal intercourse, where oil-based lubricants increase rates of breakage and water-based lubricants decrease rates of breakage (Russell-Brown et al. 1992; Steiner et al. 1994). In contrast to vaginal intercourse, water-based lubricants do not increase rates of slippage during anal intercourse (A. M. Smith et al. 1998). The use of oil-based lubricants has also long been known to increase risk of latex condom breakage by decreasing tensile strength and increasing permeability, whereas water-based lubricants do not have this effect (Voeller et al. 1989; White et al. 1988). No studies were found that specifically evaluate the effectiveness of the ability of lubricants to decrease transmission of HIV during anal intercourse, likely because preventing men from using lubricants during sex would not be feasible or ethical. However, where evaluated, levels of use of appropriate lubricants by MSM in LMICs have been low. For example, in one study of MSM in Botswana, Malawi, and Namibia, less than 13 percent of men who reported always using condoms during anal intercourse reported using water-based lubricants. Approximately three times more MSM in this study reported always using condoms with oil-based lubricants (Baral et al. 2009). Inappropriate use of lubricants among MSM is not a new phenomenon and was observed in high-income settings nearly two decades ago (Martin 1992). However, a study completed at an STI clinic in Jamaica among presumed heterosexual men demonstrated that education can be an effective intervention to decrease condom breakage rates among men (Steiner et al. 2007). Studies evaluating lubricant preference for MSM have seen a resurgence given the potential for an effective rectal microbicide in preventing HIV transmission. These studies have consistently demonstrated that use of lubricants among MSM is common and acceptable (Carballo-Dieguez 2000). A few major barriers exist to the increased use of these lubricants among MSM in LMICs, including cost, access, and lack of knowledge. In lieu of appropriate lubricants, MSM in these settings are using whatever is available, including body creams, Vaseline, and saliva (Baral et al. 2009). Saliva has been implicated in the transmission of numerous pathogens, including cytomegalovirus, hepatitis B virus (HBV), and Kaposi sarcoma–associated herpesvirus among MSM (Butler et al. 2009). Hence, although no distinct efficacy data exist for the inclusion of lubricants in CHPIs, biological plausibility suggests that including water-based lubricants in prevention strategies targeting MSM is an important component of a comprehensive strategy. Thus, the provision and effective distribution—including education—of appropriate lubricants has been given a Grade 1, or strong, recommendation.

Thickness of condoms has also been found to be an important determinant of condom breakage; thicker European condoms have been found to be less likely to break than thinner standard condoms used elsewhere (Benton et al. 1997). In a randomized trial of 92 men reporting both vaginal and anal intercourse, Australian and Swiss condoms were compared for rates of breakage. In this study, the thinner Australian condoms were nearly five times more likely to break during anal sex (relative risk [RR] = 4.84, 95 percent CI 1.07–21.8, $p < 0.05$) than thicker Swiss condoms, whereas no difference was seen for vaginal sex (Benton et al. 1997). However, in a double-blind randomized controlled study of a standard versus a thicker condom, no significant difference was seen between failure rates, including breakage and slippage, for these two types of condoms after adjusting for inappropriate use (Golombok, Harding, and Sheldon 2001). Given high rates of condom failure among MSM, thicker condoms plausibly would confer additional protection, but studies on this subject have yielded inconsistent results (Silverman and Gross 1997). Thicker condoms have been given a Grade 2b, or possible, rating for inclusion in CHPIs because further evaluation is needed.

The female condom was designed as a barrier method for the receptive partner independent of the insertive partner. Because these condoms provide a physical barrier against genital secretions, evaluating the efficacy of female condoms placed rectally to prevent transmission associated with rectal intercourse was considered important. Theoretically, these condoms would be an excellent alternative because they obviate the need for effective condom negotiation skills, which is a major limitation to the consistent use of condoms among both receptive female and receptive male partners. In addition, because female condoms are not latex based, they would theoretically be safe to use with oil-based lubricants, which are much more easily accessible than water-based lubricants in LMICs. However, early studies among MSM have demonstrated higher rates of slippage (odds ratio [OR] 2.7, 95 percent CI 1.2–5.8 for receptive partners and OR 34.1, 95 percent CI 13.8–84.1 for insertive partners), and pain and discomfort (OR 5.0, 95 percent CI, 2.6–9.4) compared to male latex condoms (Renzi et al. 2003). Data from Population Services International have suggested high rates of acceptability among MSM in Myanmar and Thailand for a nearly identical female condom when marketed under the name Feel Condoms—although less is known about the relative efficacy of these condoms in preventing infection (Khan 2008). Although data describing the efficacy of female condoms for MSM have been inconsistent, numerous community groups from Asia and Africa have had significant success in distribution and use of female condoms because they circumvent the need for condom negotiation. This factor is especially relevant in the context of transactional sex where MSM may have more difficulty negotiating condom use for the insertive partner. Moreover, biological plausibility exists for the efficacy of this method of barrier protection. As such, female condoms have been given a Grade of 2b, or possible, for inclusion in CHPIs. In certain settings, female condoms may be an important component of CHPIs, but their use is context-specific and these condoms require significant further design improvements before they can be recommended for use among all MSM.

Interventions to decrease unprotected anal intercourse. Although the proposed HIV prevention package among MSM focuses on LMICs, the majority of data regarding prevention is derived from high-income settings, which may limit the generalizability of these studies to lower-income settings. The latest evidence suggests that unprotected anal intercourse (UAI), although less prevalent than in the earlier phases of the HIV pandemic, remains common, especially among HIV-positive MSM. Of 20 cross-sectional studies of sexual risk behavior among MSM in high-income settings, 14 studies demonstrated that UAI is significantly more common among HIV-positive men than among HIV-negative men or those never tested (van Kesteren, Hospers, and Kok 2007). Given high levels of serosorting resulting in HIV-positive men having sex with other seropositive MSM, these practices may not drive a majority of new infections; rather, they may be responsible for treatment failures and HIV progression (Bouhnik et al. 2007). However, levels of UAI are also high among serodiscordant-couples and status-unknown couples. These results are not limited to any one region: consistent prevalence of sexual risk behaviors are observed in Europe, North America, and Australia. In a study of nearly 5,000 MSM in Amsterdam, being HIV-negative or never having been tested for HIV were both strongly associated with lower odds of UAI at last sexual encounter: OR 0.24, 95 percent CI 0.14–0.42, and OR 0.1, 95 percent CI 0.11–0.32, respectively. Notably, even after correction for known serosorting, HIV-positive men were more likely to have UAI. Other statistically significant determinants of UAI at last sexual encounter were being less educated, not being of Dutch origin, and being younger (Hospers et al. 2005). Similar results were seen among more than 10,000 MSM from San Francisco, California, and subgroup analysis demonstrated that, among HIV-positive MSM, higher odds of UAI were predicted by being white (OR 1.8, 95 percent CI 1.3–2.5) and being older than 30 (OR 1.9, 95 percent CI 1.3–2.7). Being white was also associated with higher odds of UAI among HIV-negative MSM, although notably the prevalence of UAI was increasing among both HIV-positive and HIV-negative MSM (Chen et al. 2003).

Highly active antiretroviral therapy (HAART) has been tremendously successful in managing the clinical manifestations of HIV infection, and in places with consistent access to these medications, this trend of increasing UAI and hence decreased risk avoidance has been seen. Since 1996, the Brazilian public health care infrastructure has worked to ensure universal access to medications needed to treat HIV, resulting in huge improvements in the quality and length of life of those affected. With this decreased HIV-related morbidity and mortality, high-risk groups in Brazil, including MSM, have seen increased optimism. A recent cross-sectional study from São Paulo demonstrated that the most optimistic study participants were nearly two times more likely to have had UAI than the least optimistic MSM (da Silva et al. 2005).

The fact that UAI is common among MSM—and becoming more common, according to self-reported use data among MSM—suggests a need for intensifying specific prevention strategies aimed at increasing condom use among MSM. Although some uncertainty still exists about which interventions are most efficacious at increasing condom use, the increasing number of new HIV infections among MSM in both high- and low-income settings suggests limited effectiveness of these interventions (Sullivan et al. 2009). The failure to curb the HIV epidemic is likely multifactorial and includes the suboptimal coverage for these programs among MSM in many lower-income settings. Theories underlying these interventions have a complex taxonomy that has been well summarized by the Joint United Nations Programme on HIV/AIDS (see box 8.1 for more information).

Since the 1990s, a number of randomized controlled trials have evaluated both individual- and community-level interventions for MSM (Koblin, Chesney, and Coates 2004). Project EXPLORE was one of the more recent randomized controlled trials focusing on individual-level interventions. It analyzed 4,295 MSM in six U.S.-based sites randomized to the experimental group, which included a more intensive intervention

Box 8.1

Theories Supporting Behavior-Change Interventions

Briefly, theories supporting individual-level interventions include the health belief model theory of reasoned action, stages of change, and social cognitive theory (learning theory or cognitive behavior theory).

Those interventions targeting social or network factors include diffusion of innovation, social inoculation theory, social network theory, and empowerment models.

Finally, the theory supporting structural interventions includes the social-ecological model, theories of gender and power, and social capital theory (Share-Net 2003).

that consisted of 10 core counseling modules delivered one-on-one and then maintenance counseling every three months until the end of the study. The control group received standard risk reduction counseling based on the U.S. Centers for Disease Control and Prevention (CDC) Project RESPECT model. Retention in this study was excellent, with rates of above 83 percent in the experimental group and above 87 percent in the control group after four years of follow-up. In multivariate analysis, the ratio for HIV infection in the group receiving the intervention was 0.84 (95 percent CI 0.66–1.08), which equates to a trend toward a 16 percent decrease in HIV incidence (95 percent CI 8–34 percent)—although not reaching statistical significance. Established causal determinants of HIV risk such as UAI decreased significantly by an additional 13.2 percent (95 percent CI 4.8–20.9) in the intervention group, as did UAI with an HIV-positive partner (14.8 percent, 95 percent CI 6.5–22.4) and unprotected receptive anal intercourse with an HIV-positive partner (22.5 percent, 95 percent CI 13.3–30.7) (Koblin, Chesney, and Coates 2004). This study demonstrated effectiveness in terms of behavioral outcomes, but it did not meet significance in the less sensitive outcome of HIV incidence. Notably, Project EXPLORE targeted individuals, which facilitated its evaluation but limited its scalability, especially in lower-income settings.

A relatively recent systematic review and meta-analysis including 16,224 men in 38 experimental and observational studies demonstrated that compared to controls with no interventions, study groups reduced self-reported UAI by 27 percent (95 percent CI 15–37 percent) (Herbst et al. 2005; Johnson et al. 2005). In an additional 16 studies where MSM were given targeted prevention strategies, UAI decreased by 17 percent (95 percent CI 5–27 percent) more than for MSM who received standard HIV prevention measures. These reviews found that prevention strategies tend to work better when targeting networks or communities of MSM rather than individuals and function equally well independent of the proportion of minorities included. For example, the Mpowerment Project intervention targeted communities of MSM with social cognitive theories based on peer influence and diffusion of innovations (Kegeles, Hays, and Coates 1996). Mpowerment was a multicomponent intervention including two types of formal outreach, informal outreach, peer-led small groups, and an ongoing publicity campaign. The Mpowerment results demonstrated a 27 percent decrease in UAI after eight months with a 45 percent decrease in UAI with casual partners in the communities that received the intervention and no difference in the prevalence of UAI in communities without these interventions (Hays, Rebchook, and Kegeles 2003). HIV infection was not used as an outcome in this study, but cost-effectiveness evaluations have demonstrated that Mpowerment was a cost-effective strategy for preventing HIV among MSM (Kahn et al. 2001). A more recent example is the Bruthas Project targeting communities of black MSM in the United States (Operario et al. 2010). This study demonstrated efficacy in decreasing UAI and number of partners among African American MSM when community outreach was included in addition to risk reduction counseling as part of a comprehensive prevention strategy. Community-level interventions are more difficult to evaluate using traditional randomized controlled trials but are likely easier to scale up to meet the needs of MSM not already covered by individual-level interventions.

Each of the studies included in the two systematic reviews was analyzed by this group (Herbst et al. 2005; Johnson et al. 2008). The majority of these studies were small randomized controlled trials using social cognitive theory in the form of peer education or a transtheoretical model in the form of risk reduction counseling. Globally, between 5 percent and 10 percent of MSM have access to programs such as these, and even then the majority of these programs are in high-income countries (UNAIDS and WHO 2005). However, where studies of interventions targeting MSM have been completed in LMIC settings, they have consistently demonstrated both need and efficacy (Amirkhanian et al. 2003, 2005; Choi, McFarland, and Kihara 2004; Operario et al. 2005). One study completed in St. Petersburg, Russian Federation, and Sofia, Bulgaria, evaluated the efficacy of a social network HIV intervention focused on training social influence leaders to decrease HIV-related risk among MSM. After four months, a pre- and postintervention comparison showed the intervention was successful in increasing the level of comfort in discussing issues of HIV/AIDS prevention, increasing knowledge within the network about HIV, and increasing condom use among members of the network in 14 different social and sexual networks (Amirkhanian et al. 2003). A follow-up randomized trial of this social network intervention was completed in the same sites. This study included a total of 52 sites, randomizing 27 to the intervention with 25 social networks as control. This two-arm randomized controlled trial found that reported UAI decreased from 71.8 percent to 48.4 percent at three months ($p < 0.05$). At 12 months, the results were attenuated but still significant when compared to the control groups (Amirkhanian et al. 2005).

As for MSM in higher-income countries, data from LMICs suggest that interventions should target networks or communities rather than individuals to potentiate increased condom use (Choi et al. 2006). Although prevention strategies targeting MSM have been shown to be effective across a number of country income levels, the benefit of episodic or one-time interventions has been shown to be subject to decay over time. At approximately 12 months, the beneficial results of cross-sectional or one-time behavioral interventions tend to be significantly attenuated. Generally because of funding limitations, the efficacy of few of these interventions has been measured past 12 months of follow-up, but one can safely assume that the attenuation of efficacy continues to highlight the need for ongoing or episodic boosters of community-level behavioral interventions if these interventions are to sustainably contribute to curbing HIV epidemics. These data as well as plausibility of the need for sustained interventions mean that sustained interventions focused on decreasing UAI for MSM in CHPIs are given a strong, or Grade 1, recommendation.

The preceding data represent mixed results for individually tailored behavioral interventions for MSM. Given these results, one can reasonably conclude that individualized risk reduction counseling is an important component that is a necessary but not sufficient component of CHPIs. It is thus given a Grade 2a, or probable, recommendation. The evidence for the use of health promotion theories including social cognitive theory, transtheoretical model, and theory of reasoned action is stronger than that for didactic teaching alone. In some settings, didactic teaching may play a role, including settings in which levels of education are very low or no well-established peer education system exists. Therefore, it is given a recommendation of Grade 2b, or possible (Chesney et al. 2003; Chin-Hong et al. 2005). The evidence for brief, client-focused counseling is inconsistent, but significant community experience with this strategy exists as well as plausibility that addressing individual drivers of high-risk behaviors would facilitate behavior change. As such, brief, client-focused counseling is given a probable, or Grade 2a, assessment. An increasing body of literature describes the added value of community engagement when implementing prevention strategies. This finding is also consistent with well-established health promotion theory that empowering communities is a core component of a comprehensive intervention (Hays, Rebchook, and Kegeles 2003; Kahn et al. 2001; Kegeles, Hays, and Coates 1996). Moreover, it is also plausible that engaging the community of people at risk in developing an intervention will improve the reach and efficacy of that intervention. As such, community-level interventions to reduce UAI among MSM are given a strong, or Grade 1, recommendation for inclusion in CHPIs.

Conversion or reparative therapy. Conversion therapy (CT), also known as reparative therapy or reorientation therapy, refers to a set of interventions or treatments designed to change the sexual orientations of homosexual or bisexual persons to that of heterosexual. These therapies are predicated on a view of homosexuality as a mental illness, despite the American Psychiatric Association having removed homosexuality from its list of mental disorders in 1973. Given the dearth of scientifically sound studies demonstrating the efficacy of CT and considerable concern about its potential harms and ethicality, many international health organizations have issued statements rejecting the use of conversion or reparative therapies. Nevertheless, some mental health counselors—many of whom are connected to the evangelical Christian right ex-gay movement—continue to give these therapies scholarly and clinical support.

Cramer and colleagues' (2008) stringent review of existing literature on the empirical efficacy of CT reports that most of it fails to meet the American Psychological Association's criteria for evidence-based treatment. Studies by Nicolosi, Byrd, and Potts (2000a, 2000b) and Byrd, Nicolosi, and Potts (2008) purportedly demonstrated that participants in CT experienced "positive" changes to their sexual orientation. Yet these studies were plagued by "serious methodological limitations" and not published in peer-reviewed journals. Also of interest, Nicolosi and Byrd are currently listed as officers in the National Association for Research and Therapy of Homosexuality. Although the organization describes itself as a "professional, scientific organization that offers hope to those who struggle with unwanted homosexuality," it is considered an organization outside the mainstream that puts a pseudo-scientific façade on an anti-gay political and religious agenda (http://www.narth.com/menus/mission.html).

In 2003, Spitzer (2003) reported that a majority of survey respondents indicated a change from primarily homosexual orientation before therapy to primarily heterosexual orientation in the year before being interviewed. This study generated intense controversy; it was lauded by those in the ex-gay movement seeking scientific support of CT's efficacy and simultaneously critiqued for its flawed methodology by Spitzer's professional peers. Among other biases, "43 percent of the 200 participants learned about the study from ex-gay religious ministries and 23 percent from the National Association for Research and Therapy of

Homosexuality" (Spitzer 2003, 415). Furthermore, only 11 percent of men and 37 percent of women reported that they completely changed their sexual orientation. Even Spitzer commented: "it would be a serious mistake for me to conclude from my study that any highly motivated homosexual can change his or her sexual orientation" (Cianciotto and Cahill 2006, 63).

A year earlier, Shidlo and Schroeder (2002) had published results of a highly regarded seven-year retrospective investigation of 202 clients who participated in CT. The authors reported that a significant minority of participants changed their sexual orientations. Of the 26 (13 percent) who believed they had a self-perceived successful change from a homosexual to heterosexual orientation, 18 experienced behavioral "slips" or relied on coping mechanisms to control their same-sex attractions. Thus, only 8 (4 percent) could be classified as having made an actual shift in sexual orientation (Shidlo and Schroeder 2002).

Beckstead and Morrow's report, regarded as "one of the most in-depth outcome investigations of CT to date," also documents a failure to show significant change in same-sex attraction as the result of reparative therapy (Beckstead and Morrow 2004; Cramer et al. 2008, 98). Among 50 Mormons who participated in CT, some perceived the benefits of therapy to include feelings of fitting in, a decreased sense of loneliness, or relief. Yet the study offers no empirical evidence for the efficacy of CT in altering one's sexual orientation.

Moreover, Beckstead and Morrow's (2004) study reveals multiple negative consequences of CT, including increased self-hatred, depression, and thoughts of suicide. Many other studies conducted in the United States and Europe similarly report harmful psychological and physical effects of CT that include, but are not limited to, long-term sexual dysfunction, increased anxiety or aggression, decreased self-esteem, social isolation, and loss of family and spirituality (Haldeman 1994, 2004; Johnston and Jenkins 2006; King and Bartlett 1999; Shidlo and Schroeder 2002; Steigerwald and Janson 2003; Tozer and McClanahan 1999). Deaths have even been reported among those who suffocated on their own vomit during aversive therapy (King and Bartlett 1999).

As Cramer and colleagues (2008, 110) conclude, "based on the failure to meet (empirically supported treatments) standards and the multitude of reports denoting the harmful effects of CTs, CT appears to not only lack an empirical basis as a treatment option but also call[s] into question the ethical rationale for its inclusion in clinical practice." Most CT is conducted by ex-gay programs (for example, "Refuge" by Exodus International, "Love Won Out" by Focus on the Family, "The Source" by Love in Action) that market themselves as religious ministries. Consequently, the "treatment" these programs provide falls outside the jurisdiction of professional and regulatory organizations that impose ethical standards and enforce accountability. Essentially, these programs are providing mental health services without a license and in violation of standard practice guidelines.

Because of the lack of data supporting the efficacy of CT, multiple reports of its potential harmful effects, and the subsequent ethical implications of conducting therapies that clearly contradict accepted professional guidelines, many professional organizations have issued policy statements denouncing CT and prejudicial or devaluing treatment of homosexuals. The American Psychiatric Association has openly opposed CT for years because of the lack of sound scientific data to support its efficacy and because it is "at odds with the scientific position of the American Psychiatric Association which has maintained, since 1973, that homosexuality per se, is not a mental disorder" (http://www.psych.org/Departments/EDU/Library/APAOfficialDocumentsandRelated/Position Statements/200001.aspx).

The American Psychological Association released a technical report documenting the consensus of major medical and mental health professions that any effort to change sexual orientation through therapy is inherently flawed and potentially harmful (1999). This publication was endorsed by the American Academy of Pediatrics and the National Association of Social Workers, among others. The American Medical Association (http://www.ama-assn.org/meetings/public/annual00/reports/refcome/506.rtf) and the American Association of Physician Assistants (http://www.aapa.org/advocacy-and-practice-resources/clinical-issues/diversity) also reject CT on similar grounds.

In the United Kingdom, the Royal College of Nursing has denounced CT (Ryan and Rivers 2003), and the Royal College of Psychiatrists issued a position statement (http://www.rcpsych.ac.uk/pdf/PS01_2010x.pdf) declaring "that lesbian, gay, and bisexual people are and should be regarded as valued members of society who have exactly similar rights and responsibilities as all other citizens." This includes "a right to protection from therapies that are potentially damaging, particularly those that purport to change sexual orientation."

Quite recently, the Psychological Society of South Africa (http://www.psyssa.com/documents/PsySSA%20statement%20-%20UN%20Vote.pdf)

released a statement declaring that "there is no reliable evidence that sexual orientation is subject to redirection, 'conversion' or any significant influence from efforts by psychological or other interventions." The society invites other organizations representing mental health professionals, especially those in Africa, to endorse its statement as a means of promoting human well-being. Through its statement, the Psychological Society of South Africa joins the international community of professional organizations who have reviewed the extant literature on the efficacy of CT and rejected it as an ineffective, unnecessary, potentially harmful, and ethically controversial intervention. On the basis of expert consensus in combination with a lack of biologic plausibility and efficacy data, reparative or corrective therapy is given a Grade 4 or inappropriate for inclusion in CHPIs.

Antiretroviral therapy as primary and secondary prevention. HAART has been well established in effectively managing HIV-positive individuals, treating postexposure prophylaxis, and preventing vertical transmission of HIV from mother to child. A growing body of evidence and consensus exists that HAART can also prevent sexual transmission of HIV by lowering per coital act transmission rates (Vernazza et al. 2008). Driving this hypothesis are observations that lower plasma viral loads secondary to HAART correlate well to lower risk of HIV transmission. In a prospective cohort study in Rakai, Uganda, after adjustment for a series of HIV-related determinants, each log increment of plasma viral load was associated with a 2.45 times RR of HIV transmission (95 percent CI 1.85–3.26) (Quinn et al. 2000; Wawer et al. 2005). In addition, a study was completed comparing prevalent HIV infections in HIV-negative partners in long-term heterosexual serodiscordant relationships before and after the development of HAART. The results demonstrated that after adjusting for key factors, the HIV-negative partners were 86 percent less likely to become HIV infected if their partner was being treated with HAART (OR 0.14, 95 percent CI 0.03–0.66). More recent data from a prospective cohort analysis evaluating HIV transmission among heterosexual couples is congruent with this study, characterizing an adjusted 92 percent reduction for those under treatment, or incidence rate ratio of 0.08 (95 percent CI 0.00–0.57, $p < 0.01$) (Donnell et al. 2010). Evidence also suggests that the ability to lower genital viral loads is antiretroviral-agent specific: tenofovir, lamivudine, emtricitabine, zidovudine, and maraviroc are much better than lopinavir, atazanavir, and efavirenz at decreasing viral loads in genital fluids (Pao, Pillay, and Fisher 2009). The vast majority of these data are derived from heterosexual transmission. No evidence indicates that the efficacy of HAART varies by route of exposure, suggesting that these results should be generalizable to sex among men. However, a recent case study demonstrated, using phylogenetic analysis, transmission of HIV in a serodiscordant male couple where the HIV-positive partner had an undetectable viral load (Sturmer et al. 2008). Even in the context of this case report, significant biologic plausibility exists that lowering viral loads will decrease the transmission of HIV among MSM at the population level. Moreover, providing treatment for HIV-positive men is important to alter the natural history of HIV infection, including opportunistic infections and death. A secondary benefit is that engaging HIV-positive men to provide treatment is a useful and practical opportunity to provide risk reduction counseling aiming to decrease high-risk sexual practices. In the previously described systematic reviews of behavioral interventions to decrease HIV transmission among MSM, many of the studies included in the meta-analysis were evaluating HIV-positive men, demonstrating efficacy in this group (Herbst et al. 2005; Johnson et al. 2008). In fact, these studies suggest a tendency for improved efficacy of risk reduction counseling among HIV-positive men compared to status-unknown or HIV-negative men with low risk perception (Johnson et al. 2008). Plausibly, increasing safe-sex practices of HIV-positive men will decrease transmission to HIV-negative men. Therefore, HAART for secondary prevention is given a Grade 1, or strong, recommendation for inclusion in CHPIs.

Ongoing trials are assessing the efficacy of treatment as prevention, but mathematical models have yielded conflicting results. One model focused on low-income settings predicted that even though HAART could avert individual HIV infection, it would not mitigate the HIV epidemic at a population level irrespective of level of coverage (Baggaley, Garnett, and Ferguson 2006; Walensky et al. 2009). Moreover, increasing ART coverage could result in the development of increased drug-resistant strains of HIV. An epidemiological model calibrated to Sub-Saharan Africa evaluated the efficacy of increasing HAART coverage or increasing coverage of combined HIV prevention strategies in reducing HIV infections and mortality (Baggaley, Ferguson, and Garnett 2005; J. A. Salomon et al. 2005). After adjusting for potential changes in sexual practices, this study found that increasing treatment coverage would slow HIV epidemic growth from 10 percent per year to declines in cases per year of 6 percent. However, a strategy focused on comprehensive prevention would result in a 36 percent decrease in HIV incidence, although population-level benefit would be delayed by more than a decade after implementation. Effective implementation of a combination of treatment and prevention has the most potential and could result in 29 million averted infections (55 percent decrease) and 10 million averted deaths (27 percent); it is also the most cost-effective strategy in the long term. (J. A. Salomon et al. 2005)

A more recent model developed in British Columbia, Canada, by Lima and colleagues (2008) calculated potential averted infections using a series of different treatment scenarios stratified by coverage and adherence rates. This model proposes early treatment of HIV-positive patients to maximize the primary preventive benefit of HAART. The recommendation of early treatment is congruent with the changes to the adult HIV treatment guidelines published in 2009, which recommend initiating HAART before CD4 levels drop below 350 cells per microliter (DHHS Panel on Antiretroviral Guidelines for Adults and Adolescents 2009). Specifically, in patients with 350 CD4 cells per microliter or more, HAART can be initiated based on individual risk for progression to AIDS as well as a high plasma viral load and relatively rapid decline of CD4 cell count (over 100 per microliter per year) (Hammer et al. 2008). In its most optimistic scenario with 100 percent coverage, the model of Lima and colleagues (2008) predicts potentially reducing prevalence of HIV by 70-fold in 45 years. These results were congruent with a more recent modeling exercise evaluating the effect of universal HAART coverage of the heterosexual HIV epidemic in South Africa (Granich et al. 2009). Cost-efficacy analysis completed as part of a Canadian study demonstrates that this approach would be cost-effective in the long run given averted treatment costs (Lalani and Hicks 2007; Lima et al. 2008; Walensky et al. 2009). However, even if one were able to achieve 100 percent coverage with HAART, it cannot displace other preventive tools such as condom use. Wilson and colleagues (2008) developed a model that evaluated replacing condom use with the effective clinical management of HIV and predicted a fourfold increase in HIV incidence among MSM as a result. Last, a model focused on transmission among MSM predicted no benefit in decreasing transmission rates based on effective HAART treatment in the absence of effective prevention strategies (McCormick et al. 2007).

For treatment to function as an effective means of primary prevention, (a) making an early diagnosis, (b) minimizing treatment optimism, and (c) increasing treatment adherence are key determinants of success (Lima et al. 2009; Pao, Pillay, and Fisher 2009). If HIV-positive MSM being managed with HAART engage in higher-risk sexual practices, then the preventive benefit of HAART will likely be offset. Moreover, treatment optimism has been well characterized in multiple populations including MSM, in a variety of different settings, but not universally (Kalichman et al. 2007; Kennedy et al. 2007; Rowniak 2009). Outcomes of increased high-risk sexual practices among HIV-positive MSM include the potential of HAART failure secondary to acquisition of resistant strains and increased risk for other STIs, such as syphilis (Ostrow et al. 2008). Although treatment optimism is an important phenomenon to consider when designing HIV prevention strategies for MSM, it is not the only driver of high-risk sexual practices among MSM who have been appropriately educated about these risks. The previously described Project EXPLORE, as well as other key observational studies, has allowed the evaluation of a series of determinants of HIV risk practices as well as burden of disease among MSM. Such determinants include substance use, childhood sexual abuse, and mood disorders (Halkitis et al. 2005; Mimiaga et al. 2009; Reisner, Mimiaga, Case et al. 2009; Reisner, Mimiaga, Skeer et al. 2009; E. A. Salomon et al. 2009). Substance use has consistently been demonstrated to be associated with higher-risk sexual practices and HIV seroconversion among MSM (Buchbinder et al. 2005; Colfax et al. 2004, 2005; Mimiaga et al. 2008; Woody et al. 1999). In Project EXPLORE, amphetamines, alkyl nitrates (poppers), and sniffed cocaine were statistically significantly associated with unprotected receptive anal intercourse with a serodiscordant partner (Colfax et al. 2004). Alcohol has also been established as a marker of high-risk sexual practices in multiple settings among MSM including LMICs. In a follow-up study of 425 men who reported selling sex, levels of HIV knowledge were very low, and alcohol was associated with lower rates of condom use during transactional sex (Geibel et al. 2008; Lane et al. 2008). In the United States, alcohol has been found to increase unprotected sex with casual male partners but had no effect on sexual risk practices among regular male partners (Vanable et al. 2004). Given the role of substance use in promoting higher-risk sexual practices, addressing substance use issues, including alcohol, should likely be included as a component of CHPIs and is given a Grade 2a, or probable, recommendation.

Significant overlap exists between the risk factors for low rates of condom use with all partners, unprotected sex with serodiscordant partners, and suboptimal adherence to prevention and treatment strategies among MSM. Notably, these determinants seem to vary greatly by region and level of economic development. In many of the lowest-income countries of the world, basic educational interventions targeting MSM have been lacking; consequently, many MSM do not appreciate the risk of anal intercourse in the acquisition and transmission of HIV (Baral et al. 2008, 2009). However, in settings where comprehensive, evidence-based, and culturally appropriate educational programs have been developed, focus should increase not only on continued sexual health education, but also on mood disorders, self-esteem, and substance use (Elam et al. 2008). The efficacy of HAART as assessed by effective viral suppression is suboptimal in 30 percent to 70 percent of HIV-positive patients (Kalichman 2008). Furthermore, inadequate compliance is not limited to HAART; rather, it is also an issue for many biomedical and behavioral prevention strategies (Stirratt and Gordon 2008). To date, interventions targeting increased adherence to HAART have been of limited success, and similar to other behavioral interventions, the beneficial effect of these interventions decays with time (Simoni et al. 2006). In addition, the identification of mental health issues as a heightened risk factor for risky sexual practices and decreased compliance with interventions or treatment suggests the need for comprehensive approaches targeting HIV risk among MSM, including addressing mental health issues. In improving sexual practices, biologic plausibility is associated with addressing mental health disorders including depression and poor self-esteem, and a probable, or Grade 2a, recommendation is made for inclusion of these services in CHPIs for MSM.

Multiple models have been developed to explain and potentially predict individual behaviors and risk practices, including the health belief model, the theory of planned action, the ecological model, and the transtheoretical model of behavior change (DiClemente, Crosby, and Kegler 2002). Efficacious interventions, including those among MSM, have tended to be cognitive behavioral approaches with regular maintenance, such as was used in the herpes simplex virus 2 (HSV-2) suppression trial among MSM and Project EXPLORE (Celum et al. 2008; Healthy Living Project Team 2007; Koblin, Chesney, and Coates 2004). These counseling approaches aim to understand what the underlying thinking processes are among MSM and then support men to change behaviors associated with these self-justification processes either to increase condom use or to adhere to HAART (Gold 2000). In addition to being effective in increasing adherence, counseling has been determined to be cost-effective in HIV prevention among MSM (Zaric et al. 2008). Modified directly observed therapy has also been used with success to improve adherence to HAART. This method not only draws on lessons learned from the successes of directly observed therapy in the management of tuberculosis but also engages members of the community, family, and nontraditional health care workers. Engaging and training the community to provide additional counseling and support in a method akin to peer support is likely a beneficial strategy to increase adherence both to HAART and to more traditional prevention strategies (Goggin, Liston, and Mitty 2007; Simoni et al. 2007).

Post- and preexposure prophylaxis with ARVs. Using ART as HIV prophylaxis is based on consistent findings in animal models that these medications can be given before exposure to reduce risk of acquisition (preexposure prophylaxis) as well as after exposure (postexposure prophylaxis) with the same goal (Garcia-Lerma et al. 2008; Otten et al. 2000). Although to date little is known of the potential population-level benefit of postexposure prophylaxis in preventing HIV acquisition after sexual transmission among MSM, a study in two U.S. sites is currently evaluating its potential benefit as a prevention strategy (Lalani and Hicks 2007).

Preexposure prophylaxis or chemoprophylaxis would function by inhibiting HIV directly with medications that already exist and are in mass production. This strategy does not rely on effective negotiation skills of the receptive partner and may have an advantage over postexposure prophylaxis, especially where high-risk exposures may not have been recognized secondary to lack of status disclosure, substance use, or even denial (Elam et al. 2008; Weatherburn et al. 1998). However, little is known about the potential side effects, which include drug resistance, long-term adverse effects of the drugs, and treatment optimism. New results on preexposure prophylaxis in MSM were presented at the 2010 International AIDS Conference in Vienna. Specifically, a safety assessment was completed for once-daily oral tenofovir among MSM in Atlanta, Boston, and San Francisco. The study enrolled 400 HIV-negative MSM and allocated these men into four study arms: taking either 300 milligrams of oral tenofovir or placebo once daily, starting either at the time of enrollment or with a nine-month delay. Of the 400 men, 373 started treatment and 323 completed treatment for a retention rate of 86 percent. Although this trial was not powered to ascertain efficacy, results suggested that this strategy may work. Seven people seroconverted during follow-up, none of whom were on active treatment with tenofovir. Reported sexual risk behavior of the participants did not change significantly in either arm during the trial. Other studies are ongoing, including preexposure prophylaxis with a combination of tenofovir plus emtricitabine, and early preclinical studies are suggesting that this combination is more effective than tenofovir monotherapy (Grohskopf et al. 2010). These trials among MSM in Africa, Asia, and the Americas are under way, and efficacy results were made available in November 2010 (http://www.nejm.org/doi/pdf/10.1056/NEJMoa1011205). The Preexposure Prophylaxis Initiative (iPrEx) trial included a random assignment of 2,499 HIV-seronegative MSM to treatment with emtricitabine and tenofovir disoproxil fumarate (FTC–TDF) or placebo once daily. All study participants received behavioral HIV prevention measures including HIV testing, risk reduction counseling, condoms, and management of STIs. Analysis included 3,324 person-years of follow-up with a median follow-up of 1.2 years. In total, 64 infections occurred in the placebo group, and 36 infections in the experimental group, indicating a 44 percent reduction in HIV incidence (95 percent CI 15–63, $p < 0.01$). Further analyses highlighted significant increases in efficacy with improved adherence. However, adherence among study participants was limited in the context of controlled trial conditions and significant available resources. If this strategy is to be operationalized, clearly it would have to be coupled with appropriate and regularly maintained counseling and education to minimize high-risk sexual practices and maximize adherence (Gray 2009). The iPrEx trial has demonstrated feasibility and early evidence of efficacy, although confirmatory trials are being planned, including the VOICE (Vaginal and Oral Interventions to Control the Epidemic) trial, which will include vaginal and oral chemoprophylaxis for HIV (http://www.mtnstopshiv.org/node/70). With early evidence of efficacy and ongoing trials, primary prevention of HIV with antivirals or chemoprophylaxis is given a Grade 2b, or probable, recommendation for inclusion in CHPIs.

Voluntary counseling and testing. Although certain domains of voluntary counseling and testing (VCT) remain controversial, knowing one's status and associated counseling are generally accepted as associated with decreased high-risk sexual practices (Holtgrave and McGuire 2007). Marks and colleagues (2005) systematically reviewed and analyzed data from the United States, finding, on average, that people who knew their HIV-positive status were 53 percent (95 percent CI 45–60) less likely to have unprotected anal or vaginal intercourse than people who were unaware of their status. In assessing unprotected sex with HIV-negative people specifically, people who knew their status were 68 percent

(95 percent CI 59–76) less likely to report these sexual encounters, compared to people with unknown status. Notably, no statistical difference was found between risk reduction in men and women (Marks et al. 2005). This finding is congruent with data highlighting that most new infections in the United States are secondary to acquisition from HIV-positive people who were unaware of their status (Holtgrave and Pinkerton 2007). However, serosorting among MSM, or the practice of having sex with only seroconcordant partners, has been aptly termed "seroguessing," given the high levels of MSM who are unaware of their serostatus. Thus, this is likely not an effective means of HIV prevention (Eaton et al. 2007; Morin et al. 2008; Zablotska et al. 2009).

The updated 2006 CDC HIV testing guidelines encouraged increased testing for all people 13–64 years of age, with little emphasis on pre- and posttest counseling. The concept driving this change to the guidelines was the theory that the risk reduction associated with VCT was secondary mainly to the testing rather than to the counseling component (Holtgrave and McGuire 2007). However, HIV testing provides an excellent opportunity for individual client-focused risk reduction counseling—and for many this session may act as their first such counseling session. Project EXPLORE demonstrated that high-quality regular counseling can significantly reduce risk practices among MSM (Koblin, Chesney, and Coates 2004). Before this, Project RESPECT demonstrated that even brief individualized risk reduction counseling sessions were superior to didactic teaching in decreasing STI risk and increasing condom use, thus implying benefit for HIV-negative men (Kamb et al. 1998). Results such as these highlight the need to capitalize on opportunities for client-focused risk reduction counseling mediated by VCT visits. Because VCT provides an important engagement point between MSM and health care providers, in the context of a plausible prevention strategy and moderate efficacy data, it is given a Grade 1, or strong, recommendation for inclusion in CHPIs for MSM.

A need exists to further develop definitive testing protocols that include rapid HIV testing for MSM in LMICs because of the high rates of loss to follow-up after HIV testing (Lane et al. 2009). Rapid HIV testing can be completed with finger-prick-based serum or whole-blood kits, urine, or oral fluid. Oral fluid rapid HIV tests can be used to provide point-of-care test results in the diagnosis of HIV-1/2 infection and are classified as minimal complexity, diminishing the need for laboratory infrastructure. This testing method has been licensed by the U.S. Food and Drug Administration, and kits have sensitivities approaching 99.1 percent for oral fluid (compared to 99.7 percent with serum) and a specificity of 99.6 percent with oral fluid (compared to 99.9 percent with serum) (Delaney et al. 2006; Rietmeijer and Thrun 2006). Notably, saliva testing for HIV has been used previously with success as a minimally invasive and well-accepted testing method in lower-income settings (Holm-Hansen, Nyombi, and Nyindo 2007). A recent WHO review found that use of rapid HIV tests has grown exponentially from 2.4 million kits in 2004 to 39.7 million in 2008 (WHO, UNAIDS, and UNICEF 2009). In combination with effective risk reduction counseling, point-of-care testing for HIV with rapid kits has the potential to play a major role in reducing high-risk practices among MSM and is given a Grade 2a, or probable, recommendation for inclusion in CHPIs.

In LMICs, a major limitation to VCT sites tends to be the stigma associated with disclosing sexual orientation to VCT counselors. Studies from Botswana, Malawi, and Namibia demonstrated that disclosure by MSM of sexual orientation to family members was significantly associated with blackmail, and disclosure to a health care provider was significantly associated with having been denied health care. In addition, those who reported blackmail were less likely to have been tested for HIV in the last six months (Baral et al. 2009). These factors limit the efficacy of VCT as an HIV prevention intervention for MSM in LMICs. Hence, even though LMICs have drastically scaled up their provision of VCT services, and 31 countries reported serving 30 percent of MSM with VCT in the preceding 12 months, a need exists to ensure that VCT services can adequately serve the needs of lesbian, gay, bisexual, and transgendered (LGBT) persons (WHO, UNAIDS, and UNICEF 2009). Health sector interventions are discussed in more detail later, but highlighting the need for VCT counselors to be sensitized to the specific needs of MSM as well as educated about specific markers of risk and methods of providing targeted risk reduction counseling is important. As previously mentioned, completing the test is likely necessary but not sufficient in decreasing risk practices—appropriate risk reduction counseling is also a core component (Holtgrave and McGuire 2007). Although no specific efficacy data were found for sensitization of VCT sites to LGBT needs, a testing site providing nonstigmatizing care is more likely to have higher acceptance and uptake rates among the community (Liverpool VCT and Parkinson 2007). Furthermore, consistent implementation science data have highlighted that LGBT sensitization improves HIV testing rates for MSM in LMICs. Thus, this intervention is given a Grade 1, or Strong, recommendation for inclusion in CHPIs.

Circumcision. The protective effect of adult male circumcision has been demonstrated for heterosexual men in three trials in East and South Africa that used immediate versus delayed circumcision designs (Auvert et al. 2005; Bailey et al. 2007; Gray et al. 2007). The first trial was halted when interim analysis showed RR reduction of 0.40, or 60 percent protection against HIV ($p < .0001$) (Auvert et al. 2005). Later trials in Kenya and Uganda demonstrated similar levels of protection against HIV (Bailey et al. 2007; Gray et al. 2007). Adverse events in these trials were managed successfully without long-term complications (Auvert et al. 2005; Bailey et al. 2007; Gray et al. 2007; Krieger et al. 2007). A more recent evaluation of real-world effectiveness was completed among serodiscordant couples in which the male was the HIV-positive partner. In this study, a trend occurred toward a 40 percent decreased risk of transmission of HIV to the HIV-negative female, thereby demonstrating that circumcision may be valuable in preventing transmission of HIV infection (Baeten, Celum, and Coates 2009; Baeten et al. 2010). The protective effect of circumcision may be mediated by a reduction of risk for STIs or more directly by removing HIV target cells on the mucosal surface of the foreskin or by reducing microtrauma of the foreskin mucosal surface. WHO and the Joint United Nations Programme on HIV/AIDS have recommended that male circumcision should constitute a component of comprehensive prevention strategies for heterosexually acquired HIV infection in men (UNAIDS and WHO 2007).

Less is known about the protective potential of circumcision in anal sex and among MSM. Although the rectal mucosa is thought to be the primary site of infection for receptive partners, it is biologically plausible that those biologic mechanisms that lead to acquisition risks for men in vaginal intercourse hold true for insertive men in anal intercourse. In the recent STEP Study of the Merck trivalent adenovirus serotype 5 vectored HIV candidate, uncircumcised MSM with evidence of prior natural infection with adenovirus serotype 5 at enrollment were over four times as likely to acquire HIV if they received vaccine (Robertson et al. 2008). Currently, these results are incompletely and poorly understood, but they do underscore that uncircumcised men were at substantial risk for HIV acquisition.

To date, evidence from observational studies regarding circumcision status and HIV risk in MSM has been contradictory, and more research is needed in this area (Millett et al. 2008; Vermund and Qian 2008). A U.S. study of 3,257 MSM demonstrated increased risk of HIV infection among uncircumcised men after adjusting for sexual practices and drug use (adjusted OR 2.0, 95 percent CI 1.1–3.7) (Buchbinder et al. 2005). An earlier study conducted among U.S. MSM also suggested that circumcision was protective, but a recent cross-sectional study in 1,154 U.S. black and Hispanic MSM found no protection for men reporting unprotected insertive anal intercourse (Kreiss and Hopkins 1993; Millett et al. 2007). In a recent prospective cohort in Sydney, Australia, no difference was found in HIV incidence between circumcised and uncircumcised MSM (Templeton et al. 2007). Specifically, in the multivariate analysis controlling for a variety of HIV-related risk factors, circumcision was not associated with a significant reduction of HIV seroincidence (hazard ratio [HR] 0.78, 95 percent CI 0.42–1.45, p = 0.4). However, in a reanalysis of these data focusing on the one-third of participants who reported higher insertivity ratios (a preference for being the insertive partner), circumcision was associated with a significant decrease in HIV seroincidence after adjustment for other HIV-related risk factors including UAI (HR 0.11, 95 percent CI 0.03–0.8, p = 0.04) (Templeton et al. 2009). In addition, this same study demonstrated a decrease in risk of syphilis acquisition among predominantly insertive MSM.

In low-income regions with lower prevalence of circumcision, a few studies have evaluated circumcision, including a cross-sectional observational study completed in Peru and Ecuador (Guanira et al. 2007). Here, among MSM reporting only insertive anal sex, there was a trend (p = 0.07) for lower HIV prevalence among circumcised men, although power was limited by small sample size. The only study evaluating circumcision among MSM in the African context was completed in South Africa by Lane and colleagues (2009). This cross-sectional study of MSM demonstrated a significantly lower HIV prevalence among those who were circumcised (adjusted OR 0.2, 95 percent CI 0.1–0.2), although most of these men also had female sexual partners. A systematic review summarized some of these and older data and did not find a statistically significant decrease in HIV prevalence based on circumcision status, even when focusing on MSM with high insertivity ratios (Millett et al. 2008). In addition, an evaluation of circumcision as a risk factor among MSM in Seattle, Washington, did not demonstrate any added value of circumcision (Jameson et al. 2010). Although the data from observational studies in MSM are not as compelling as those for heterosexual men, MSM who are predominantly insertive and those who also have female sexual partners do seem to benefit from circumcision. This population of MSM has a shared biologic basis for protection, which arguably supports the need for an interventional trial of circumcision in MSM. Because circumcision has proven efficacious in three trials among heterosexual men, an argument can be made for a trial among MSM in the context of combination HIV prevention services. Circumcision may be an appropriate intervention for MSM who are predominantly insertive during anal intercourse or those with multiple female partners. Given the current status of efficacy results among MSM as well as a lack of community experience with this prevention strategy, circumcision is given a Grade 2b, or possible, recommendation, with a focus on MSM who report a high level of bisexual concurrency and high insertivity ratios as almost exclusively the insertive partner during anal sex with men. For these men, circumcision may function to decrease HIV acquisition risks in a manner similar to what has been observed among heterosexual men.

Syndromic STI treatment. Screening and management of curable STIs has been evaluated with limited success, predominantly in heterosexual populations and to a lesser extent among MSM (Padian et al. 2008). These trials were developed in response to the well-demonstrated causal role of genital ulcerative diseases in increasing the acquisition and transmission of HIV. A case-control study of HIV-positive MSM not on ART for at least three months found that active urethritis secondary to gonorrhea and chlamydia increased seminal viral load levels (Sadiq et al. 2005). Earlier randomized controlled trials focused on active management of curable infectious genital diseases, including syphilis, gonorrhea and chlamydia, chancroid, and trichomoniasis, with little effect on HIV seroincidence in self-reported heterosexual populations. No trial was found evaluating efficacy of HIV prevention secondary to the active management of curable STIs among MSM.

A trial of HSV-2 suppression was completed among MSM in multiple sites in Peru and the United States in the context of a larger randomized controlled trial including high-risk women in Africa. This trial was developed in response to the finding that HSV-2 infection was consistently associated with higher risk for HIV infection and higher levels of HIV viral load in plasma and genital samples of both men and women (E. L. Brown et al. 2006). Furthermore, suppression of HSV-2 in HIV-positive men had demonstrated the capacity to decrease HIV viral loads and seminal levels of HIV (Zuckerman et al. 2007, 2009). A randomized controlled trial of 3,172 participants including 1,358 women in Sub-Saharan Africa and 1,814 MSM in Peru and the United States was effective in preventing all clinically diagnosed genital ulcers by 47 percent (RR 0.53, 95 percent CI 0.46–0.62) and efficacious in preventing HSV-2 ulcers by 63 percent (RR 0.37, 95 percent CI 0.31–0.45) (Celum et al. 2008). Although adherence to both acyclovir and the control drug was over 90 percent, a nonstatistically significant trend of increased risk of HIV incidence was seen in the treatment arm. Specifically, the HR was 1.16 (95 percent CI 0.83–1.62) with an incidence rate of 3.9 in the acyclovir arm and an incidence rate of 3.3 in the placebo group. Among MSM in both of these sites, no benefit to HSV-2 suppression was seen, with an HR of 1.09 (95 percent CI 0.36–3.24) in the United States and an HR of 0.82 (0.48–1.41) among MSM in Peru. A more recent study demonstrated that although acyclovir is able to effect a significant reduction of HIV-1 RNA and decrease genital ulcers attributable to HSV-2 by 73 percent, HIV transmission is not affected (Celum et al. 2010). With consistent data of lack of effect, HSV-2 suppression is given a Grade IV.

Using these data, one cannot conclude that syndromic STI surveillance and treatment is sufficient to curb HIV spread among MSM. However, given the consistently demonstrated causal role of STIs in HIV acquisition and transmission, effectively managing these infectious diseases should constitute a component of CHPIs. Moreover, treating symptomatic STIs provides an opportunity to engage and provide risk reduction counseling, which have been shown to decrease high-risk sexual practices. Thus, treating STIs is given a Grade 2a, or probable, recommendation for inclusion in CHPIs for MSM in LMICs.

Vaccination. MSM are at high risk for several vaccine-preventable infections including hepatitis A virus (HAV), HBV, and human papillomavirus (HPV). Traditionally, HAV has been a well-documented public health problem generally limited to LMICs with transmission secondary to fecal-oral contact or ingestion of contaminated food or water (Jacobsen and Koopman 2004). Although incidence of HAV is decreasing in many parts of the developing world because of improved water sanitation facilities, seroincidence secondary to sexual transmission remains high among MSM in high-income countries (Ferson, Young, and Stokes 1998). Current estimates suggest that HBV has infected nearly 2 billion people worldwide, of whom 350 million have evidence of chronic infection that carries similar risks to hepatitis C infection of complications such as cirrhosis and liver cancer (Kane 1995, 1996; Lin and Kirchner 2004; Poland and Jacobson 2004). As with HAV, an effective vaccine has been available for HBV for more than two decades (Hutchinson et al. 2004). The viral hepatitidies remain major public health concerns for MSM given the significant disease burden as well as the role of HBV in potentiating HIV-related morbidity, which is why the CDC recommends all MSM be vaccinated for both infections (Kahn 2002). Thus, although vaccinating MSM for HBV and HAV is key for comprehensive health care, no evidence was found that the viral hepatitidies increase the risk of HIV acquisition and transmission.

HPV is a nonenveloped double-stranded DNA virus that WHO has classified as a definitive biological carcinogen causing squamous intraepithelial lesions and squamous cell cancers (Bosch et al. 2002). It is most commonly seen as an STI and is spread by both penile-vaginal and penile-anal penetrative intercourse as well as digital-genital penetration. It is most commonly associated with cervical cancer in women but is also an important component of squamous cell anal cancers in men (Snijders et al. 2006). Infection is usually asymptomatic and transient, but approximately 10 percent of women and a yet-to-be-determined proportion of men develop persistent infection that is a prerequisite for cancer (L. A. Herrera et al. 2005). In immunocompetent men, cancer is a less common outcome with benign papillomas, or genital warts, which are observed more frequently (van der Snoek et al. 2003). However, more than 100 serotypes of HPV have been identified, and some of these serotypes have been typed as high risk because they are more commonly associated with progression to squamous intraepithelial lesions and squamous cell cancers. Anal cancers are relatively rare in the general population of men; however, MSM are at significantly increased risk of developing anal cancer with estimates ranging from 44 to 50 times higher rates than the general population (Friedman et al. 1998). The relationship between HPV and HIV initially focused on the nearly 30 times incidence of anal cancer in HIV-positive people, with the highest risk among MSM compared to injecting drug users or sex workers (Grulich et al. 2007). Moreover, data from MACS demonstrated that HIV-positive MSM are nearly five times as likely to develop anal cancer compared to HIV-negative MSM (RR 4.7, 95 percent CI 1.3–17) (D'Souza et al. 2008). Because less than 1 percent of men infected with HPV will develop genital warts, screening for this infection and dysplastic changes using anal pap smears has the potential to alter the natural history of this disease (Palefsky et al. 1998).

More recent evidence has linked HPV infection with increased risk of HIV acquisition among both heterosexual men and MSM. Specifically, a study assessing the relationship between prevalent HPV infection and HIV infection demonstrated an HR of 1.8 (95 percent CI 1.1–2.9) after adjusting for numerous confounders including circumcision status,

HSV-2 infection, and sexual and sociodemographic factors (J. Smith et al. 2010). Similar results among heterosexual men were observed in South Africa with increased risk being associated with high-risk serotypes of HPV—those men infected had an adjusted incidence rate ratio of 3.8 (95 percent CI 2.0–9.8) compared with uninfected men (Auvert et al. 2009). The first study to assess the relationship between HPV and HIV among MSM was reported in 2009 and showed that infection with one HPV serotype was associated with an HR of 2.8 (95 percent CI 1.0–7.4, $p = 0.04$) for HIV seroconversion among MSM in four U.S. cities after adjusting for potential confounders. Furthermore, infection with two or more serotypes of HPV was associated with an HR of 3.6 (95 percent CI 1.5–8.4) for HIV seroconversion among MSM (Chin-Hong et al. 2009). In Project EXPLORE, HPV DNA was found in the anal canal of 57 percent of MSM study participants; risk factors included receptive anal intercourse (OR 2.0, $p < 0.0001$) and more than five male partners in the preceding six months (OR 1.5, $p < 0.001$) (Chin-Hong et al. 2005). Notably, data from MACS demonstrated that condom use does not seem to protect against the development of HPV infection or secondary anal condylomas (Wiley et al. 2005). Because when using more sensitive methods, HPV DNA has been observed in as many as 78 percent of HIV-negative MSM and 92 percent of HIV-positive MSM, HPV infection may play a significant role in HIV epidemics among MSM (Friedman et al. 1998). HPV may be especially important for HIV acquisition and transmission among MSM given that, unlike the heterosexual men assessed in these studies, MSM have both penile and anal exposures to HPV.

The recently developed and marketed quadrivalent vaccine that protects against HPV 6/11/16/18 has been integrated into vaccination in numerous high-income countries. This vaccine has also shown significant efficacy in protecting against HPV infection in men and the development of anogenital warts (Franceschi and De Vuyst 2009). The standard of clinical care of MSM should include appropriate screening and management of anal papillomas with anal pap smears; however, no evidence was found indicating that this strategy can decrease the risk of HIV acquisition. In some high-income settings, boys are now included as target groups for HPV vaccination because of its role in preventing associated anal cancers. Although no research is yet available on the role of HPV vaccination in preventing HIV infection, HPV's role in promoting HIV acquisition and transmission among MSM creates an expectation that the HPV vaccine may play a significant role in comprehensive HIV prevention for MSM. Further research among MSM is necessary, but the HPV vaccine may be an important component of primary HIV prevention among populations practicing receptive anal intercourse such as MSM. Therefore, HPV vaccination has been designated as a Grade 2a, or probable, intervention for MSM.

Rectal microbicides. Microbicides, including gels, films, and suppositories, are currently being developed as an alternate HIV prevention strategy for women, especially those who have difficulty negotiating condom use with their male partners. Despite some concern about heightened risk of HIV acquisition with regular vaginal application of these products, the concept has been extrapolated to rectal use of these products in HIV prevention for MSM.

The first gel to be significantly evaluated was nonoxynol-9 (N-9), a detergent ingredient previously thought to have microbicidal properties that was included as an ingredient in numerous sexual lubricants, condoms, gels, and spermicidal products (Gross et al. 1998; Roddy et al. 2002). Throughout these trials, it became increasingly clear that N-9 was not protective against gonorrhea or chlamydia infection, caused disruption of the rectal mucosa in humans, and potentially increased the risk for HIV (Mansergh et al. 2003). No microbicide to date has shown efficacy in HIV prevention vaginally among women or rectally among MSM, but a new generation of antiretroviral-loaded gels is currently under development (C. Herrera et al. 2009). Recent preclinical data have been encouraging and demonstrate the potential efficacy of tenofovir-loaded rectal microbicides in preventing rectal transmission of SIV in macaques (Cranage et al. 2008). Microbicides have high acceptability among MSM, especially in the form of gels and ideally as long-acting agents rather than coitally dependent (Carballo-Dieguez et al. 2008). Rectal microbicides are currently being evaluated in Phase 1/2 studies in the United States and are potentially of benefit to populations at risk for HIV acquisition secondary to unprotected receptive intercourse. The recently presented CAPRISA 004 trial demonstrated efficacy of a vaginal gel containing 1 percent tenofovir in significantly reducing a woman's risk of being infected with HIV or genital herpes. The tenofovir gel, used both before and after intercourse, reduced the risk of HIV acquisition by 39 percent in the primary intent-to-treat analysis. The absolute risk difference in incident HIV infections between the two groups was 35 infections per 100 person-years. HSV-2 infection was also decreased by 51 percent by using the 1 percent tenofovir gel. Notably, improved adherence of the gel was associated with an absolute rate reduction of 54 percent for

HIV infection (Abdool Karim et al. 2010). Given early evidence of efficacy among women, an equipoise argument exists that a tenofovir gel may reduce the risk of HIV acquisition among MSM who are at risk secondary to unprotected anal intercourse. This argument is potentiated by evidence that several antiretroviral agents have demonstrated an affinity for cevicovaginal and rectal tissue, including tenofovir, emtricitabine, and maraviroc (K. Brown et al. 2010; Dumond et al. 2009; Patterson et al. 2010). Groups such as the International Rectal Microbicide Advocates (http://www.rectalmicrobicides.org/) have demonstrated broad interest in rectal microbicide development among MSM populations in the United States, Latin America, Asia, and Africa. Because rectal microbicides will likely continue to be evaluated in clinical trials, MSM in LMICs must be engaged and offered participation in these research studies. Participation in research studies facilitates the access to combination HIV prevention services offered to all participants and increases community-level knowledge of the risks of HIV and prevention strategies. As the basic science of these gels continues to improve, assessing both the willingness to take part in these studies and attitudes toward rectal microbicides among MSM in all LMICs will be key. Because of the lack of current efficacy data, rectal microbicides are given a Grade 2c, or pending, recommendation for inclusion in CHPIs.

Targeting Structural Risk

An increasing body of evidence highlights that structural drivers working at levels above and around the individual are a primary determinant of the dynamics of infectious disease epidemics. Structural drivers of risk contextualize individual-level risks. Furthermore, structural factors determine where, how, and whether individuals will engage in any HIV-related interventions. Without a better understanding of high-order risk factors, attempts to mitigate HIV spread will likely be of limited success (Kippax 2008; Rhodes et al. 1999). In a seminal systematic review by Wellings and colleagues (2006) detailing the global context of sexual practices, higher-order levels of risk were reinforced as key determinants of sexual practices. HIV-related risk factors for MSM are presented here using a modified ecological model that provides a framework for displaying individual-level HIV risk in the context of network, community, public policy, and stage of HIV epidemic factors and describing the interactions between these levels (McLeroy et al. 1988). *Individual risks* are those biologic or behavioral characteristics and practices that have been shown to be associated with a higher probability of HIV infection.

Individual-level acquisition risks have focused on the highest probability exposure: UAI—specifically, correlates of receptive anal intercourse (Koblin et al. 2006). Use of party drugs such as methamphetamines and alkyl nitrates (poppers) has been associated with heightened sexual exposure among MSM in several settings (Beyrer et al. 2005; Koblin et al. 2006; Mansergh et al. 2008). As with men who report sex with women only, HIV transmission in MSM is associated with being infected with genitourinary disease, being uncircumcised, having a high frequency of male partners, and having a high lifetime number of male partners (Buchbinder et al. 2005). Finally, in developed-country settings, being a black or minority ethnic MSM is associated with higher risk of HIV in comparison with white MSM (Harawa et al. 2004). A critical review of the evidence examining the racial differential seen in the HIV epidemic among MSM suggested the increased HIV prevalence seen among black MSM is most likely caused by a decreased proportion of that population having been tested and knowing their HIV status and having higher rates of STIs that facilitate HIV transmission (Millett et al. 2006). A similar trend among minorities, though of lesser magnitude, has been observed in other high-income countries including Canada and the United Kingdom.

Networks of MSM are defined as groups of people who have a higher probability of exposure to infectious disease from each other mediated through sexual exposure. Sexual networks are not necessarily bound by geography, socioeconomic status, or cultural, racial, and religious lines, and such networks may not even share a common social identity or language. At the same time, sexual networks may share locations for social and sexual interactions or practices and norms of sexual practices and drug use. Network levels of risk include both biologic and behavioral factors that potentiate the spread of infectious disease among the individual members of that network. Social network analysis has been a key tool in understanding transmission patterns of HIV. However, these analyses tend to be limited by the long latency period and subclinical characteristics of HIV infection. Recently developed tools allow the use of molecular phylodynamics to better describe transmission patterns and HIV epidemic dynamics. In addition, phylogenetics will provide data to describe whether strains of HIV circulating among MSM overlap with dominant strains in the general population, including women. Network social and sexual dynamics such as having particularly high-risk individuals (for example, male sex workers and transgendered individuals) in a sexual network will put all the members of that network at increased risk of infection (Beyrer et al. 2005). And a high prevalence of STIs will increase the probability of HIV transmission within the network.

Few countries are homogenous in terms of their cultural and demographic makeup; rather, countries are composed of a set of communities. These communities are bounded by cultural, economic, religious, or geographic lines; prison walls; or any combination of these. With some notable exceptions, communities in a country tend to be centrally governed by a common set of laws and policies whose interpretation and implementation differ greatly. These differences create a situation that either increases or mitigates the risk level for infection of MSM in a particular community. Hence, at the community level, access to preventive services, VCT, and ARVs contributes to the level of risk of any particular community of MSM. Stigma and discrimination limit access to comprehensive health and preventive care programming by affected communities. Furthermore, sexuality-based violence targeting MSM can result in MSM being afraid to walk in their own communities, which may limit access to appropriate health care (Baral et al. 2009). In contexts of stigma and discrimination, blackmail is more common, and opportunities for gainful employment can be limited if one is identified as gay or bisexual, which again limits access to care.

The laws and policies of any state provide the general framework for defining the risk status of high-risk subsets of the population as well as the general population. These policies either promote or decrease the community's ability to provide preventive or harm reduction services to its constituents by enacting laws criminalizing populations or interventions, or by disrupting funding mechanisms supporting evidenced-based HIV prevention and treatment programs. Homosexuality remains criminalized in more than 80 member states of the United Nations, with punishments ranging from jail time to the death penalty. Criminalization and other limits on human freedom and bodily integrity likely play roles in structural risks for HIV and STIs. Repressive legal contexts limit access for these men to appropriate STI and HIV services, including prevention, treatment, and care. In these environments, even if funding were available for state-of-the-art combination HIV prevention and care packages for MSM, they would likely be of limited value because men in such settings are quite justified in not seeking care. It has been anecdotally suggested that criminalization of same-sex practices limits them and in turn limits the absolute amount of UAI that takes place within a country. A detailed analysis of this suggestion has not been completed for this book, but a brief overview of the data presented here contradicts the assumption that criminalization limits the development of same-sex practices or limits UAI among MSM. In fact, these data support the hypothesis that criminalization plays no role in the development of same-sex practices and likely potentiates high-risk practices among MSM by limiting the provision and uptake of HIV prevention, treatment, and care services. If one compares the data on number of MSM in LMICs to number of MSM in many high-income countries, the trend shows proportionally more MSM in LMICs than in high-income countries where laws criminalizing same-sex practices are rare (Cáceres et al. 2006). Within the country scenarios modeled in this book, same-sex practices are criminalized in Kenya but not in Peru, Ukraine, or Thailand. Although disproportionate condom use is caused by many factors, reported consistent condom use among MSM was lowest in Kenya at 32.1 percent, compared with 80.4 percent in Ukraine, 39.5 percent in Thailand, and 42.0 percent in Peru. Similar trends of higher rates of UAI in countries that criminalize same-sex practices have been observed, although complete analyses are pending at the writing of this book.

Ultimately, the stage of the epidemic in the network, the community, and the country determines the risk of disease acquisition for the individual. No sexual practice, policy or law, community determinant, network attribute, or individual characteristic can create infectious disease; rather, these can only create conditions that either increase or decrease the probability of acquisition or transmission of an already prevalent disease. Thus, any of these factors should be considered as high risk only in the context of a high prevalence level of an infectious disease.

All the individual interventions described so far, both biomedical and behavioral, have one thing in common: they are designed to address the needs of high-risk individuals rather than to target the population as a whole. Structural interventions are intended to do just that—target the entire population in a community or country by attempting to modify social, economic, political, and environmental factors (Gupta et al. 2008). Using the principles of health promotion, these interventions should enable MSM to increase control over, and to improve, their health. This outcome implies reaching a state of complete physical, mental, and social well-being, which is accomplished by the ability to identify and to realize aspirations, to satisfy needs, and to change or cope with the environment. With this approach, health is not the objective of living; rather, it is intended to act as a resource for everyday life. Health promotion defines health as a positive concept emphasizing social and personal resources as well as physical capacities. Thus, these interventions cannot simply target the health sector but instead must address all facets of society to go beyond encouraging health lifestyles for MSM and encourage well-being (WHO 1986).

The vast majority of HIV intervention studies to date have evaluated the efficacy and effectiveness of interventions targeting individual risk factors. Few studies of biomedical interventions have been completed among MSM, and interventions that have been evaluated have seen little success. Biomedical interventions that may hold promise for MSM include pre- and postexposure prophylaxis, syndromic STI treatment, rectal microbicides, circumcision, and ultimately HIV vaccines. Similarly, behavioral change interventions have tended to focus on individual-level risk factors, including rates of UAI, with a dearth of focus on the social determinants of health that contextualize those practices (Beyrer 2007). The recognition of the need to develop CHPIs that address structural risks has been highlighted in a series of consultations and key reports (Global HIV Prevention Working Group 2004, 2007; Kippax 2008; WHO, UNAIDS, and UNICEF 2009). Addressing structural drivers of risk implies targeting the entire population rather than just those at the highest risk, which means that evaluating these interventions is more complicated. In addition, changes in structural drivers of risk such as stigma and discrimination result in social change rather than changes in sexual practices, which again complicates the assessment of the effectiveness of these interventions. Although CHPIs should be developed in response to evidence (Wilson and Halperin 2008), the limitations in generating evidence of the efficacy of structural drivers must be appreciated, given that benefit is upstream and distributed across a population rather than concentrated among high-risk individuals. To develop this package, this book includes interventions targeting the structural risk factors for HIV infection among MSM discussed previously. Although most of these approaches have not been adequately evaluated, evaluative research can be completed after implementation to assess which components of CHPIs are most efficacious and cost-effective. Finally, because individual risks for HIV infection among MSM are likely shared by men worldwide, interventions targeting these drivers of risk will likely work in numerous settings as long as they are culturally appropriate. Structural approaches are more complicated because they have to be tailored to the prevailing structural risks in the targeted community, region, or country.

Health promotion encourages the building of healthy public policy, which implies identifying obstacles to the adoption of healthy public policies in nonhealth sectors and developing ways to remove them. As previously mentioned, same-sex practices are criminalized in more than 80 member countries of the United Nations, which limits the ability to adopt other healthy public policies targeting MSM. As such, advocacy campaigns targeting decriminalization, where applicable, should be a component of CHPIs. However, in few places in the world is significant stigma targeting LGBT communities not a reality, highlighting the potential disconnect between constitutional protections and real-life experiences for sexual minorities (Burrell et al. 2008; Cáceres 2002). Australia has had numerous successes in avoiding epidemics of HIV among vulnerable populations, including, to some extent, MSM. This outcome was accomplished by adopting supportive policies, appropriately resourcing affected communities, developing dedicated research centers, and taking collective ownership of the epidemic (Gupta et al. 2008). An important example from LMICs was the Brazilian government's development and sponsorship of the policy "Brazil without Homophobia," which focused on decreasing population-based stigma targeting LGBT populations and included a school-based component to decrease homophobia in the public schools and increase self-esteem and self-efficacy for LGBT youth as an HIV preventive intervention (Altman 2005).

Mass media strategies have been used in difficult contexts to spread HIV-related education targeting MSM in Senegal (Diouf et al. 2004). Given the ability to target large populations using popular media sources, developing region-specific media strategies is an important component of CHPIs.

The World Bank has evaluated larger, multicountry approaches targeting MSM in challenging contexts in the form of the Multi-Country HIV/AIDS Program, which took place in Burkina Faso, Senegal, and The Gambia. The program was deemed successful in increasing access to HIV/AIDS prevention, care, support, and treatment programs for MSM—especially among those who engaged in commercial male-to-male sexual contact (Niang et al. 2004). Finally, male engagement programs focusing on changing perceptions of straight-identified men and women have demonstrated success in decreasing stigma against LGBT populations (Ehrhardt et al. 2009). Programs providing education to challenge gender norms, such as those offered by Sonke Gender Justice in South Africa, may be generalizable to other settings and be an important component of CHPIs (Peacock et al. 2009).

Health promotion also calls for strengthening community action by drawing on existing human resources and focusing on the development of community-based resources to enhance self-help and social support. The initial collective response to the HIV epidemic was led by people living with HIV, their caregivers, and communities at risk (Merson, O'Malley et al. 2008). Community systems strengthening remains a core component of HIV prevention strategies and should be given further resources. As an example, building social capital has functioned in the development and dissemination of education for MSM in Ghana (Porter et al. 2006). In difficult contexts, constructive research collaborations with local sexual minority rights groups can build community capacity in HIV research, outreach, and prevention and in advocacy for inclusion of MSM in national AIDS programs and plans. Research institutions bring technical expertise, while local community-based organizations bring credibility within communities, allowing study accrual of an otherwise hidden population. Moreover, these collaborations will be critical in testing the efficacy of preventive biomedical and behavioral HIV interventions among MSM in many LMICs. Capacity building through transfer of knowledge and skills is a core focus of this type of collaboration and will further function to strengthen the responses of civil society organizations in addressing the needs of MSM. These research projects can be used to characterize, from the community perspective, how best to implement outreach and targeted health and preventive services for MSM in a particular setting. Studies such as these are needed to inform prevention, including deciding between mainstreaming of health care for MSM or providing men's health clinics specifically serving the needs of MSM or alternatively a combined approach. If a men's health clinic has a role, further evaluative research will be needed to determine the optimal mode of service delivery, including deciding between a storefront model and mobile services, pending feedback from community members. These strategies of community capacity building for local groups have been shown to be essential to increase community penetration of HIV prevention packages, build community social capital, and improve advocacy for inclusion of MSM (Latkin and Knowlton 2005; Roehr 2008). As previously described, data demonstrating the value of using community-based approaches for decreasing high-risk sexual practices are encouraging, including the Bruthas and Mpowerment studies in the United States (Hays, Rebchook, and Kegeles 2003; Operario et al. 2010).

Also crucial is that the health sector be appropriately educated and provided with adequate resources to address the specific needs of MSM. Determining the optimal model for VCT for MSM in settings with significant stigma and discrimination is vital. Sensitivity training on LGBT health and rights issues for existing VCT sites, thereby making them LGBT-friendly, may significantly increase willingness among the community of MSM to use these clinics and would strengthen local capacity to provide care in the future. Training for clinicians could range from social services including couples-based counseling for MSM to clinical skills such as anoscopy evaluating anal papillomas or anal cancer. An excellent training module called the *Guide to Lesbian, Gay, Bisexual and Transgender Health* has been developed by Makadon and colleagues (2008) and methods of dissemination of products such as these in LMICs, including learning collaboratives, should be evaluated (Roehr 2008). A learning collaborative could mean training 10–15 clinicians about the specific health care needs of MSM and then supporting them to do outreach to hospitals, medical and nursing schools, and large clinics. Although structural interventions much transcend the health sector alone, investing adequate attention and resources in behavior change toward LGBT individuals in doctors, nurses, and VCT counselors as part of CHPIs is vital.

No significant body of literature describes the efficacy of decreasing high-risk sexual practices secondary to structural interventions, in part because the majority of interventions have taken place in high-income settings where overt stigma and discrimination targeting MSM are often illegal. Moving forward, assessments of stigma among MSM in LMICs should include comprehensive analyses of multiple facets of stigma including upstream and downstream factors. These data are needed to inform not only interventions targeting MSM to improve levels of same-sex condom use but also interventions targeting health care staff—and society more broadly—to decrease levels of discrimination targeting MSM, thereby facilitating their access to available health care services (Chakrapani et al. 2007). In the absence of convincing efficacy data, a growing body of literature links structural risk with increased rates of individual risk for HIV infection among MSM (Ayala et al. 2010). Moreover, public health plausibility exists that improving contexts for MSM will facilitate HIV service provision and service uptake among MSM, as has been demonstrated in several conceptual frameworks. Last, a consistent consensus exists in community groups of MSM that structural interventions are an important component of CHPIs for MSM in LMICs. As such, structural interventions are collectively given a strong, or Grade 1, recommendation for inclusion in CHPI (table 8.2). The use of HASTE in the evaluation of implementation

Table 8.2 Strength of Recommendations for Inclusion of Specific Prevention Components in CHPI Package for MSM

Intervention	*Components*	*HASTE level*	*Strength of recommendation*
Condoms and water- or silicone-based lubricants	Effective distribution	Grade 1	Strong
	Counseling and education about condoms and lubricants	Grade 1	Strong
	Thicker condoms	Grade 2b	Possible
	Female condoms	Grade 2b	Possible
Behavioral interventions	Individualized risk-reduction counseling	Grade 2a	Probable
	Conversion or reparative therapy	Grade 4	Inappropriate
	Didactic teaching	Grade 2b	Possible
	Brief client-focused counseling	Grade 2a	Probable
Intervention characteristics	Sustained interventions	Grade 1	Strong
	Community-level interventions	Grade 1	Strong
HAART and ARV agent–based prevention modes	Method of secondary prevention	Grade 1	Strong
	Primary prevention	Grade 2b	Probable
	Address substance use and mental health disorders to increase adherence	Grade 2a	Probable
	Chemoprophylaxis (preexposure prophylaxis)	Grade 2a	Probable
Voluntary counseling and testing	HIV testing	Grade 1	Strong
	Rapid testing for HIV	Grade 2a	Probable
	LGBT sensitization	Grade 1	Strong
Circumcision	n.a.	Grade 2b	Possible
Syndromic STI treatment	Herpes simplex virus-2 suppression	Grade 4	Inappropriate
	Screening and treatment of all genital ulcerative diseases	Grade 2a	Probable
Vaccination	HPV	Grade 2a	Probable
Rectal microbicides	n.a.	Grade 2c	Pending
Structural interventions	Decriminalization, government-sponsored antihomophobia policy, mass media engagement, male engagement programs, community systems strengthening, health sector interventions	Grade 1	Strong

Source: Stefan Baral, Chris Beyrer, and Andrea Wirtz.

Note: n.a. = not applicable. The Recommendations generated here employed the HASTE system described in this chapter. This system integrates with equal weight efficacy data from RCTs, implementation science data, and public health plausibility. The inclusion of implementation science data facilitates Strong Recommendations in the absence of RCT data.

science data facilitates the ability to give a strong recommendation for structural approaches in the absence of convincing efficacy data generated from randomized controlled trials caused by the difficulties in operationalizing meaningful randomized controlled trials of these interventions.

Discussion: Implications of Diversity and Consistency

Decreasing the relative burden of disease among MSM will require a concerted effort and a strategic approach that is specifically adapted to each epidemic scenario. This book suggests that any such strategy should include at least three main components: comprehensive surveillance, enhanced research, and targeted prevention programs. The four different scenarios highlight that HIV risk among MSM is significantly affected by the dynamics of contextualizing HIV epidemics.

Countries belonging to scenario 1, by definition, generally have a greater understanding of HIV risk among MSM, and current research focus has transitioned to characterizing effective modes of HIV prevention and active and passive surveillance systems for HIV infection, behavioral outcomes, and syndromic and laboratory-based surveillance for STIs among MSM. In scenario 2 epidemic countries, HIV risk among MSM is generally not well accepted, and research remains focused on parenteral risks. Moreover, research is complicated by the combined risk of injecting drug use among MSM in the context of HIV epidemics driven by such drug use. Some evidence is emerging about effective surveillance and prevention programs for MSM, but very little evaluative data concerns ongoing HIV prevention programs targeting MSM. In the generalized epidemic countries of scenario 3, data about HIV risk among MSM remain limited, with few exceptions, to prevalence studies based on convenience samples, and attention is still focused on heterosexual and vertical transmission. Very few data exist about effective HIV prevention for MSM because research is complicated by increasing stigma and criminalization of sexual minorities. Data from scenario 4 countries have shown that MSM are at high risk, but the attributable fraction has not been well defined. In a few of these settings, such as India and Thailand, research has moved past epidemiologic studies and is focused on prevention studies.

The levels of knowledge of HIV risk among MSM by epidemic scenario highlight the trends in the types of research studies that either have been completed or are needed in these countries. In countries or regions with no bio-behavioral data about MSM, rapid appraisal techniques are needed that focus on quantitatively and qualitatively characterizing HIV risk. Such appraisals would include studies of disease burden and estimations of population size with the goal of demonstrating HIV risk and population attributable fraction; moreover, they would help "fill in the map." Nevertheless, studies of HIV risk among MSM in one country would likely not be generalizable to others. The results of these studies have been used for regional, domestic, and international advocacy and highlight the need for targeted HIV prevention expenditures even in generalized epidemics. These studies also are important in capacity building among local community-based organizations, in fostering partnerships with local academia, and in developing the knowledge base on how to accrue local MSM populations for implementation of prevention studies. Next in the evolution of research would be completion of cohort studies, in part to demonstrate the feasibility of implementing prevention strategies. These studies would also not be generalizable to other countries. If following MSM in often stigmatizing settings is possible, then appropriately powered HIV prevention studies could be put in motion to demonstrate efficacy. Finally, evaluative and outcome studies could be completed to characterize effectiveness among MSM in real-world settings. The results from HIV prevention studies, especially if completed in LMICs, should be somewhat generalizable to other countries with similar social contexts.

Although the science of HIV prevention has made significant progress, consensus has yet to be reached on an effective package of CHPIs for MSM. To some extent, the problem is that a single package of preventive programs will be unable to address the needs of MSM in the varied settings represented by the different epidemic scenarios. Rather, CHPIs would have to be locally adapted based on individual and structural drivers of HIV risk as well as sociocultural contexts.

In broad terms, three levels of CHPIs are available: (a) to address individual-level risks, (b) to target structural risks, and (c) to focus on health sector interventions. All three levels of the CHPI program should be directed to the local needs of MSM.

The individual-level CHPI should include the following elements:

- Outreach and education using a peer-based approach
- VCT targeting individualized risk reduction counseling to reduce sexual risks with both male and female partners

- Behavioral change interventions aimed at increasing condom use, reducing risks in bisexual concurrency, and negotiating condom use with male partners
- STI screening and treatment with a specific focus on STIs of importance to MSM (genital and also oropharyngeal and ano-rectal STIs)
- Referral to care for HIV-positive MSM
- Evaluation of acceptability of participation in research to assess the efficacy of unproven HIV prevention technologies for MSM such as preexposure prophylaxis, circumcision, HIV vaccines, and rectal microbicides

Health care–level interventions should focus on VCT and STI clinic centers and include clinical training and sensitization for health care providers and testing counselors to reduce barriers to appropriate VCT and STI services for MSM. Finally, community systems strengthening is needed to facilitate increased capacity among community-based organizations to increase community penetration of HIV prevention packages, build community social capital, and improve advocacy for inclusion of MSM.

> In countries without laws to protect sex workers, drug users and men who have sex with men, only a fraction of the population has access to prevention. Conversely, in countries with legal protection and the protection of human rights for these people, many more have access to services. As a result, there are fewer infections, less demand for antiretroviral treatment and fewer deaths. Not only is it unethical not to protect these groups; it makes no sense from a health perspective. It hurts all of us.
>
> *Ban Ki-moon, Secretary-General of the United Nations, August 2008*
> (UNAIDS 2009, 1)

An important question that should to be addressed in each epidemic scenario is whether preventive services for MSM should be mainstreamed with HIV prevention programs targeting the general population or should be designed in parallel to these existing structures. Although mainstreaming would likely increase the cost-efficacy of these interventions, significant social stigma and criminalization would limit their efficacy because men in such settings are quite justified in not seeking care. In settings where MSM do not feel safe in seeking care, models of care need to be designed in response to these structural barriers.

References

Abdool Karim, Q., S. S. Abdool Karim, J. A. Frohlich, A. C. Grobler, C. Baxter, L. E. Mansoor, A. B. M. Kharsany, S. Sibeko, K. P. Mlisana, Z. Omar, et al. 2010. "Effectiveness and Safety of Tenofovir Gel, an Antiretroviral Microbicide, for the Prevention of HIV Infection in Women." *Science* 329 (5996): 1168–74.

Altman, D. 2005. "Rights Matter: Structural Interventions and Vulnerable Communities." *Health and Human Rights* 8 (2): 203–13.

Amirkhanian, Y. A., J. A. Kelly, E. Kabakchieva, A. V. Kirsanova, S. Vassileva, J. Takacs, W. J. DiFranceisco, T. L. McAuliffe, R. A. Khoursine, and L. Mocsonaki. 2005. "A Randomized Social Network HIV Prevention Trial with Young Men Who Have Sex with Men in Russia and Bulgaria." *AIDS* 19 (16): 1897–905.

Amirkhanian, Y. A., J. A. Kelly, E. Kabakchieva, T. L. McAuliffe, and S. Vassileva. 2003. "Evaluation of a Social Network HIV Prevention Intervention Program for Young Men Who Have Sex with Men in Russia and Bulgaria." *AIDS Education and Prevention* 15 (3): 205–20.

Ansari, M. T., A. Tsertsvadze, and D. Moher. 2009. "Grading Quality of Evidence and Strength of Recommendations: A Perspective." *PLoS Med* 6 (9): e1000151.

Auvert, B., P. Lissouba, E. Cutler, K. Zarca, A. Puren, and D. Taljaard. 2009. "Is Genital Human Papillomavirus Infection Associated with HIV Incidence?" Presentation at the 5th International AIDS Conference on HIV Pathogenesis, Treatment and Prevention, Cape Town, South Africa, July 19–22.

Auvert, B., D. Taljaard, E. Lagarde, J. Sobngwi-Tambekou, R. Sitta, and A. Puren. 2005. "Randomized, Controlled Intervention Trial of Male Circumcision for Reduction of HIV Infection Risk: The ANRS 1265 Trial." *PLoS Med* 2 (11): e298.

Ayala, G., J. Beck, K. Lauer, R. Reynolds, and M. Sundararaj. 2010. *Social Discrimination against Men Who Have Sex with Men (MSM): Implications for HIV Policy and Programs*. MSMGF Policy Brief. Oakland, CA: Global Forum on MSM & HIV (MSMGF).

Baeten, J. M., C. Celum, and T. J. Coates. 2009. "Male Circumcision and HIV Risks and Benefits for Women." *Lancet* 374 (9685): 182–84.

Baeten, J. M., D. Donnell, S. H. Kapiga, A. Ronald, G. John-Stewart, M. Inambao, R. Manongi, B. Vwalika, C. Celum, and Partners in Prevention HSV/HIV Transmission Study Team. 2010. "Male Circumcision and Risk of Male-to-Female HIV-1 Transmission: A Multinational Prospective Study in African HIV-1-Serodiscordant Couples." *AIDS* 24 (5): 737–44.

Baggaley, R. F., N. M. Ferguson, and G. P. Garnett. 2005. "The Epidemiological Impact of Antiretroviral Use Predicted by Mathematical Models: A Review." *Emerging Themes in Epidemiology* 2: 9.

Baggaley, R. F., G. P. Garnett, and N. M. Ferguson. 2006. "Modelling the Impact of Antiretroviral Use in Resource-Poor Settings." *PLoS Med* 3 (4): 124.

Bailey, R. C., S. Moses, C. B. Parker, K. Agot, I. Maclean, J. N. Krieger, C. F. M. Williams, R. T. Campbell, and J. O. Ndinya-Achola. 2007. "Male Circumcision for HIV Prevention in Young Men in Kisumu, Kenya: A Randomised Controlled Trial." *Lancet* 369 (9562): 643–56.

Baral, S., F. Dausab, N. F. Masenior, S. Iipinge, and C. Beyrer. 2008. "A Systematic Review of HIV Epidemiology and Risk Factors among MSM in Sub-Saharan Africa." Presentation at "AIDS 2008": XVII International AIDS Conference, Mexico City, Mexico, August 3–8.

Baral, S., G. Trapence, F. Motimedi, E. Umar, S. Iipinge, F. Dausab, and C. Beyrer. 2009. "HIV Prevalence, Risks for HIV Infection, and Human Rights among Men Who Have Sex with Men (MSM) in Malawi, Namibia, and Botswana." *PLoS One* 4 (3): e4997.

Beckstead, A. L., and S. L. Morrow. 2004. "Mormon Clients' Experiences of Conversion Therapy: The Need for a New Treatment Approach." *Counseling Psychologist* 32 (5): 651–90.

Begg, C., M. Cho, S. Eastwood, R. Horton, D. Moher, I. Olkin, R. Pitkin, D. Rennie, K. F. Schulz, D. Simel, et al. 1996. "Improving the Quality of Reporting of Randomized Controlled Trials: The CONSORT Statement." *JAMA* 276 (8): 637–39.

Benton, K. W., D. Jolley, A. M. Smith, J. Gerofi, and R. Moodie. 1997. "An Actual Use Comparison of Condoms Meeting Australian and Swiss Standards: Results of a Double-Blind Crossover Trial." *International Journal of STD and AIDS* 8 (7): 427–31.

Beyrer, C. 2007. "HIV Epidemiology Update and Transmission Factors: Risks and Risk Contexts—16th International AIDS Conference Epidemiology Plenary." *Clinical Infectious Diseases* 44 (7): 981–87.

Beyrer, C., T. Sripaipan, S. Tovanabutra, J. Jittiwutikarn, V. Suriyanon, T. Vongchak, N. Srirak, S. Kawichai, M. H. Razak, and D. D. Celentano. 2005. "High HIV, Hepatitis C and Sexual Risks among Drug-Using Men Who Have Sex with Men in Northern Thailand." *AIDS* 19 (14): 1535–40.

Bosch, F. X., A. Lorincz, N. Muñoz, C. J. Meijer, and K. V. Shah. 2002. "The Causal Relation between Human Papillomavirus and Cervical Cancer." *Journal of Clinical Pathology* 55 (4): 244–65.

Bouhnik, A. D., M. Préau, M. A. Schiltz, F. Lert, Y. Obadia, and B. Spire. 2007. "Unprotected Sex in Regular Partnerships among Homosexual Men Living with HIV: A Comparison between Sero-nonconcordant and Seroconcordant Couples (ANRS-EN12-VESPA Study)." *AIDS* 21 (Suppl. 1): S43–48.

Briss, P. A., S. Zaza, M. Pappaioanou, J. Fielding, L. Wright-De Agüero, B. I. Truman, D. P. Hopkins, P. D. Mullen, R. S. Thompson, S. H. Woolf, et al. 2000. "Developing an Evidence-Based Guide to Community Preventive Services—Methods." *American Journal of Preventive Medicine* 18 (Suppl. 1): 35–43.

Brown, E. L., A. Wald, J. P. Hughes, R. A. Morrow, E. Krantz, K. Mayer, S. Buchbinder, B. Koblin, and C. Celum. 2006. "High Risk of Human Immunodeficiency Virus in Men Who Have Sex with Men with Herpes Simplex Virus Type 2 in the EXPLORE Study." *American Journal of Epidemiology* 164 (8): 733–41.

Brown, K., K. Patterson, S. Malone, N. Shaheen, H. Prince, J. Dumond, M. Spacek, P. Heidt, M. Cohen, and A. Kashuba. 2010. "Antiretrovirals for Prevention: Maraviroc Exposure in the Semen and Rectal Tissue of Healthy Male Volunteers after Single and Multiple Dosing." Presentation at the 17th Conference on Retroviruses and Opportunistic Infections, San Francisco, CA, February 16–19.

Buchbinder, S. P., E. Vittinghoff, P. J. Heagerty, C. L. Celum, G. R. Seage, III, F. N. Judson, D. McKirnan, K. H. Mayer, and B. A. Koblin. 2005. "Sexual Risk, Nitrite Inhalant Use, and Lack of Circumcision Associated with HIV Seroconversion in Men Who Have Sex with Men in the United States." *Journal of Acquired Immune Deficiency Syndromes* 39 (1): 82–89.

Burrell, E., S. Baral, C. Beyrer, R. Wood, and L. G. Bekker. 2008. "Exploratory Study to Determine Rights Violations and HIV Prevalence among Township Men Who Have Sex with Men (MSM) in Cape Town, South Africa." Presentation at "AIDS 2008": XVII International AIDS Conference, Mexico City, Mexico, August 3–8.

Butler, L. M., D. H. Osmond, A. G. Jones, and J. N. Martin. 2009. "Use of Saliva as a Lubricant in Anal Sexual Practices among Homosexual Men." *Journal of Acquired Immune Deficiency Syndromes* 50 (2): 162–67.

Byrd, A. D., J. Nicolosi, and R. W. Potts. 2008. "Clients' Perceptions of How Reorientation Therapy and Self-Help Can Promote Changes in Sexual Orientation." *Psychological Reports* 102 (1): 3–28.

Cáceres, C. F. 2002. "HIV among Gay and Other Men Who Have Sex with Men in Latin America and the Caribbean: A Hidden Epidemic?" *AIDS* 16 (Suppl. 3): S23–33.

Cáceres, C., K. Konda, M. Pecheny, A. Chatterjee, and R. Lyerla. 2006. "Estimating the Number of Men Who Have Sex with Men in Low and Middle Income Countries." *Sexually Transmitted Infections* 82 (Suppl. 3): iii3–iii9.

Carballo-Dieguez, A., C. Dolezal, J. A. Bauermeister, W. O'Brien, A. Ventuneac, and K. Mayer. 2008. "Preference for Gel over Suppository as Delivery Vehicle for a Rectal Microbicide: Results of a Randomised, Crossover Acceptability Trial among Men Who Have Sex with Men." *Sexually Transmitted Infections* 84 (6): 483–87.

Carballo-Dieguez, A., Z. Stein, H. Saez, C. Dolezal, L. Nieves-Rosa, and F. Diaz. 2000. "Frequent Use of Lubricants for Anal Sex among Men Who Have Sex with Men: The HIV Prevention Potential of a Microbicidal Gel." *American Journal of Public Health* 90 (7): 1117–21.

Celum, C., A. Wald, J. Hughes, J. Sanchez, S. Reid, S. Delany-Moretlwe, F. Cowan, M. Casapia, A Ortiz, J Fuchs, et al. 2008. "Effect of Aciclovir on HIV-1 Acquisition in Herpes Simplex Virus 2 Seropositive Women and Men Who Have Sex with Men: A Randomised, Double-Blind, Placebo-Controlled Trial." *Lancet* 371 (9630): 2109–19.

Celum, C., A. Wald, J. R. Lingappa, A. S. Magaret, R. S. Wang, N. Mugo, A. Mujugira, J. M. Baeten, J. I. Mullins, J. P. Hughes, et al. 2010. "Acyclovir and Transmission of HIV-1 from Persons Infected with HIV-1 and HSV-2." *New England Journal of Medicine* 362 (5): 427–39.

Chakrapani, V., P. A. Newman, M. Shunmugam, A. McLuckie, and F. Melwin. 2007. "Structural Violence against Kothi-Identified Men Who Have Sex with Men in Chennai, India: A Qualitative Investigation." *AIDS Education and Prevention* 19 (4): 346–64.

Chen, S. Y., S. Gibson, D. Weide, and W. McFarland. 2003. "Unprotected Anal Intercourse between Potentially HIV-Serodiscordant Men Who Have Sex with Men, San Francisco." *Journal of Acquired Immune Deficiency Syndromes* 33 (2): 166–70.

Chesney, M. A., B. A. Koblin, P. J. Barresi, M. J. Husnik, C. L. Celum, G. Colfax, K. Mayer, D. McKirnan, F. N. Judson, et al. 2003. "An Individually Tailored Intervention for HIV Prevention: Baseline Data from the EXPLORE Study." *American Journal of Public Health* 93 (6): 933–38.

Chin-Hong, P. V., M. Husnik, R. D. Cranston, G. Colfax, S. Buchbinder, M. Da Costa, T. Darragh, D. Jones, F. Judson, B. Koblin, et al. 2009. "Anal Human Papillomavirus Infection Is Associated with HIV Acquisition in Men Who Have Sex with Men." *AIDS* 23 (9): 1135–42.

Chin-Hong, P. V., E. Vittinghoff, R. D. Cranston, L. Browne, S. Buchbinder, G. Colfax, M. Da Costa, T. Darragh, D. J. Benet, F. Judson, et al. 2005. "Age-Related Prevalence of Anal Cancer Precursors in Homosexual Men: The EXPLORE Study." *Journal of the National Cancer Institute* 97 (12): 896–905.

Choi, K. H., W. McFarland, and M. Kihara. 2004. "HIV Prevention for Asian and Pacific Islander Men Who Have Sex with Men: Identifying Needs for the Asia Pacific Region." *AIDS Education and Prevention* 16 (1): v–vii.

Choi, K. H., Q. Pan, Z. Ning, and S. Gregorich. 2006. "Social and Sexual Network Characteristics Are Associated with HIV Risk among Men Who Have Sex with Men (MSM) in Shanghai, China." Presentation at "AIDS 2006": XVI International AIDS Conference, Toronto, Canada, August 13–18.

Cianciotto, J., and S. Cahill. 2006. *Youth in the Crosshairs: The Third Wave of Ex-Gay Activism.* Washington, DC: National Gay and Lesbian Taskforce

Policy Institute. http://www.thetaskforce.org/downloads/reports/reports/YouthInTheCrosshair.pdf.

Clarke, M. 2000. "The QUORUM Statement." *Lancet* 355 (9205): 756–57.

Coates, T. J., L. Richter, and C. Cáceres. 2008. "Behavioural Strategies to Reduce HIV Transmission: How to Make Them Work Better." *Lancet* 372 (9639): 669–84.

Colfax, G., T. J. Coates, M. J. Husnik, Y. Huang, S. Buchbinder, B. Koblin, M. Chesney, E. Vittinghoff and the EXPLORE Study Team. 2005. "Longitudinal Patterns of Methamphetamine, Popper (Amyl Nitrite), and Cocaine Use and High-Risk Sexual Behavior among a Cohort of San Francisco Men Who Have Sex with Men." *Journal of Urban Health* 82 (Suppl. 1): i62–i70.

Colfax, G., E. Vittinghoff, M. J. Husnik, D. McKirnan, S. Buchbinder, B. Koblin, C. Celum, M. Chesney, Y. Huang, K. Mayer, S. Bozeman, et al. 2004. "Substance Use and Sexual Risk: A Participant- and Episode-Level Analysis among a Cohort of Men Who Have Sex with Men." *American Journal of Epidemiology* 159 (10): 1002–12.

Cramer, R. J., F. D. Golom, C. T. LoPresto, and S. M. Kirkley. 2008. "Weighing the Evidence: Empirical Assessment and Ethical Implications of Conversion Therapy." *Ethics and Behavior* 18 (1): 93–114.

Cranage, M., S. Sharpe, C. Herrera, A. Cope, M. Dennis, N. Berry, C. Ham, J. Heeney, N. Rezk, A. Kashuba, et al. 2008. "Prevention of SIV Rectal Transmission and Priming of T Cell Responses in Macaques after Local Pre-exposure Application of Tenofovir Gel." *PLoS Med* 5 (8): e157.

da Silva, C. G., D. A. Gonçalves, J. C. Pacca, E. Merchan-Hamann, and N. Hearst. 2005. "Optimistic Perception of HIV/AIDS, Unprotected Sex and Implications for Prevention among Men Who Have Sex with Men, São Paulo, Brazil." *AIDS* (Suppl. 4): S31–36.

Delaney, K. P., B. M. Branson, A. Uniyal, P. R. Kerndt, P. A. Keenan, K. Jafa, A. D. Gardner, D. J. Jamieson, and M. Bulterys. 2006. "Performance of an Oral Fluid Rapid HIV-1/2 Test: Experience from Four CDC Studies." *AIDS* 20 (12): 1655–60.

DHHS Panel on Antiretroviral Guidelines for Adults and Adolescents. 2009. *Guidelines for the Use of Antiretroviral Agents in HIV-1-Infected Adults and Adolescents. December 1, 2009*. Washington DC: Department of Health and Human Services. http://www.aidsinfo.nih.gov/ContentFiles/AdultandAdolescentGL.pdf.

DiClemente, R. J., R. A. Crosby, and M. C. Kegler, eds. 2002. *Emerging Theories in Health Promotion Practice and Research: Strategies for Improving Public Health*. San Francisco, CA: John Wiley & Sons.

Diouf, D., A. Moreau, C. Castle, G. Engelberg, and P. Tapsoba. 2004. "Working with the Media to Reduce Stigma and Discrimination towards MSM in Senegal." Presentation at the XV International AIDS Conference, Bangkok, Thailand, July 14–16.

Donnell, D., J. M. Baeten, J. Kiarie, K. K. Thomas, W. Stevens, C. R. Cohen, J. McIntyre, J. R Lingappa, and C. Celum for the Partners in Prevention HSV/ HIV Transmission Study Team. 2010. "Heterosexual HIV-1 Transmission after Initiation of Antiretroviral Therapy: A Prospective Cohort Analysis." *Lancet* 375 (9731): 2092–98.

D'Souza, G., D. J. Wiley, X. Li, J. S. Chmiel, J. B. Margolick, R. D. Cranston, and L. P. Jacobson. 2008. "Incidence and Epidemiology of Anal Cancer in the Multicenter AIDS Cohort Study." *Journal of Acquired Immune Deficiency Syndromes* 48 (4): 491–99.

Dumond, J. B., K. B. Patterson, A. L. Pecha, R. E. Werner, E. Andrews, B. Damle, R. Tressler, J. Worsley, and A. D. Kashuba. 2009. "Maraviroc Concentrates in the Cervicovaginal Fluid and Vaginal Tissue of HIV-Negative Women." *Journal of Acquired Immune Deficiency Syndromes* 51 (5): 546–53.

Eaton, L. A., S. C. Kalichman, D. N. Cain, C. Cherry, H. L. Stearns, C. M. Amaral, J. A. Flanagan, and H. L. Pope. 2007. "Serosorting Sexual Partners and Risk for HIV among Men Who Have Sex with Men." *American Journal of Preventive Medicine* 33 (6): 479–85.

Ehrhardt, A. A., S. Sawires, T. McGovern, D. Peacock, and M. Weston. 2009. "Gender, Empowerment, and Health: What Is It? How Does It Work?" *Journal of Acquired Immune Deficiency Syndromes* 51 (Suppl. 3): S96–105.

Elam, G., N. Macdonald, F. C. Hickson, J. Imrie, R. Power, C. A. McGarrigle, K. A. Fenton, V. L. Gilbart, H. Ward, and B. G. Evans. 2008. "Risky Sexual Behaviour in Context: Qualitative Results from an Investigation into Risk Factors for Seroconversion among Gay Men Who Test for HIV." *Sexually Transmitted Infections* 84 (6): 473–77.

Ferson, M. J., L. C. Young, and M. L. Stokes. 1998. "Changing Epidemiology of Hepatitis A in the 1990s in Sydney, Australia." *Epidemiology and Infection* 121 (3): 631–36.

Franceschi, S., and H. De Vuyst. 2009. "Human Papillomavirus Vaccines and Anal Carcinoma." *Current Opinion in HIV and AIDS* 4 (1): 57–63.

Friedman, H., A. J. Saah, M. Sherman, A. Busseniers, W. Blackwelder, R. Kaslow, A. M. Ghaffari, R. W. Daniel, and K. V. Shah. 1998. "Human Papillomavirus, Anal Squamous Intraepithelial Lesions, and Human Immunodeficiency Virus in a Cohort of Gay Men." *Journal of Infectious Diseases* 78 (1): 45–52.

Garcia-Lerma, J. G., R. A. Otten, S. H. Qari, E. Jackson, M. E. Cong, S. Masciotra, W. Luo, C. Kim, D. R. Adams, M. Monsour, et al. 2008. "Prevention of Rectal

SHIV Transmission in Macaques by Daily or Intermittent Prophylaxis with Emtricitabine and Tenofovir." *PLoS Med* 5 (2): e28.

Geibel, S., S. Luchters, N. King'ola, E. Esu-Williams, A. Rinyiru, and W. Tun. 2008. "Factors Associated with Self-Reported Unprotected Anal Sex among Male Sex Workers in Mombasa, Kenya." *Sexually Transmitted Diseases* 35 (8): 746–52.

Global HIV Prevention Working Group. 2004. *HIV Prevention in the Era of Expanded Treatment Access.* Kaiser Family Foundation. http://www.globalhivprevention.org/pdfs/Prevention%20in%20Era%20of%20Treatment.pdf.

———. 2007. *Bringing HIV Prevention to Scale: An Urgent Global Priority.* http://www.globalhivprevention.org/pdfs/PWG-HIV_prevention_report_FINAL.pdf.

Goggin, K., R. J. Liston, and J. A. Mitty. 2007. "Modified Directly Observed Therapy for Antiretroviral Therapy: A Primer from the Field." *Public Health Reports* 22 (4): 472–81.

Gold, R. S. 2000. "AIDS Education for Gay Men: Towards a More Cognitive Approach." *AIDS Care* 12 (3): 267–72.

Golombok, S., R. Harding, and J. Sheldon. 2001. "An Evaluation of a Thicker versus a Standard Condom with Gay Men." *AIDS* 15 (2): 245–50.

Granich, R. M., C. F. Gilks, C. Dye, K. M. De Cock, and B. G. Williams. 2009. "Universal Voluntary HIV Testing with Immediate Antiretroviral Therapy as a Strategy for Elimination of HIV Transmission: A Mathematical Model." *Lancet* 73 (9657): 48–57.

Gray, R. H. 2009. "Methodologies for Evaluating HIV Prevention Intervention (Populations and Epidemiologic Settings)." *Current Opinion in HIV and AIDS* 4 (4): 274–78.

Gray, R. H., G. Kigozi, D. Serwadda, F. Makumbi, S. Watya, F. Nalugoda, N. Kiwanuka, L. H. Moulton, M. A. Chaudhary, M. Z. Chen, et al. 2007. "Male Circumcision for HIV Prevention in Men in Rakai, Uganda: A Randomised Trial." *Lancet* 369 (9562): 657–66.

Grohskopf, L. A., R. Gvetadze, S. Pathak, B. O'Hara, K. Mayer, A. Liu, K. Chillag, S. Buchbinder, M. Ackers, L. Paxton, et al. 2010. "Preliminary Analysis of Biomedical Data from the Phase II Clinical Safety Trial of Tenofovir Disoproxil Fumarate (TDF) for HIV-1 Pre-exposure Prophylaxis (PrEP) among U.S. Men Who Have Sex with Men (MSM)." Presentation at the XVIII International AIDS Conference, Vienna, Austria, July 18–23.

Gross, M., S. P. Buchbinder, C. Celum, P. Heagerty, and G. R. Seage III. 1998. "Rectal Microbicides for U.S. Gay Men. Are Clinical Trials Needed? Are They Feasible? HIVNET Vaccine Preparedness Study Protocol Team." *Sexually Transmitted Diseases* 25 (6): 296–302.

Grulich, A. E., M. T. van Leeuwen, M. O. Falster, and C. M. Vajdic. 2007. "Incidence of Cancers in People with HIV/AIDS Compared with Immunosuppressed Transplant Recipients: A Meta-Analysis." *Lancet* 370 (9581): 59–67.

Guanira, J., J. R. Lama, P. Goicochea, P. Segura, O. Montoya, and J. Sanchez. 2007. "How Willing Are Gay Men to 'Cut Off' the Epidemic? Circumcision among MSM in the Andean Region." Presentation at the 4th IAS Conference on HIV Pathogenesis, Treatment and Prevention, Sydney, Australia, July 22–25.

Gupta, G. R., J. O. Parkhurst, J. A. Ogden, P. Aggleton, and A. Mahal. 2008. "Structural Approaches to HIV Prevention." *Lancet* 372 (9640): 764–75.

Guyatt, G. H., A. D. Oxman, G. E. Vist, R. Kunz, Y. Falck-Ytter, P. Alonso-Coello, and H. J. Schünemann for the GRADE Working Group. 2008. "GRADE: An Emerging Consensus on Rating Quality of Evidence and Strength of Recommendations." *BMJ* 336 (7650): 924–26.

Haldeman, D. C. 1994. "The Practice and Ethics of Sexual Orientation Conversion Therapy." *Journal of Consulting and Clinical Psychology* 62 (2): 221–27.

———. 2004. "When Sexual and Religious Orientation Collide: Considerations in Working with Conflicted Same-Sex Attracted Male Clients." *Counseling Psychologist* 32 (5): 691–715.

Halkitis, P. N., K. A. Green, R. H. Remien, M. J. Stirratt, C. C. Hoff, R. J. Wolitski, and J. R. Parsons. 2005. "Seroconcordant Sexual Partnerings of HIV-Seropositive Men Who Have Sex with Men." *AIDS* 19 (Suppl. 1): S77–86.

Hammer, S. M., J. J. Eron Jr., P. Reiss, R. T. Schooley, M. A. Thompson, S. Walmsley, P. Cahn, M. A. Fischl, J. M. Gatell, M. S. Hirsch, et al. 2008. "Antiretroviral Treatment of Adult HIV Infection: 2008 Recommendations of the International AIDS Society-USA Panel." *JAMA* 300 (5): 555–70.

Harawa, N. T., S. Greenland, T. A. Bingham, D. F. Johnson, S. D. Cochran, W. E. Cunningham, D. D. Celentano, B. A. Koblin, M. Lalota, D. Mackellar, et al. 2004. "Associations of Race/Ethnicity with HIV Prevalence and HIV-Related Behaviors among Young Men Who Have Sex with Men in 7 Urban Centers in the United States." *Journal of Acquired Immune Deficiency Syndromes* 35 (5): 526–36.

Hays, R. B., G. M. Rebchook, and S. M. Kegeles. 2003. "The Mpowerment Project: Community-Building with Young Gay and Bisexual Men to Prevent HIV1." *American Journal of Community Psychology* 31 (3–4): 301–12.

Healthy Living Project Team. 2007. "Effects of a Behavioral Intervention to Reduce Risk of Transmission among People Living with HIV: The Healthy Living Project Randomized Controlled Study." *Journal of Acquired Immune Deficiency Syndromes* 44 (2): 213–21.

Herbst, J. H., R. T. Sherba, N. Crepaz, J. B. Deluca, L. Zohrabyan, R. D. Stall, and C. M. Lyles. 2005. "A Meta-Analytic Review of HIV Behavioral Interventions for Reducing Sexual Risk Behavior of Men Who Have Sex with Men." *Journal of Acquired Immune Deficiency Syndromes* 39 (2): 228–41.

Herrera, C., C. Cranage, I. McGowan, P. Anton, and R. J. Shattock. 2009. "Reverse Transcriptase Inhibitors as Potential Colorectal Microbicides." *Antimicrobial Agents and Chemotherapy* 53 (5): 1797–807.

Herrera, L. A., L. Benítez-Bribiesca, A. Mohar, and P. Ostrosky-Wegman. 2005. "Role of Infectious Diseases in Human Carcinogenesis." *Environmental and Molecular Mutagenesis* 45 (2–3): 284–303.

Hill, A. B. 1965. "The Environment and Disease: Association or Causation?" *Proceedings of the Royal Society of Medicine* 58: 295–300.

Holm-Hansen, C., B. Nyombi, and M. Nyindo. 2007. "Saliva-Based HIV Testing among Secondary School Students in Tanzania Using the OraQuick Rapid HIV1/2 Antibody Assay." *Annals of the New York Academy of Sciences* 1098: 461–66.

Holtgrave, D. R., and J. McGuire. 2007. "Impact of Counseling in Voluntary Counseling and Testing Programs for Persons at Risk for or Living with HIV Infection." *Clinical Infectious Diseases* 45(Suppl. 4): S240–43.

Holtgrave, D. R., and S. D. Pinkerton. 2007. "Can Increasing Awareness of HIV Seropositivity Reduce Infections by 50 Percent in the United States?" *Journal of Acquired Immune Deficiency Syndromes* 44 (3): 360–63.

Hospers, H. J., G. Kok, P. Harterink, and O. de Zwart. 2005. "A New Meeting Place: Chatting on the Internet, E-Dating and Sexual Risk Behaviour among Dutch Men Who Have Sex with Men." *AIDS* 19 (10): 1097–101.

Hutchinson, S. J., S. Wadd, A. Taylor, S. M. Bird, A. Mitchell, D. S. Morrison, S. Ahmed, and D. J. Goldberg. 2004. "Sudden Rise in Uptake of Hepatitis B Vaccination among Injecting Drug Users Associated with a Universal Vaccine Programme in Prisons." *Vaccine* 23 (2): 210–14.

Jacobsen, K. H., and J. S. Koopman. 2004. "Declining Hepatitis A Seroprevalence: A Global Review and Analysis." *Epidemiology and Infecttion* 132 (6): 1005–22.

Jameson, D. R., C. L. Celum, L. Manhart, T. W. Menza, and M. R. Golden. 2010. "The Association between Lack of Circumcision and HIV, HSV-2, and Other Sexually Transmitted Infections among Men Who Have Sex with Men." *Sexually Transmitted Diseases* 37 (3): 147–52.

Johnson, W. D., R. M. Diaz, W. D. Flanders, M. Goodman, A. N. Hill, D. Holtgrave, R. Malow, and W. M. McClellan. 2008. "Behavioral Interventions to Reduce Risk for Sexual Transmission of HIV among Men Who Have Sex with Men." *Cochrane Database of Systematic Reviews (Online)* (3): CD001230.

Johnson, W. D., D. R. Holtgrave, W. M. McClellan, W. D. Flanders, A. N. Hill, and M. Goodman. 2005. "HIV Intervention Research for Men Who Have Sex with Men: A 7-Year Update." *AIDS Education and Prevention* 17 (6): 568–89.

Johnston, L. B., and D. Jenkins. 2006. "Lesbians and Gay Men Embrace Their Sexual Orientation after Conversion Therapy and Ex-Gay Ministries: A Qualitative Study." *Social Work in Mental Health* 4 (3): 61–82.

Kahn, J. 2002. "Preventing Hepatitis A and Hepatitis B Virus Infections among Men Who Have Sex with Men." *Clinical Infectious Diseases* 35 (11): 1382–87.

Kahn, J. G., S. M. Kegeles, R. Hays, and N. Beltzer. 2001. "Cost-Effectiveness of the Mpowerment Project, a Community-Level Intervention for Young Gay Men." *Journal of Acquired Immune Deficiency Syndromes* 27 (5): 482–91.

Kaldor, J. M., R. J. Guy, and D. Wilson. 2008. "Efficacy Trials of Biomedical Strategies to Prevent HIV Infection. *Current Opinion in HIV and AIDS* 3 (4): 504–8.

Kalichman, S. C. 2008. "Co-occurrence of Treatment Nonadherence and Continued HIV Transmission Risk Behaviors: Implications for Positive Prevention Interventions." *Psychosomatic Medicine* 70 (5): 593–97.

Kalichman, S. C., L. Eaton, D. White, C. Cherry, H. Pope, D. Cain, and M. O. Kalichman. 2007. "Beliefs about Treatments for HIV/AIDS and Sexual Risk Behaviors among Men Who Have Sex with Men, 1997–2006." *Journal of Behavioral Medicine* 30 (6): 497–503.

Kamb, M. L., M. Fishbein, J. M. Douglas Jr., F. Rhodes, J. Rogers, G. Bolan, J. Zenilman, T. Hoxworth, C. K. Malotte, M. Iatesta, et al. 1998. "Efficacy of Risk-Reduction Counseling to Prevent Human Immunodeficiency Virus and Sexually Transmitted Diseases: A Randomized Controlled Trial. Project RESPECT Study Group." *JAMA* 280 (13): 1161–67.

Kane, M. A. 1995. "Epidemiology of Hepatitis B Infection in North America." *Vaccine* 13 (Suppl. 1): S16–17.

———. 1996. "Global Status of Hepatitis B Immunisation." *Lancet* 348 (9029): 696.

Kegeles, S. M., R. B. Hays, and T. J. Coates. 1996. "The Mpowerment Project: A Community-Level HIV Prevention Intervention for Young Gay Men." *American Journal of Public Health* 86 (8): 1129–36.

Kennedy, C., K. O'Reilly, A. Medley, and M. Sweat. 2007. "The Impact of HIV Treatment on Risk Behaviour in Developing Countries: A Systematic Review." *AIDS Care* 19 (6): 707–20.

Khan, S. 2008. *Second National Country Consultation and Training Meeting on Male Sexual Health in Myanmar: A PSI/Myanmar Workshop; 10th–12th September 2008 Final Technical Report*. Rangoon, Myanmar: PSI/Myanmar.

King, M., and A. Bartlett. 1999. "British Psychiatry and Homosexuality." *British Journal of Psychiatry* 175 (2): 106–13.

Kippax, S. 2008. "Understanding and Integrating the Structural and Biomedical Determinants of HIV Infection: A Way Forward for Prevention." *Current Opinion in HIV and AIDS* 3 (4): 489–94.

Koblin, B. A., M. Chesney, and T. Coates. 2004. "Effects of a Behavioural Intervention to Reduce Acquisition of HIV Infection among Men Who Have Sex with Men: The EXPLORE Randomised Controlled Study." *Lancet* 364 (9428): 41–50.

Koblin, B. A., M. J. Husnik, G. Colfax, Y. Huang, M. Madison, K. Mayer, P. J. Barresi, T. J. Coates, M. A. Chesney, and S. Buchbinder. 2006. "Risk Factors for HIV Infection among Men Who Have Sex with Men." *AIDS* 20 (5): 731–39.

Kreiss, J. K., and S. G. Hopkins. 1993. "The Association between Circumcision Status and Human Immunodeficiency Virus Infection among Homosexual Men." *Journal of Infectious Diseases* 168 (6): 1404–8.

Krieger, J. N., R. C. Bailey, J. C. Opeya, B. O. Ayieko, F. A. Opiyo, D. Omondi, K. Agot, C. Parker, J. O. Ndinya-Achola, S. Moses, et al. 2007. "Adult Male Circumcision Outcomes: Experience in a Developing Country Setting." *Urologia Internationalis* 78 (3): 235–40.

Lalani, T., and C. Hicks. 2007. "Does Antiretroviral Therapy Prevent HIV Transmission to Sexual Partners?" *Current Opinion in HIV and AIDS* 4 (2): 80–85.

Lane, T., H. F. Raymond, S. Dladla, J. Rasethe, H. Struthers, W. McFarland, and J. McIntyre. 2009. "High HIV Prevalence among Men Who Have Sex with Men in Soweto, South Africa: Results from the Soweto Men's Study." *AIDS and Behavior* August 7 [Epub ahead of print].

Lane, T., S. B. Shade, J. McIntyre, and S. F. Morin. 2008. "Alcohol and Sexual Risk Behavior among Men Who Have Sex with Men in South African Township Communities." *AIDS and Behavior* 12 (4 Suppl.): S78–85.

Latkin, C. A., and A. R. Knowlton. 2005. "Micro-social Structural Approaches to HIV Prevention: A Social Ecological Perspective." *AIDS Care* 17 (Suppl. 1): S102–13.

Lima, V. D., R. Harrigan, D. R. Bangsberg, R. S. Hogg, R. Gross, B. Yip, et al. 2009. "The Combined Effect of Modern Highly Active Antiretroviral Therapy Regimens and Adherence on Mortality over Time." *Journal of Acquired Immune Deficiency Syndromes* 50 (5): 529–36.

Lima, V. D., K. Johnston, R. S. Hogg, A. R. Levy, P. R. Harrigan, A. Anema, and J. S. G. Montaner. 2008. "Expanded Access to Highly Active Antiretroviral Therapy: A Potentially Powerful Strategy to Curb the Growth of the HIV Epidemic." *Journal of Infectious Diseases* 198 (1): 59–67.

Lin, K. W., and J. T. Kirchner. 2004. "Hepatitis B." *American Family Physician* 69 (1): 75–82.

Liverpool VCT and A. Parkinson. 2007. *Reducing HIV and STI Transmission among Men Who Have Sex with Men in Kenya*. Nairobi: Liverpool VCT.

Makadon, H. J., K. H. Mayer, J. Potter, and H. Goldhammer, eds. 2008. *Fenway Guide to Lesbian, Gay, Bisexual and Transgender Health*. Philadelphia, PA: American College of Physicians.

Mansergh, G., S. Flores, B. Koblin, S. Hudson, D. McKirnan, and G. N. Colfax. 2008. "Alcohol and Drug Use in the Context of Anal Sex and Other Factors Associated with Sexually Transmitted Infections: Results from a Multi-City Study of High-Risk Men Who Have Sex with Men in the USA." *Sexually Transmitted Infections* 84 (6): 509–11.

Mansergh, G., G. Marks, M. Rader, G. N. Colfax, and S. Buchbinder. 2003. "Rectal Use of Nonoxynol-9 among Men Who Have Sex with Men." *AIDS* 17 (6): 905–9.

Marks, G., N. Crepaz, J. W. Senterfitt, and R. S. Janssen. 2005. "Meta-analysis of High-Risk Sexual Behavior in Persons Aware and Unaware They Are Infected with HIV in the United States: Implications for HIV Prevention Programs." *Journal of Acquired Immune Deficiency Syndromes* 39 (4): 446–53.

Martin, D. J. 1992. "Inappropriate Lubricant Use with Condoms by Homosexual Men." *Public Health Reports* 107 (4): 468–73.

McCormick, A. W., R. P. Walensky, M. Lipsitch, E. Losina, H. Hsu, M. C. Weinstein, A. D. Paltiel, K. A. Freedberg, and G. R. Seage III. 2007. "The Effect of Antiretroviral Therapy on Secondary Transmission of HIV among Men Who Have Sex with Men." *Clinical Infectious Diseases* 44 (8): 1115–22.

McLeroy, K. R., D. Bibeau, A. Steckler, and K. Glanz. 1988. "An Ecological Perspective on Health Promotion Programs." *Health Education Quarterly* 15 (4): 351–77.

McQueen, D. V. 2002. "The Evidence Debate." *Journal of Epidemiology and Community Health* 56 (2): 83–84.

Merson, M. H., J. O'Malley, D. Serwadda, and C. Apisuk. 2008. "The History and Challenge of HIV Prevention." *Lancet* 372 (9637): 475–88.

Merson, M., N. Padian, T. J. Coates, G. R. Gupta, S. M. Bertozzi, P. Piot, P. Mane, M. Bartos, and Lancet HIV Prevention Series Authors. 2008. "Combination HIV Prevention." *Lancet* 372 (9652): 1805–6.

Millett, G. A., H. Ding, J. Lauby, S. Flores, A. Stueve, T. Bingham, A. Carballo-Dieguez, C. Murrill, K. L. Liu, D. Wheeler, et al. 2007. "Circumcision Status and HIV Infection among Black and Latino Men Who Have Sex with Men in 3 US Cities." *Journal of Acquired Immune Deficiency Syndromes* 46 (5): 643–50.

Millett, G. A., S. A. Flores, G. Marks, J. B. Reed, and J. H. Herbst. 2008. "Circumcision Status and Risk of HIV and Sexually Transmitted Infections among Men Who Have Sex with Men: A Meta-Analysis." *JAMA* 300 (14): 1674–84.

Millett, G. A., J. L. Peterson, R. J. Wolitski, and R. Stall. 2006. "Greater Risk for HIV Infection of Black Men Who Have Sex with Men: A Critical Literature Review." *American Journal of Public Health* 96 (6): 1007–19.

Mimiaga, M. J., A. D. Fair, K. H. Mayer, K. Koenen, S. Gortmaker, A. M. Tetu, J. Hobson, and S. A. Safren. 2008. "Experiences and Sexual Behaviors of HIV-Infected MSM Who Acquired HIV in the Context of Crystal Methamphetamine Use." *AIDS Education and Prevention* 20 (1): 30–41.

Mimiaga, M. J., E. Noonan, D. Donnell, S. A. Safren, K. C. Koenen, S. Gortmaker, C. O'Cleirigh, M. A. Chesney, T. J. Coates, B. A. Koblin, et al. 2009. "Childhood Sexual Abuse Is Highly Associated with HIV Risk-Taking Behavior and Infection among MSM in the EXPLORE Study." *Journal of Acquired Immune Deficiency Syndromes* 51 (3): 340–48.

Morin, S. F., S. B. Shade, W. T. Steward, A. W. Carrico, R. H. Remien, M. J. Rotheram-Borus, J. A. Kelly, E. D. Charlebois, M. O. Johnson, M. A. Chesney, et al. 2008. "A Behavioral Intervention Reduces HIV Transmission Risk by Promoting Sustained Serosorting Practices among HIV-Infected Men Who Have Sex with Men." *Journal of Acquired Immune Deficiency Syndromes* 49 (5): 544–51.

Niang, C., A. Moreau, K. Kostermans, H. Binswanger, C. Compaore, M. Diagne, et al. 2004. "Men Who Have Sex with Men in Burkina Faso, Senegal, and The Gambia: The Multi-Country HIV/AIDS Program Approach." Presentation at the XV International AIDS Conference, Bangkok, Thailand, July 14–16.

Nicolosi, J., A. D. Byrd, and R. W. Potts. 2000a. "Beliefs and Practices of Therapists Who Practice Sexual Reorientation Psychotherapy." *Psychological Reports* 86 (2): 689–702.

———. 2000b. "Retrospective Self-Reports of Changes in Homosexual Orientation: A Consumer Survey of Conversion Therapy Clients." *Psychological Reports* 86 (3 Pt 2): 1071–88.

Operario, D., T. Nemoto, T. Ng, J. Syed, and M. Mazarei. 2005. "Conducting HIV Interventions for Asian Pacific Islander Men Who Have Sex with Men: Challenges and Compromises in Community Collaborative Research." *AIDS Education and Prevention* 17 (4): 334–46.

Operario, D., C. D. Smith, E. Arnold, and S. Kegeles. 2010. "The Bruthas Project: Evaluation of a Community-Based HIV Prevention Intervention for African American Men Who Have Sex with Men and Women." *AIDS Education and Prevention* 22 (1): 37–48.

Ostrow, D. G., M. J. Silverberg, R. L. Cook, J. S. Chmiel, L. Johnson, X. Li, L. P. Jacobson, and the Multicenter AIDS Cohort Study. 2008. "Prospective Study of Attitudinal and Relationship Predictors of Sexual Risk in the Multicenter AIDS Cohort Study." *AIDS and Behavior* 12 (1): 127–38.

Otten, R. A., D. K. Smith, D. R. Adams, J. K. Pullium, E. Jackson, C. N. Kim, H. Jaffe, R. Janssen, S. Butera, and T. M. Folks. 2000. "Efficacy of Postexposure Prophylaxis after Intravaginal Exposure of Pig-Tailed Macaques to a Human-Derived Retrovirus (Human Immunodeficiency Virus Type 2)." *Journal of Virology* 74 (20): 9771–75.

Padian, N. S., A. Buve, J. Balkus, D. Serwadda, and W. Cates Jr. 2008. "Biomedical Interventions to Prevent HIV Infection: Evidence, Challenges, and Way Forward." *Lancet* 372 (9638): 585–99.

Palefsky, J. M., E. A. Holly, M. Ralston, and N. Jay. 1998. "Prevalence and Risk Factors for Human Papillomavirus Infection of the Anal Canal in Human Immunodeficiency Virus (HIV)-Positive and HIV-Negative Homosexual Men." *Journal of Infectious Diseases* 77 (2): 361–67.

Pao, D., D. Pillay, and M. Fisher. 2009. "Potential Impact of Early Antiretroviral Therapy on Transmission." *Current Opinion in HIV and AIDS* 4 (3): 215–21.

Patterson, K. P. H., E. Kraft, A. Jones, S. Paul, N. Shaheen, M. Spacek, P. Heidt, S. Reddy, J. Rooney, M. Cohen, et al. 2010. "Extracellular and Intracellular Tenofovir DF and Emtricitabine Exposure in Mucosal Tissue after a Single Dose of Fixed-Dose TDF/FTC: Implications for Pre-exposure Prophylaxis." Presentation at XVIII International AIDS Conference, Vienna, Austria, July 18–23.

Peacock, D., L. Stemple, S. Sawires, and T. J. Coates. 2009. "Men, HIV/AIDS, and Human Rights." *Journal of Acquired Immune Deficiency Syndrome* 51 (Suppl. 3): S119–25.

Petticrew, M., and H. Roberts. 2003. "Evidence, Hierarchies, and Typologies: Horses for Courses." *Journal of Epidemiology and Community Health* 57 (7): 527–29.

Piot, P., M. Bartos, H. Larson, D. Zewdie, and P. Mane. 2008. "Coming to Terms with Complexity: A Call to Action for HIV Prevention." *Lancet* 372 (9641): 845–59.

Poland, G. A., and R. M. Jacobson. 2004. "Clinical Practice: Prevention of Hepatitis B with the Hepatitis B Vaccine." *New England Journal of Medicine* 351 (27): 2832–38.

Porter, R., M. D. Cobbina, K. Hanson, J. D. Dupree, G. Akanlu, and M. Kaplan. 2006. "An Exploratory Study of MSM Social Networks in Urban Ghana." Presentation at "AIDS 2006": XVI International AIDS Conference, Toronto, Canada, August 13–18.

Quinn, T. C., M. J. Wawer, N. Sewankambo, D. Serwadda, C. Li, F. Wabwire-Mangen, M. O. Meehan, T. Lutalo, and R. H. Gray. 2000. "Viral Load and Heterosexual Transmission of Human Immunodeficiency Virus Type 1. Rakai Project Study Group." *New England Journal of Medicine* 342 (13): 921–29.

Reisner, S. L., M. J. Mimiaga, P. Case, C. V. Johnson, S. A. Safren, and K. H. Mayer. 2009. "Predictors of Identifying as a Barebacker among High-Risk New England HIV Seronegative Men Who Have Sex with Men." *Journal of Urban Health* 86 (2): 250–62.

Reisner, S. L., M. J. Mimiaga, M. Skeer, D. Bright, K. Cranston, D. Isenberg, S. Bland, T. A. Barker, and K. H. Mayer. 2009. "Clinically Significant Depressive Symptoms as a Risk Factor for HIV Infection among Black MSM in Massachusetts." *AIDS and Behavior* 13 (4): 798–810.

Renzi, C., S. R. Tabet, J. A. Stucky, N. Eaton, A. S. Coletti, C. M. Surawicz, S. N. Agoff, P. J. Heagerty, M. Gross, and C. L. Celum. 2003. "Safety and Acceptability of the Reality Condom for Anal Sex among Men Who Have Sex with Men." *AIDS* 17 (5): 727–31.

Rhodes, T., G. V. Stimson, N. Crofts, A. Ball, K. Dehne, and L. Khodakevich. 1999. "Drug Injecting, Rapid HIV Spread, and the 'Risk Environment': Implications for Assessment and Response." *AIDS* 13 (Suppl. A): S259–69.

Rietmeijer, C. A., and M. W. Thrun. 2006. "Mainstreaming HIV Testing." *AIDS* 20 (12): 1667–68.

Robertson, M., D. Mehrotra, D. Fitzgerald, A. Duerr, D. Casimiro, J. McElrath, D. Lawrence, and S. Buchbinder. 2008. "Efficacy Results from the STEP Study (Merck V520 Protocol 023/HVTN 502): A Phase II Test-of-Concept Trial of the MRKAd5 HIV-1 Gag/Pol/Nef Trivalent Vaccine." Presentation at the 15th Conference on Retroviruses and Opportunistic Infections (abstract no. 88LB), Boston, MA, February 3–6.

Roddy, R. E., L. Zekeng, K. A. Ryan, U. Tamoufe, and K. G. Tweedy. 2002. "Effect of Nonoxynol-9 Gel on Urogenital Gonorrhea and Chlamydial Infection: A Randomized Controlled Trial." *JAMA* 287 (9): 1117–22.

Roehr, B. 2008. "The Invisible Epidemic." *BMJ* 337: a2566.

Rose, G. 1985. "Sick Individuals and Sick Populations." *International Journal of Epidemiology* 14 (1): 32–38.

Rowniak, S. 2009. "Safe Sex Fatigue, Treatment Optimism, and Serosorting: New Challenges to HIV Prevention among Men Who Have Sex with Men." *Journal of the Association of Nurses in AIDS Care* 20 (1): 31–38.

Russell-Brown, P., C. Piedrahita, R. Foldesy, M. Steiner, and J. Townsend. 1992. "Comparison of Condom Breakage during Human Use with Performance in Laboratory Testing." *Contraception* 45 (5): 429–37.

Ryan, C., and I. Rivers. 2003. "Lesbian, Gay, Bisexual, and Transgender Youth: Victimization and Its Correlates in the USA and UK." *Culture, Health and Sexuality* 5 (2): 103–19.

Rychetnik, L., M. Frommer, P. Hawe, and A. Shiell. 2002. "Criteria for Evaluating Evidence on Public Health Interventions." *Journal of Epidemiology and Community Health* 56 (2): 119–27.

Sadiq, S. T., S. Taylor, A. J. Copas, J. Bennett, S. Kaye, S. M. Drake, S. Kirk, D. Pillay, and I. Weller. 2005. "The Effects of Urethritis on Seminal Plasma HIV-1 RNA Loads in Homosexual Men Not Receiving Antiretroviral Therapy." *Sexually Transmitted Infections* 81 (2): 120–23.

Salomon, E. A., M. J. Mimiaga, M. J. Husnik, S. L. Welles, M. W. Manseau, A. B. Montenegro, S. A. Safren, B. A. Koblin, M. A. Chesney, and K. H. Mayer. 2009. "Depressive Symptoms, Utilization of Mental Health Care, Substance Use and Sexual Risk among Young Men Who Have Sex with Men in EXPLORE: Implications for Age-Specific Interventions." *AIDS and Behavior* 13 (4): 811–21.

Salomon, J. A., D. R. Hogan, J. Stover, K. A. Stanecki, N. Walker, P. D. Ghys, and B. Schwartländer. 2005. "Integrating HIV Prevention and Treatment: From Slogans to Impact." *PLoS Med* 2 (1): e16.

Share-Net (Netherlands Network on Sexual & Reproductive Health and AIDS). 2003. Sexual Behaviour Change and HIV/AIDS: Challenges and Experiences. Amsterdam: Share-Net—Netherlands Network on Sexual & Reproductive Health and AIDS.

Shidlo, A., and M. Schroeder. 2002. "Changing Sexual Orientation: A Consumers' Report." *Professional Psychology: Research and Practice* 33 (3): 249–59.

Silverman, B. G., and T. P. Gross. 1997. "Use and Effectiveness of Condoms during Anal Intercourse: A Review." *Sexually Transmitted Diseases* 24 (1): 11–17.

Simoni, J. M., D. W. Pantalone, M. D. Plummer, and B. Huang. 2007. "A Randomized Controlled Trial of a Peer Support Intervention Targeting Antiretroviral Medication Adherence and Depressive Symptomatology in HIV-Positive Men and Women." *Journal of Health Psychology* 26 (4): 488–95.

Simoni, J. M., C. R. Pearson, D. W. Pantalone, G. Marks, and N. Crepaz. 2006. "Efficacy of Interventions in Improving Highly Active Antiretroviral Therapy Adherence and HIV-1 RNA Viral Load: A Meta-Analytic Review of Randomized Controlled Trials." *Journal of Acquired Immune Deficiency Syndromes* 43 (Suppl. 1): S23–35.

Smith, A. M., D. Jolley, J. Hocking, K. Benton, and J. Gerofi. 1998. "Does Additional Lubrication Affect Condom Slippage and Breakage?" *International Journal of STD and AIDS* 9 (6): 330–35.

Smith, J., S. Moses, M. G. Hudgens, C. Parker, K. Agot, I. Maclean, J. O. Ndinya-Achola, P. J. F. Snijders, C. J. L. M. Meijer, and R. C. Bailey. 2010. "Increased Risk of HIV Acquisition among Kenyan Men with Human Papillomavirus Infection." *Journal of Infectious Diseases* 201 (11): 1677–85.

Snijders, P. J., R. D. Steenbergen, D. A. Heideman, and C. J. Meijer. 2006. "HPV-Mediated Cervical Carcinogenesis: Concepts and Clinical Implications." *Journal of Pathology* 208 (2): 152–64.

Spitzer, R. L. 2003. "Can Some Gay Men and Lesbians Change Their Sexual Orientation? 200 Participants Reporting a Change from Homosexual to Heterosexual Orientation." *Archives of Sexual Behavior* 32 (5): 403–17.

Steigerwald, F., and G. R. Janson. 2003. "Conversion Therapy: Ethical Considerations in Family Counseling." *Family Journal* 11 (1): 55–59.

Steiner, M., C. Piedrahita, L. Glover, C. Joanis, A. Spruyt, and R. Foldesy. 1994. "The Impact of Lubricants on Latex Condoms during Vaginal Intercourse." *International Journal of STD and AIDS* 5 (1): 29–36.

Steiner, M. J., D. Taylor, T. Hylton-Kong, N. Mehta, J. P. Figueroa, D. Bourne, M. Hobbs, and F. Behets. 2007. "Decreased Condom Breakage and Slippage Rates after Counseling Men at a Sexually Transmitted Infection Clinic in Jamaica." *Contraception* 75 (4): 289–93.

Stirratt, M. J., and C. M. Gordon. 2008. "Adherence to Biomedical HIV Prevention Methods: Considerations Drawn from HIV Treatment Adherence Research." *Current HIV/AIDS Reports* 5 (4): 186–92.

Stroup, D. F., J. A. Berlin, S. C. Morton, I. Olkin, G. D. Williamson, D. Rennie, D. Moher, B. J. Becker, T. A. Sipe, and S. B. Thacker.. 2000. "Meta-analysis of Observational Studies in Epidemiology: A Proposal for Reporting. Meta-analysis of Observational Studies in Epidemiology (MOOSE) Group." *JAMA* 2283 (15): 2008–12.

Sturmer, M., H. W. Doerr, A. Berger, and P. Gute. 2008. "Is Transmission of HIV-1 in Non-viraemic Serodiscordant Couples Possible?" *Antiviral Therapy* 13 (5): 729–32.

Sullivan, P. S., O. Hamouda, V. Delpech, J. E. Geduld, J. Prejean, C. Semaille, et al. 2009. "Reemergence of the HIV Epidemic among Men Who Have Sex with Men in North America, Western Europe, and Australia, 1996–2005." *Annals of Epidemiology* 19 (6): 423–31.

Tang, K. C., B. C. K. Choi, and R. Beaglehole. 2008. "Grading of Evidence of the Effectiveness of Health Promotion Interventions." *Journal of Epidemiology and Community Health* 62 (9): 832–34.

Templeton, D. J., F. Jin, L. Mao, G. P. Prestage, B. Donovan, J. Imrie, S. Kippax, J. M. Kaldor, and A. E. Grulich. 2009. "Circumcision and Risk of HIV Infection in Australian Homosexual Men." *AIDS* 23 (17): 2347–51.

Templeton, D. J., F. Jin, G. P. Prestage, B. Donovan, J. Imrie, S. C. Kippax, J. M. Kaldor, and A. E. Grulich. 2007. "Circumcision Status and Risk of HIV Seroconversion in the HIM Cohort of Homosexual Men in Sydney (Abstract WEAC103)." Presented at the 4th IAS Conference on HIV Pathogenesis, Treatment and Prevention, Sydney, Australia, July 22–25.

Tozer, E. E., and M. K. McClanahan. 1999. "Treating the Purple Menace: Ethical Considerations of Conversion Therapy and Affirmative Alternatives." *Counseling Psychologist* 27 (5): 722–42.

UNAIDS (Joint United Nations Programme on HIV/AIDS). 2009. *UNAIDS Action Framework: Universal Access for Men Who Have Sex with Men and Transgender People*. UNAIDS/09.22E/JC1720E. Geneva: UNAIDS.

UNAIDS (Joint United Nations Programme on HIV/AIDS) and WHO (World Health Organization). 2005. *AIDS Epidemic Update: December 2005; Special Report on HIV Prevention*. Geneva: UNAIDS and WHO.

———. 2007. *New Data on Male Circumcision and HIV Prevention: Policy and Programme Implications*. Geneva: UNAIDS and WHO.

UNDP (United Nations Development Programme), ASEAN (Association of Southeast Asian Nations), WHO WPRO and SEARO (World Health Organization Western Pacific Region and Regional Office for South-East Asia), UNESCO (United Nations Educational, Scientific, and Cultural Organization), UNAIDS (Joint United Nations Programme on HIV/AIDS), APCOM (Asia Pacific Coalition on Male Sexual Health), and USAID (U.S. Agency for International Development)/Asia. 2009. *Developing a Comprehensive Package of Services to Reduce HIV among Men Who Have Sex with Men (MSM) and Transgender (TG) Populations in Asia and the Pacific: Regional Consensus Meeting*. Colombo, Sri Lanka: Regional HIV and Development Programme for Asia and the Pacific, UNDP Regional Centre for Asia Pacific.

Vanable, P. A., D. J. McKirnan, S. P. Buchbinder, B. N. Bartholow, J. M. Douglas Jr., F. N. Judson, and K. M. MacQueen. 2004. "Alcohol Use and High-Risk Sexual Behavior among Men Who Have Sex with Men: The Effects of Consumption Level and Partner Type." *Health Psychology* 23 (5): 525–32.

van der Snoek, E. M., H. G. Niesters, P. G. Mulder, G. J. van Doornum, A. D. Osterhaus, and W. I. van der Meijden. 2003. "Human Papillomavirus Infection in Men Who Have Sex with Men Participating in a Dutch Gay-Cohort Study." *Sexually Transmitted Diseases* 30 (8): 639–44.

van Kesteren, N. M., H. J. Hospers, and G. Kok. 2007. "Sexual Risk Behavior among HIV-Positive Men Who Have Sex with Men: A Literature Review." *Patient Education and Counseling* 65 (1): 5–20.

Vermund, S. H., K. L. Allen, and Q. A. Karim. 2009. "HIV-Prevention Science at a Crossroads: Advances in Reducing Sexual Risk." *Current Opinion in HIV and AIDS* 4 (4): 266–73.

Vermund, S. H., and H. Z. Qian. 2008. "Circumcision and HIV Prevention among Men Who Have Sex with Men: No Final Word." *JAMA* 300 (14): 1698–700.

Vernazza, P., B. Hirschel, E. Bernasconi, and M. Flepp. 2008. "HIV Transmission under Highly Active Antiretroviral Therapy." *Lancet* 372 (9652): 1806–7.

Vittinghoff, E., J. Douglas, F. Judson, D. McKirnan, K. MacQueen, and S. P. Buchbinder. 1999. "Per-Contact Risk of Human Immunodeficiency Virus Transmission between Male Sexual Partners." *American Journal of Epidemiology* 150 (3): 306–11.

Voeller, B., A. H. Coulson, G. S. Bernstein, and R. M. Nakamura. 1989. "Mineral Oil Lubricants Cause Rapid Deterioration of Latex Condoms." *Contraception* 39 (1): 95–102.

Walensky, R. P., L. L. Wolf, R. Wood, M. O. Fofana, K. A. Freedberg, N. A. Martinson, A. D. Paltiel, X. Anglaret, M. C. Weinstein, and E. Losina for the CEPAC (Cost-Effectiveness of Preventing AIDS Complications)-International Investigators. 2009. "When to Start Antiretroviral Therapy in Resource-Limited Settings." *Annals of Internal Medicine* 151 (3): 157–66.

Wawer, M. J., R. H. Gray, N. K. Sewankambo, D. Serwadda, X. Li, O. Laeyendecker, N. Kiwanuka, G. Kigozi, M. Kiddugavu, T. Lutalo, et al. 2005. "Rates of HIV-1 Transmission Per Coital Act, by Stage of HIV-1 Infection, in Rakai, Uganda." *Journal of Infectious Diseases* 191 (9): 1403–9.

Weatherburn, P., F. Hickson, D. S. Reid, P. M. Davies, and A. Crosier. 1998. "Sexual HIV Risk Behaviour among Men Who Have Sex with Both Men and Women." *AIDS Care* 10 (4): 463–71.

Weller, S., and K. Davis-Beaty. 2002. "Condom Effectiveness in Reducing Heterosexual HIV Transmission." *Cochrane Database of Systematic Reviews* (1): CD003255.

Wellings, K., M. Collumbien, E. Slaymaker, S. Singh, Z. Hodges, D. Patel, and N. Bajos. 2006. "Sexual Behaviour in Context: A Global Perspective." *Lancet* 368 (9548): 1706–28.

White, N., K. Taylor, A. Lyszkowski, J. Tullett, and C. Morris. 1988. "Dangers of Lubricants Used with Condoms." *Nature* 335 (6185): 19.

WHO (World Health Organization). 1986. "Ottawa Charter for Health Promotion." WHO/HPR/HEP/95.1. Charter adopted at First International Conference on Health Promotion, Ottawa, Canada, November 21.

WHO (World Health Organization), UNAIDS (Joint United Nations Programme on HIV/AIDS), and UNICEF (United Nations Children's Fund). 2009. *Towards Universal Access: Scaling Up Priority HIV/AIDS Interventions in the Health Sector: Progress Report 2009*. Geneva: WHO.

Wiley, D. J., D. M. Harper, D. Elashoff, M. J. Silverberg, C. Kaestle, R. L. Cook, M. Heilemann, and L. Johnson. 2005. "How Condom Use, Number of Receptive Anal Intercourse Partners and History of External Genital Warts Predict Risk for External Anal Warts." *International Journal of STD and AIDS* 16 (3): 203–11.

Wilson, D., and D. T. Halperin. 2008. "'Know Your Epidemic, Know Your Response': A Useful Approach, If We Get It Right." *Lancet* 372 (9637): 423–26.

Wilson, D. P., M. G. Law, A. E. Grulich, D. A. Cooper, and J. M. Kaldor. 2008. "Relation between HIV Viral Load and Infectiousness: A Model-Based Analysis." *Lancet* 372 (9635): 314–20.

Woody, G. E., D. Donnell, G. R. Seage, D. Metzger, M. Marmor, B. A. Koblin, S. Buchbinder, M. Gross, B. Stone, and F. N. Judson. 1999. "Non-injection Substance Use Correlates with Risky Sex among Men Having Sex with Men: Data from HIVNET." *Drug and Alcohol Dependence* 53 (3): 197–205.

Zablotska, I. B., J. Imrie, G. Prestage, J. Crawford, P. Rawstorne, A. Grulich, J. Fengyi, and S. Kippax. 2009. "Gay Men's Current Practice of HIV Seroconcordant Unprotected Anal Intercourse: Serosorting or Seroguessing?" *AIDS Care* 21 (4): 501–10.

Zaric, G. S., A. M. Bayoumi, M. L. Brandeau, and D. K. Owens. 2008. "The Cost-Effectiveness of Counseling Strategies to Improve Adherence to Highly Active Antiretroviral Therapy among Men Who Have Sex with Men." *Medical Decision Making* 28 (3): 359–76.

Zuckerman, R. A., A. Lucchetti, W. L. Whittington, J. Sanchez, R. W. Coombs, A. Magaret, A. Wald, L. Corey, and C. Celum. 2009. "HSV Suppression Reduces Seminal HIV-1 Levels in HIV-1/HSV-2 Co-infected Men Who Have Sex with Men." *AIDS* 23 (4): 479–83.

Zuckerman, R. A., A. Lucchetti, W. L. Whittington, J. Sanchez, R. W. Coombs, R. Zuniga, A. S. Magaret, A. Wald, L. Corey, and C. Celum. 2007. "Herpes Simplex Virus (HSV) Suppression with Valacyclovir Reduces Rectal and Blood Plasma HIV-1 Levels in HIV-1/HSV-2-Seropositive Men: A Randomized, Double-Blind, Placebo-Controlled Crossover Trial." *Journal of Infectious Diseases* 196 (10): 1500–8.

PART III

Modeling

CHAPTER 9

Modeling MSM Populations, HIV Transmission, and Intervention Impact

Key themes:

- The population of men who have sex with men (MSM) varies in number of sexual partners and risks for HIV; as for heterosexual populations, these differences can and should be taken into account when developing and evaluating HIV prevention programs.
- By 2015, the proportion of new infections attributed to behavior of MSM in these case studies can range from 12 percent in Kenya to 95 percent in Perù if coverage of interventions for MSM remains at current levels.
- Modeling projections that include four risk groups of MSM indicate that MSM-specific interventions (community-based behavioral interventions, distribution of condoms and lubricants with risk reduction counseling, and expanded access and use of antiretrovirals [ARVs]) positively impact new infections among the general population.
- In countries where the epidemic is increasing and MSM are the predominant or significant exposure mode for HIV infection (as in Peru and Thailand, respectively), an increase in coverage of MSM-specific interventions could change the trajectory of the HIV epidemic.

Developing an evidence-based response to the HIV epidemic requires understanding of a country's epidemic features, as described by the epidemic scenarios in part I of this book; assessment of the costs for various response options; and knowledge of appropriate and effective interventions for prevention, treatment, and care. Understanding the fractions of HIV attributable to same-sex practices among men by country and region is important to understanding and responding to the HIV epidemic because a growing body of evidence suggests that MSM as a group of populations constitute a significant portion of the HIV epidemic in many low- and middle-income countries (LMICs). Such calculations can then be used in tandem with mathematical models and cost estimates to assess and estimate appropriate interventions to meet public health priorities in a selected country, which is the focus of chapter 10. Particularly for HIV interventions, mathematical models and cost analysis can be used to inform national and local programming by providing estimates of resources and funding necessary to reach targets, identifying effective combinations or alternative interventions, and identifying the achievements possible with available resources (Stover, Bollinger, and Cooper-Arnold 2003).

Adapting and Using the Goals Model to Estimate HIV Prevalence and Incidence

For this analysis, the Goals Model (see www.futuresinstitute.org/pages/Goals.aspx) was used to estimate HIV prevalence and incidence, with and without one or more interventions delivered at different levels of coverage. The Goals Model is a deterministic model that uses data in three main areas to project HIV prevalence and incidence: demography, sexual behavior, and HIV and sexually transmitted infection (STI) prevalence estimates. Before this effort, the Goals Model considered five different risk groups, stratified by gender, in the general population: MSM, injecting drug users (IDUs), high-risk heterosexuals, medium-risk heterosexuals, and low-risk heterosexuals. Recognizing the social and behavioral variations that exist among MSM and that not all MSM are inherently high risk, as the model assumed, the researchers for this book undertook a collaborative effort with the Futures Institute to revise the Goals Model to allow the input of epidemiologic data relating to four risk categories among MSM. These risk categories are now defined as follows:

- High-risk MSM, who are male sex workers who engage in sex with men
- Medium-risk MSM, who are men with more than one male sex partner in the last 12 months

- Low-risk MSM, who are men with no or one male sex partner in the last 12 months (that may be a stable relationship)
- MSM-IDU, who are MSM who also inject drugs

The adapted program now accommodates estimates of the proportion of the male population constituting MSM in each of these four risk groups and accommodates the HIV and STI prevalence estimates and behavioral inputs of each MSM risk group among the overall male populations.

To investigate the effect of implementing MSM-specific interventions on the HIV epidemic among the population of MSM as well as the general population for this book, the researchers adapted the Goals Model to include the distribution of condoms with water-based lubricants (acknowledging that water-based lubricants must be provided with condoms to maintain condom efficacy in anal intercourse) and community-based behavioral interventions. The effects of these interventions, in addition to access to ARVs, can provide insight into the effects of proven interventions and possible combinations for reaching national targets.

Using the Goals Model, this chapter also provides calculations of the fraction of all new HIV cases attributable to MSM behavior. These attributable fraction estimates are given for each of the four countries examined (that is, Kenya, Peru, Thailand, and Ukraine). The impact of these interventions is then modeled with varying coverage levels and combinations of interventions, using inputs for a country example from each epidemic scenario. Furthermore, these modeling exercises were performed to demonstrate the utility of the Goals Model to inform strategic planning and the variation in results observed across epidemic scenarios and environments.

Methods

The attributable fraction of HIV transmission with same-sex behavior and impacts of HIV interventions for MSM were estimated for representative countries using national data and updated assumptions of the Goals Model that reflect the most current research findings.

Inputs and Assumptions for the Goals Model

Because Goals is a deterministic model, it requires data in three main areas to project HIV prevalence and incidence: national data for MSM and the general population on (a) demography, (b) sexual behavior, and (c) HIV and STI prevalence (Stover, Bollinger, and Cooper-Arnold 2003). MSM-specific data were collected by communicating with country experts, whereas information specific to the general population, including HIV and STI prevalence percentages, intervention coverage, and other country background data, was collected from reports by the Joint United Nations Programme on HIV/AIDS (UNAIDS), the United Nations General Assembly Special Session (UNGASS) on HIV/AIDS, the U.S. Agency for International Development, and various ministries of health (MOHs). The assistance from in-country experts to collect MSM-specific data has allowed this book to address issues specific to the modeling work, such as variability in definitions, recall periods, and data that are collected and accessibility of data. Such collaborations ensure the accuracy and validity of country-specific data. Where MSM-specific data were not available from local experts, UNAIDS reports and peer-reviewed publications provided missing information. Other assumptions of transmission multipliers, intervention effectiveness, and time-in-infection stages were preloaded into the Goals Model from previous work (Case 2010b), and these assumptions can be found in table 9.1.

Scenario 1 focused on Peru, and reports from UNAIDS and UNGASS (UNAIDS and WHO 2008b, 2009) and the Peruvian MOH (INEI 2010; MINSA 2009, 2010) were used to obtain STI and HIV prevalence, behavioral, and intervention coverage inputs among the general population. The 2009 paper by Aldridge and colleagues (2009), who conducted similar modeling work, was used to provide any missing information.

Scenario 2 focused on Ukraine, with general population data provided by the Futures Institute and Imperial College in preparation for aids2031 (Case 2010d); IDU and MSM prevalence and behavioral data were derived from UNAIDS/MOH reports (UNAIDS and Ministry of Health of Ukraine 2008) and published papers (Amjadeen 2005; Balakiryeva et al. 2008; Kruglov et al. 2008). Data from the Russian Federation were used as a proxy for data specific to the MSM IDU category (Amirkhanian, Kelly, and Issayev 2001; Baral et al. 2010; Kelly et al. 2002; Sergeyev and Gorbachev 2008; Sifakis et al. 2008; Tyusova et al. 2009; WHO Regional Office for Europe 2007). Current MSM and ARV intervention coverage data were obtained from UNGASS/MOH reports (UNAIDS and Ministry of Health of Ukraine 2008), and data on IDU intervention coverage were drawn from a systematic review (Mathers et al. 2010).

Scenario 3 focused on Kenya with general prevalence data provided from aids2031 work (Case 2010a). Prevalence of MSM in the population was calculated using data from peer-reviewed publications (Onyango-Ouma, Birungi, and Geibel 2005; Sanders et al. 2007); prevalence of HIV

Table 9.1 Goals Model Epidemiology Inputs and Assumptions for Select Countries

Input	*Peru*	*Thailand*	*Ukraine*	*Kenya*
Relative infectiousness by stage				
Primary infection	8.000	15.500	9.000	22.000
Asymptomatic stage	1.000	1.000	1.000	1.000
Symptomatic stage (no ART)	4.000	4.000	4.000	4.000
Symptomatic stage (with ART)	0.075[a]	0.075[a]	0.075[a]	0.075[a]
Transmissibility				
Transmission of HIV per act (female to male)	0.001	0.001	0.001	0.001
Transmission multiplier for male to female	1.000	1.000	1.000	1.000
Transmission multiplier for STI	6.000	7.200	7.200	7.200
Transmission multiplier for MSM contacts	2.200	2.200	2.200	2.500
Months in primary stage	3.000	3.000	3.000	3.000
Time in asymptomatic stage (years)	8.000	8.000	8.000	8.000
Time in symptomatic stage (years)	3.000	3.000	3.000	3.000
Intervention				
Condom efficacy (0–1)	0.800	0.800	0.800	0.800
Reduction in male susceptibility when circumcised (0–100%)	60.000	60.000	60.000	60.000
Reduction in male infectiousness when circumcised (0–100%)	30.000	30.000	30.000	30.000
Microbicide effectiveness (0–1)	0.800	0.800	0.800	0.800
Preexposure prophylaxis effectiveness (0–1)	0.600	0.600	0.600	0.600
Size of initial pulse of infection (0–0.01)	0.001	0.000	0.001	0.008
Proportion of adults on ART surviving to the following year (0–1)	0.890	0.950	0.900	0.950

Source: Authors with L. Bollinger.
a. Based on a calculation of 92.5 percent reduction in infectivity while on ART reported by Donnell et al. 2010.

and STIs, and behavioral data were provided by experts from the Kenya Medical Research Institute (E. Sanders, pers. comm. with S. Baral, Kenya, 2010); and coverage of MSM-specific interventions was obtained from UNGASS/MOH reports (UNAIDS and WHO 2008a).

Finally, scenario 4 focused on Thailand; general population data were drawn from aids2031 work (Case 2010b), IDU and MSM epidemiologic and behavioral data were collected with assistance from the Bangkok MSM cohort research experts (F. van Griensven and W. Wimonsate, pers. comm. with S. Baral, C. Beyrer, and A. Wirtz, Baltimore and Bangkok, 2010) and from data published in the Asian Epidemic Model (A^2 and Thai Working Group on HIV/AIDS Projections 2008) and other publications from the U.S. Centers for Disease Control and Prevention, the Thai Red Cross, Thailand's Ministry of Public Health, and other regional experts (Beyrer et al. 2005; CDC 2006; Kunawararak et al. 1995; van

Griensven et al. 2005, 2009; Wimonsate et al. 2008). Coverage of interventions was obtained from UNGASS/MOH reports.

Regarding Goals inputs in general epidemiology, the work conducted for aids2031 contributed to most inputs on transmissibility, infectiousness, and intervention effectiveness (Case 2010c). The item "infectiousness when on ART" was updated with the recent finding by Donnell and colleagues (2010) who reported a 92.5 percent reduction in HIV transmission after ARV treatment was initiated (see table 9.1). Aids2031 also contributed to the matrices used in the Goals Model detailing impact of exposure to a prevention intervention on the following: reduction in nonuse of condoms, reduction in nontreatment of STIs, reduction in number of partners, and increase in age at first sex for the high-, medium-, and low-risk heterosexual and IDU populations. Because two new interventions for MSM were added, the effects of exposure to MSM prevention interventions were derived through systematic review of HIV prevention interventions for MSM. The results of the systematic review were added to the impact matrix for each MSM risk group (table 9.2).

For these inputs, a meta-analysis was completed to develop summary estimates of the reductions in unprotected anal intercourse or the corollary of increase in condom use rates during anal intercourse. Studies were weighted by their relative sample sizes. These summary estimates were stratified using three different variables to assess the differential benefit of interventions for MSM. The first stratum focused on the risk status of the participants in the intervention studies; high-risk participants were defined as sex workers, medium risk meant having more than one partner in the last 12 months, and low risk was having zero or one partner in the last 12 months. The second stratum focused on the level of the intervention,

Table 9.2 Goals Impact Matrix for MSM-Specific Interventions and Impacts on MSM Risk Categories: Results of a Systematic Review

	Reduction in condom nonuse			*Reduction in number of partners*		
	High risk MSM	*Medium risk MSM*	*Low risk MSM*	*High risk MSM*	*Medium risk MSM*	*Low risk MSM*
Intervention	*% reduction (range)*	*% reduction (range)*	*% reduction (range)*	*% reduction (range)*	*% reduction (range)*	*% reduction (range)*
Outreach	−19.6 (−8.1 to −29.9)	−19.6 (−8.1 to −29.9)	−19.6 (−8.1 to −29.9)	−19.0 (−0.7 to −25.0)	−19.0 (−0.7 to −25.0)	−19.0 (−0.7 to −25.0)
Provision of condoms and lubricants	−22.8 (−0.6 to −26.0)	−17.4 (−2.0 to −58.78)	−6.9 (−4.0 to −9.0)	−18.3 (−1.1 to −25.0)	−0.8 (0 to −3.8)	0

Source: Authors with L. Bollinger.
Note: Figures in parentheses represent lower and upper ranges.

differentiating between individual-level interventions (the package of condoms with lubricant and partner reduction counseling) and those implemented and evaluated at the level of communities (community-based behavioral intervention). The third stratum differentiated between those studies that explicitly discussed the inclusion and provision of lubricants as part of the intervention and those that did not. For the stratified meta-analysis, studies were again weighted by sample size.

Estimating the Attributable Fraction

Estimation of the total fraction of new HIV-positive cases attributable to same-sex behavior of MSM is nested in the overall Goals Model analyses for each of the case countries. The number of new HIV infections used for the baseline was estimated by the Goals Model in each country's current state (that is, without any interventions added to what is currently in place in 2007). Next, the HIV transmission probability for MSM was assumed to be zero so that the counterfactual could be used to estimate the number of new HIV infections *not* attributed to MSM behavior. The numerator, in turn, for the attributable fraction was calculated as the number of new HIV cases not attributed to MSM subtracted from the total number of new HIV cases; the denominator was the number of total new HIV cases. The fraction is presented for year 2015 for each case country.

Estimating Impact

MSM-specific interventions to prevent HIV infections were assessed using multiple intervention scenarios with the outcome being total new infections. MSM-specific interventions modeled were individual-level distribution of condoms with water-based lubricants coupled with partner reduction counseling, and community-based behavioral interventions. These interventions were modeled in three scenarios:

1. Null: current coverage drops to zero after 2007 for MSM-specific interventions only, all other interventions—including antiretroviral therapy (ART) for MSM and interventions for IDUs—remaining constant.
2. Current: coverage remains constant at current levels for MSM-specific community-based behavioral intervention and individual interventions, all other interventions remaining constant (including ART for MSM and interventions for IDUs).
3. Full (100 percent) coverage for MSM: community-based behavioral interventions and individual interventions increase to 100 percent

from the 2007 coverage level, and ARV coverage increases by a percentage estimated as sufficient to cover the estimated population of MSM living with HIV by 2015. The Goals Model currently does not allow targeted ARV coverage for specific risk groups; therefore, this parameter was calculated by using current ARV coverage data and then estimating the percentage of those on ARVs who may be HIV-positive MSM. The proportion of MSM with unmet need for ARV was then added to the current coverage level. *For this exercise only, the assumption is that the increase in ARVs will go strictly to the HIV-positive population of MSM.* This third scenario can be used to estimate the impact of a supportive environment in which interventions for MSM are fully provided and HIV-positive MSM have full access to ARVs.

For countries with an HIV epidemic among IDUs (Thailand and Ukraine), a fourth scenario was modeled that assessed an increase in coverage of services by 2015 to reach 100 percent coverage of interventions for MSM (scenario 3 above) plus 60 percent coverage of IDU services, including substitution therapy, harm reduction, and counseling services.

Sensitivity analyses were performed using upper and lower bounds of impacts of MSM-specific interventions determined by the systematic review described above for the most comprehensive intervention scenarios in each country (scenario 3 for Peru and Kenya and scenario 4 for Ukraine and Thailand). These sensitivity analyses are represented as "high range" and "low range" in the following modeling figures.

Results

Estimations of the proportion of new infections attributed to behavior of MSM in these case studies can range from 12 percent in Kenya to 95 percent in Peru, by 2015, if coverage of interventions for MSM remains at current levels. How to address and respond to this range of transmission can be depicted through modeling projections that include MSM populations and interventions. These projections show the impact on the general population by applying MSM-specific interventions across the range of epidemic scenarios.

Estimating the Attributable Fraction in Selected Countries

Assuming HIV prevention interventions and ARV coverage were to remain at current levels, the proportion of new HIV cases attributed to behavior of MSM in 2015 varies across the four selected countries (table 9.3 and figure 9.1). Such behavior will contribute 95.4 percent,

Table 9.3 Attributable Fraction of New HIV Infections from MSM Behavior in Selected Countries, 2015

Country	*Number of new HIV cases*	*Proportion of all new HIV cases (%)*
Peru		
Total population	19,947	100.0
Attributed to MSM behavior	19,021	95.4
Ukraine		
Total population	38,594	100.0
Attributed to MSM behavior	8,535	22.1
Kenya		
Total population	94,047	100.0
Attributed to MSM behavior	11,530	12.3
Thailand		
Total population	27,238	100.0
Attributed to MSM behavior	16,374	39.9

Source: Authors.

Figure 9.1 Percentage of New HIV Infections Attributed to MSM Behavior in Selected Countries, 2015

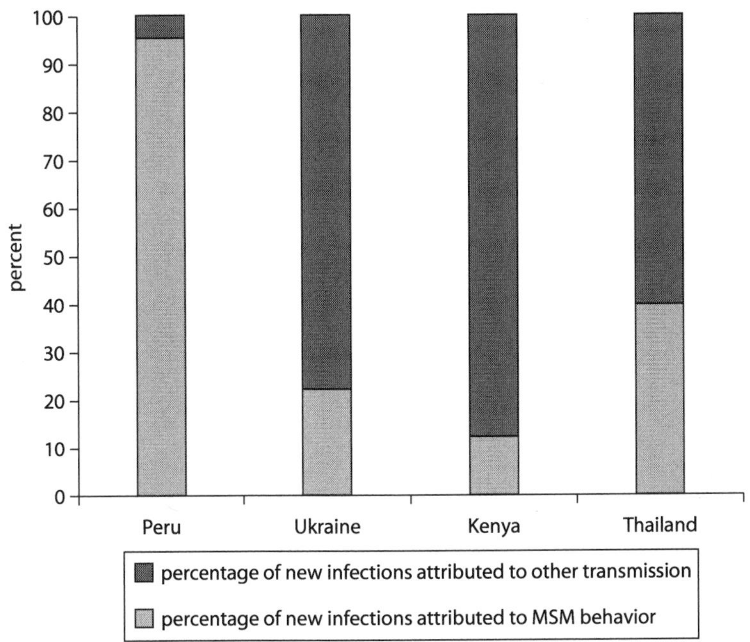

Source: Authors.

Table 9.4 New HIV Cases Attributed to MSM Behavior, by Selected Country Annually, 2010–15

Country	*2010*	*2011*	*2012*	*2013*	*2014*	*2015*
Peru						
Total new HIV cases	16,002	16,960	17,726	18,533	19,262	19,947
New HIV cases *not* attributed to MSM behavior	973	967	957	947	937	926
New HIV cases attributed to MSM behavior	15,029	15,993	16,769	17,586	18,325	19,021
Percentage attributed to MSM behavior	93.9	94.3	94.6	94.9	95.1	95.4
Ukraine						
Total new HIV cases	46,590	43,807	41,848	40,443	39,413	38,594
New HIV cases *not* attributed to MSM behavior	34,757	32,952	31,758	31,002	30,487	30,059
New HIV cases attributed to MSM behavior	11,833	10,855	10,090	9,441	8,926	8,535
Percentage attributed to MSM behavior	25.4	24.8	24.1	23.3	22.6	22.1
Kenya						
Total new HIV cases	105,689	103,637	101,425	99,027	96,549	94,047
New HIV cases *not* attributed to MSM behavior	95,526	93,205	90,706	88,052	85,311	82,517
New HIV cases attributed to MSM behavior	10,163	10,432	10,719	10,975	11,238	11,530
Percentage attributed to MSM behavior	9.6	10.1	10.6	11.1	11.6	12.3
Thailand						
Total new HIV cases	22,148	22,273	22,684	23,514	24,952	27,238
New HIV cases *not* attributed to MSM behavior	19,352	18,795	18,213	17,609	16,993	16,374
New HIV cases attributed to MSM behavior	2,796	3,478	4,471	5,905	7,959	10,864
Percentage attributed to MSM behavior	12.62	15.62	19.71	25.11	31.90	39.89

Source: Authors.

22.1 percent, 12.3 percent, and 39.9 percent of all new HIV infections in Peru, Ukraine, Kenya, and Thailand, respectively, in 2015.

These proportions include HIV infections among heterosexuals, MSM, and IDUs, where HIV transmission is attributed to same-sex behavior among men, thus accounting for bridge populations (that is, MSM who inject drugs, female IDUs, and female sex partners of bisexual men). The attributable proportion needs to be examined in relation to all other risk groups contributing to the total number of HIV cases in a given country during a given year.

As seen in table 9.4, between 2010 and 2015, the absolute number of new HIV cases attributed to behavior of MSM as well as the MSM attributable fraction is increasing in Peru and Thailand—though to a lesser degree in Thailand than in Peru—thus highlighting the predominance of MSM in these countries' overall HIV epidemics. The prevalence of HIV among IDUs in Thailand may account for a significant proportion of the remaining 60 percent of HIV that is attributed to other modes of transmission. In Ukraine, both the absolute number of new HIV cases attributed to MSM behavior and the MSM attributable fraction are slowly decreasing with time, denoting an influence of the course of the overall HIV epidemic on the course of the HIV epidemic among MSM in this country. Finally, both the absolute number of new HIV cases attributed to MSM behavior and the MSM attributable fraction are increasing in Kenya, despite a small incremental decrease in the overall HIV epidemic. This estimate may suggest that HIV infection among MSM in Kenya is emerging as a continuously significant contributor, and it may occur in relative isolation to the HIV epidemic among heterosexuals. Modeling the attributable fraction, therefore, corroborates the conceptualization of the epidemic scenarios presented in part I of this book. Ultimately, the attributable fraction can be used to allocate HIV prevention resources and target programs on the basis of contribution of risk groups to local HIV incidence.

Estimating the Impacts

Figures 9.2 to 9.5 display the projected effect of the interventions and coverage levels for the countries representing each epidemic scenario. Tables 9.5 to 9.8 show the numbers of new HIV infections for each country stratified by intervention combination.

Projections from Peru show that if coverage levels for interventions for MSM and ARVs remain constant, the number of new HIV infections in the general population will increase to reach almost 20,000 new infections by 2015. Much higher coverage of interventions for MSM will be needed to change the trajectory of HIV in Peru; increasing MSM-specific interventions to 100 percent and providing HIV-positive MSM with increased access to ARVs may begin to achieve a decrease in the epidemic or may stabilize the epidemic at the minimum.

In Ukraine, the current coverage of MSM-specific interventions is low and mirrors the effect on the general population that is observed when

Figure 9.2 Projections of the Number of New HIV Infections with Implementation of Three Intervention Scenarios for MSM, Peru, 2008–15

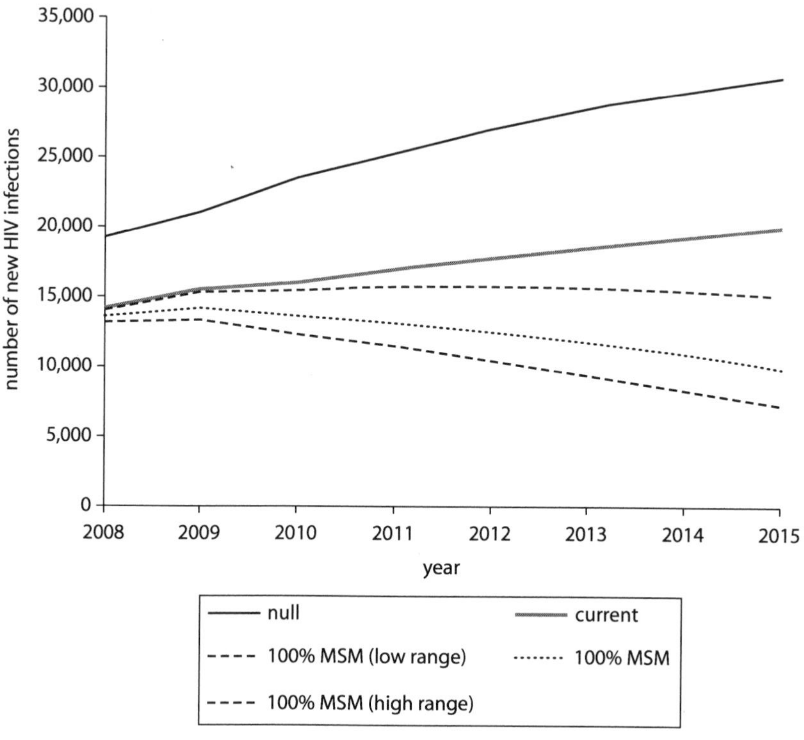

Source: Authors with L. Bollinger.

Table 9.5 Number of Estimated New HIV Infections with Implementation of Three Intervention Scenarios for MSM, Peru, 2008–15

Year	*Null*	*Current*	*100% MSM (low)*	*100% MSM*	*100% MSM (high)*
2008	19,232	14,149	14,101	13,556	13,160
2009	21,077	15,519	15,350	14,179	13,365
2010	23,499	16,002	15,387	13,521	12,274
2011	25,301	16,960	15,765	13,145	11,470
2012	27,066	17,726	15,795	12,464	10,432
2013	28,520	18,533	15,743	11,730	9,400
2014	29,772	19,262	15,501	10,886	8,340
2015	30,757	19,947	15,116	9,984	7,300

Source: Authors with L. Bollinger.

Figure 9.3 Projections of the Number of New HIV Infections with Implementation of Four Intervention Scenarios for MSM, Ukraine, 2008–15

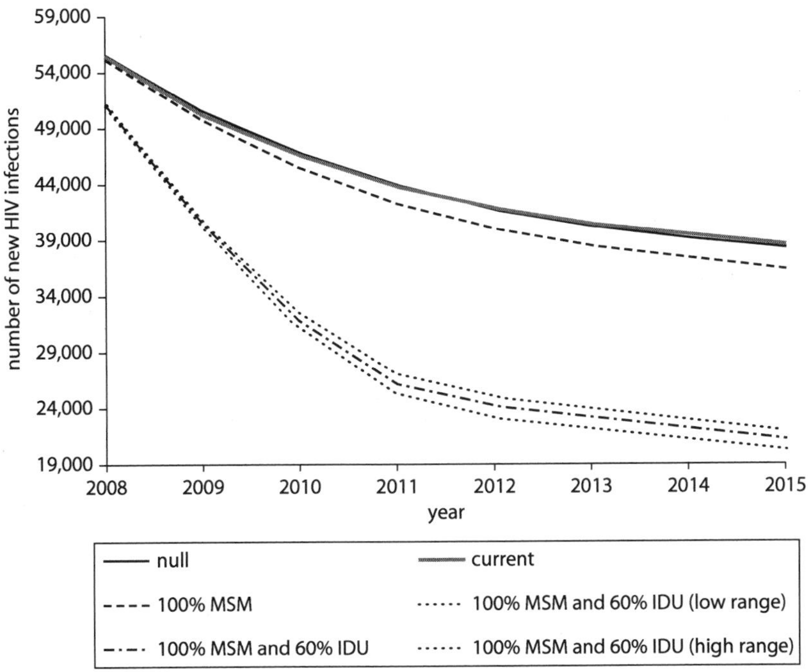

Source: Authors with L. Bollinger.

Table 9.6 Number of Estimated New HIV Infections with Implementation of Four Intervention Scenarios for MSM, Ukraine, 2008–15

Year	*Null*	*Current*	*100% MSM*	*100% MSM and 60% IDU (low)*	*100% MSM and 60% IDU*	*100% MSM and 60% IDU (high)*
2008	55,494	55,392	55,154	51,066	50,974	50,866
2009	50,602	50,202	49,732	40,913	40,551	40,125
2010	46,852	46,590	45,447	32,494	31,816	31,041
2011	43,882	43,807	42,195	26,995	26,170	25,244
2012	41,732	41,848	39,939	25,042	24,194	23,233
2013	40,200	40,443	38,390	23,811	23,008	22,056
2014	39,105	39,413	37,277	22,864	22,113	21,163
2015	38,271	38,594	36,383	21,977	21,262	20,305

Source: Authors with L. Bollinger.

Figure 9.4 Projections of the Number of New HIV Infections with Implementation of Three Intervention Scenarios for MSM, Kenya, 2008–15

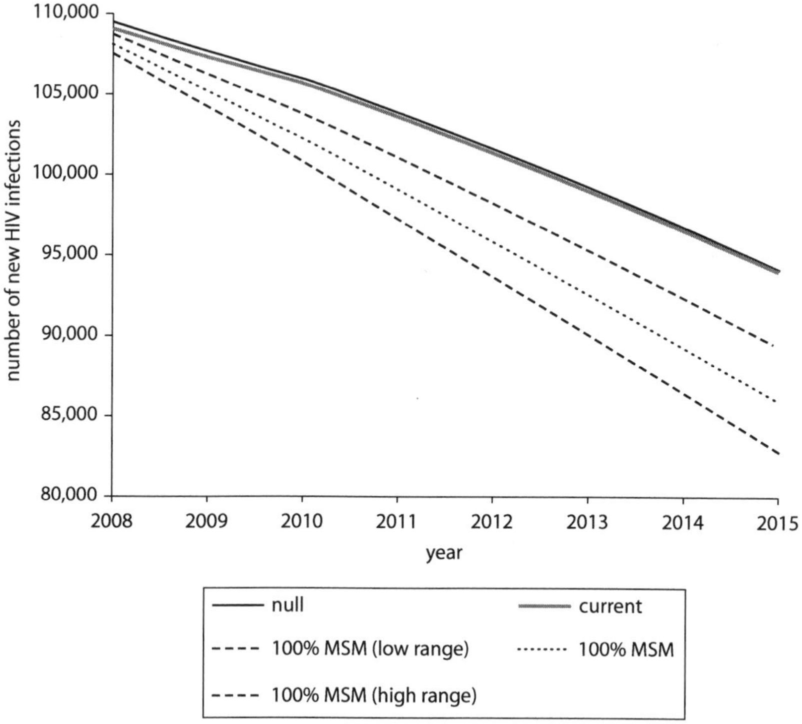

Source: Authors with L. Bollinger.

Table 9.7 Number of Estimated New HIV Infections with Implementation of Three Intervention Scenarios for MSM, Kenya, 2008–15

Year	*Null*	*Current*	*100% MSM (low)*	*100% MSM*	*100% MSM (high)*
2008	109,462	109,115	108,682	108,098	107,522
2009	107,648	107,338	106,178	105,140	104,144
2010	105,980	105,689	103,766	102,247	100,817
2011	103,869	103,637	101,037	99,092	97,287
2012	101,613	101,425	98,222	95,888	93,739
2013	99,181	99,027	95,299	92,604	90,137
2014	96,683	96,549	92,355	89,303	86,526
2015	94,170	94,047	89,431	86,003	82,922

Source: Authors with L. Bollinger.

Figure 9.5 Projections of the Number of New HIV Infections with Implementation of Four Intervention Scenarios for MSM, Thailand, 2008–15

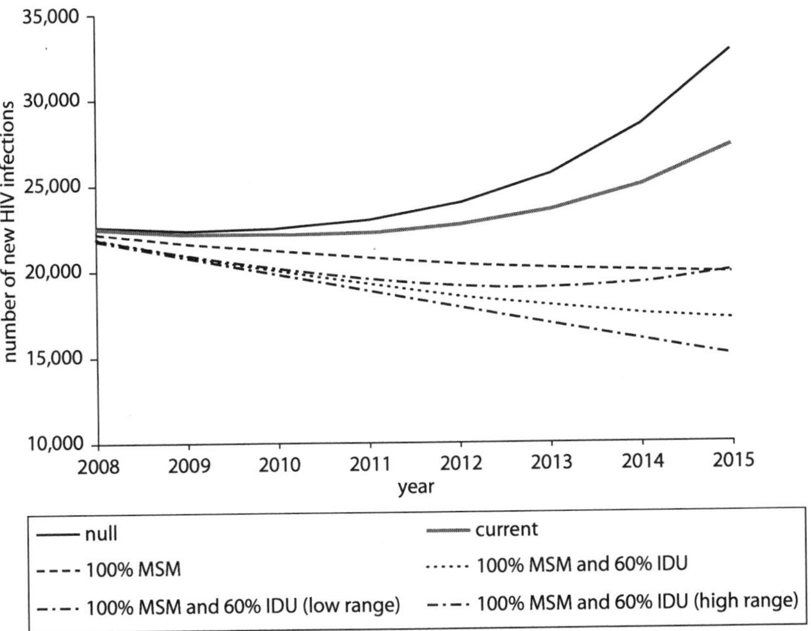

Source: Authors with L. Bollinger.

Table 9.8 Number of Estimated New HIV Infections with Implementation of Four Intervention Scenarios for MSM, Thailand, 2008–15

Year	*Null*	*Current*	*100% MSM*	*100% MSM and 60% IDU (low)*	*100% MSM and 60% IDU*	*100% MSM and 60% IDU (high)*
2008	22,574	22,470	22,216	21,861	21,839	21,810
2009	22,390	22,183	21,620	20,924	20,851	20,764
2010	22,546	22,148	21,177	20,163	19,990	19,794
2011	22,988	22,273	20,761	19,536	19,185	18,816
2012	23,927	22,684	20,411	19,133	18,484	17,857
2013	25,613	23,514	20,134	19,022	17,903	16,920
2014	28,405	24,952	19,942	19,279	17,450	16,004
2015	32,757	27,238	19,832	19,979	17,124	15,103

Source: Authors with L. Bollinger.

2007 coverage levels are dropped to zero for MSM-specific interventions (intervention scenario 1). Increasing MSM-specific interventions to 100 percent (intervention scenario 3) would affect the HIV epidemic among the general population in later years; however, combinations that support interventions targeted toward IDUs and MSM demonstrate the greatest impact.

Where HIV prevalence is high and mature among the general population, as it is in Kenya, MSM-specific interventions positively affect the general population, and although relative impact may be modest, the numbers of infections averted are considerable. As in Ukraine, the current coverage of interventions for MSM has almost the same impact as when coverage for MSM is negligible ("null" scenario); however, increasing coverage of interventions for MSM from current levels to 100 percent by 2015 would decrease the number of new infections by approximately 8,000 in 2015.

In Thailand, epidemic projections show an increase over time in the number of new infections, particularly when MSM-specific interventions are removed. As in Peru, the increase in coverage of MSM-specific interventions could change the trajectory of the epidemic. Here, as well, substantial increases in coverage of IDU interventions would have major effects on the HIV epidemic, demonstrating a difference of more than 12,135 new infections in 2015 when compared to current coverage levels.

Discussion

Although recent studies of HIV interventions among MSM have demonstrated effects among the population of MSM, these modeling projections show the additional impact of such interventions among the general population of all persons at risk for HIV in a given country. MSM-specific interventions, including community-based behavioral interventions and individual interventions of distribution of condoms and lubricants, risk reduction counseling, and expanded access and use of ARVs, positively impact new infections among MSM *and* the general population in each scenario studied. Benefits, however, vary according to each country's epidemic scenario. Countries that have actively sought to understand the epidemic among MSM and that work to prevent transmission among MSM, such as Thailand and Peru, show that including interventions for MSM in national health strategies and decreasing stigma toward MSM have benefit for both MSM and the general population. Peru has made significant progress in providing access to prevention and treatment services for vulnerable populations; however, the work by Cáceres and colleagues (2010), for example, demonstrates that despite evidence that HIV transmission occurs predominantly among MSM, as demonstrated by the attributable fraction calculation here, a substantial proportion of funding is allocated to prevention for female sex workers, where the prevalence is lower (0.5 percent) (Cáceres et al. 2010; Ugarte Ubilluz et al. 2010). In countries with IDU epidemics, such as Thailand and Ukraine, major effects in the general population can be seen when coverage of needle exchange and substitution therapy is increased. Critical to effectively decreasing transmission of HIV among MSM and the general population in all countries is enabling full access to ARVs for HIV-positive MSM. Increasing overall access to ARVs, including for MSM, has the greatest impact in countries where the HIV epidemic is generalized among the heterosexual population. For such countries where programmatic impacts have begun to plateau, implementing MSM-specific interventions and ensuring full access to ARVs for MSM may stimulate further impact.

The Goals Model was used to estimate the additional effect created by interventions for MSM among the general population of all persons at risk for HIV in a given country. A number of methodological challenges associated with the model have to be recognized. Although Goals is unique in its ability to project impacts based on varying coverage rates, the current version assumes that the intervention effects are additive; it does not currently accommodate interaction effects. This limitation is acceptable if one agrees that the interaction effects are multiplicative (because then the model estimates would be lower-bound estimates of the true impact). However, this would appear to be a strong assumption. A key component of the Goals Model is an impact matrix that indicates how behavior changes when a group of people are exposed to specific prevention interventions based on the existing literature. The developers of Goals are in the process of finishing an effort to grade all of those studies and plan to post an interactive matrix with sources and grades that will allow users to determine the level of quality they feel is necessary for assessing impact. In terms of transmission network issues, some questions remain regarding the effect of acute infection and treatment as prevention. As the Goals Model continues to be refined, estimates of impact (and cost-effectiveness, see chapter 10 of this book) should be updated, and efforts to validate the projections should be made.

As with any model, these projections rely on the data available, which vary in terms of quality and quantity, particularly in countries where underreporting may occur because of pervasive stigma toward MSM and IDUs. By systematically reviewing publications and reports and by communicating with country experts, this book attempted to obtain the most accurate and complete set of resources possible. However, this work may be subject to reporting and publication bias, particularly with respect to data on the prevalence of HIV among MSM and other more sensitive behavioral data. Policy makers who use results of epidemiologic studies and modeling projections should take into consideration other factors associated with the HIV epidemic, including identification of high-risk groups, social factors that affect risk behavior (such as alcohol and drug use), human rights considerations such as criminalization and stigmatization of behaviors or identities, and resources available for HIV services. These features were outlined for each epidemic scenario and can be adapted for application of the algorithm to determine the scenario and assist in understanding the situation of any LMIC. Finally, although this book's modeling work shows the effect of these interventions, more understanding of the costs associated with such interventions is required before policy makers can make informed decisions. LMICs are often faced with limited financial resources and have to make tough decisions about how to spend these resources among competing priorities. Cost-effectiveness analysis of these intervention scenarios would assist policy makers in making well-informed choices that meet both fiscal and public health needs. That is the topic of the next chapter.

References

A^2 (Analysis and Advocacy Project in Thailand) and Thai Working Group on HIV/AIDS Projections. 2008. *The Asian Epidemic Model (AEM) Projections for HIV/AIDS in Thailand: 2005–2025*. Bangkok, Thailand: Family Health International and Bureau of AIDS, TB and STIs, Department of Disease Control, Ministry of Public Health, Thailand.

Aldridge, R. W., D. Iglesias, C. F. Cáceres, and J. J. Miranda. 2009. "Determining a Cost Effective Intervention Response to HIV/AIDS in Peru." *BMC Public Health* 9: 352.

Amirkhanian, Y. A., J. A. Kelly, and D. D. Issayev. 2001. "AIDS Knowledge, Attitudes, and Behaviour in Russia: Results of a Population-Based, Random-Digit Telephone Survey in St Petersburg." *International Journal of STD and AIDS* 12 (1): 50–57.

Amjadeen, L. 2005. *Report on the Survey "Monitoring Behaviours of MSM as a Component of Second-Generation Surveillance"* [in Ukrainian]. Kyiv: International HIV/AIDS Alliance in Ukraine.

Balakiryeva, O. N., T. V. Bondar, M. G. Kasyanczuk, Z. R. Kis, Y. B. Leszczynski, and S. P. Sheremet-Sheremetyev. 2008. *Report on the Survey "Monitoring Behaviours of Men Having Sex with Men as a Component of Second Generation Surveillance."* Kyiv: International HIV/AIDS Alliance in Ukraine.

Baral, S., D. Kizub, N. F. Masenior, A. Peryskina, J. Stachowiak, M. Stibich, V. Moguilny, and C. Beyrer. 2010. "Male Sex Workers in Moscow, Russia: A Pilot Study of Demographics, Substance Use Patterns, and Prevalence of HIV-1 and Sexually Transmitted Infections." *AIDS Care* 22 (1): 112–18.

Beyrer, C., T. Sripaipan, S. Tovanabutra, J. Jittiwutikarn, V. Suriyanon, T. Vongchak, N. Srirak, S. Kawichai, M. H. Razak, and D. D. Celentano. 2005. "High HIV, Hepatitis C and Sexual Risks among Drug-Using Men Who Have Sex with Men in Northern Thailand." *AIDS* 19 (14): 1535–40.

Cáceres, C. F., B. de Zalduondo, T. Hallett, C. Avila, and M. Clayton. 2010. "Combination HIV Prevention: Crafting a New Standard for the Long-Term Response to HIV." Presentation at the XVIII International AIDS Conference (AIDS 2010), Vienna, Austria, July 18–23.

Case, K. 2010a. "Kenya General Population Epidemiology, Behavior, and Intervention Inputs for Goals." Unpublished data prepared for aids2031, Imperial College, London, and Futures Institute, Glastonbury, CT.

———. 2010b. "Thailand General Population Epidemiology, Behavior, and Intervention Inputs for Goals." Unpublished data prepared for aids2031, Imperial College, London, and Futures Institute, Glastonbury, CT.

———. 2010c. "Transmissibility, Infectiousness, and Intervention Effectiveness Inputs for Goals." Unpublished data prepared for aids2031, Imperial College, London, and Futures Institute, Glastonbury, CT.

———. 2010d. "Ukraine General Population Epidemiology, Behavior, and Intervention Inputs for Goals." Unpublished data prepared for aids2031, Imperial College, London, and Futures Institute, Glastonbury, CT.

CDC (U.S. Centers for Disease Control and Prevention). 2006. "HIV Prevalence among Populations of Men Who Have Sex with Men—Thailand, 2003 and 2005." *Morbidity and Mortality Weekly Report* 55 (31): 844–48.

Donnell, D., J. Baeten, J. Kiarie, K. Thomas, W. Stevens, C. Cohen, J. McIntyre, J. Lingappa, and C. Celum. 2010. "Heterosexual HIV-1 Transmission after Initiation of Antiretroviral Therapy: A Prospective Cohort Analysis." *Lancet* 375 (9731): 2092–98.

INEI (Instituto Nacional de Estadística e Informática). 2010. *Perú: Encuesta Demográfica y de Salud Familiar, ENDES Continua, 2009; Informe Principal.* Lima, Peru: INEI.

Kelly, J. A., Y. A. Amirkhanian, T. L. McAuliffe, J. V. Granskaya, O. I. Borodkina, R. V. Dyatlov, A. Kukharsky, and A. P. Kozlov. 2002. "HIV Risk Characteristics and Prevention Needs in a Community Sample of Bisexual Men in St. Petersburg, Russia." *AIDS Care* 14 (1): 63–76.

Kruglov, Y. V., Y. V. Kobyshcha, T. Salyuk, O. Varetska, A. Shakarishvili, and V. P. Saldanha. 2008. "The Most Severe HIV Epidemic in Europe: Ukraine's National HIV Prevalence Estimates for 2007." *Sexually Transmitted Infections* 84 (Suppl. 1): i37–i41.

Kunawararak, P., C. Beyrer, C. Natpratan, W. Feng, D. D. Celentano, M. de Boer, K. E. Nelson, and C. Khamboonruang. 1995. "The Epidemiology of HIV and Syphilis among Male Commercial Sex Workers in Northern Thailand." *AIDS* 9 (5): 517–21.

Mathers, B. M., L. Degenhardt, H. Ali, L. Wiessing, M. Hickman, R. P. Mattick, B. Myers, A. Ambekar, and S. A. Strathdee. 2010. "HIV Prevention, Treatment, and Care Services for People Who Inject Drugs: A Systematic Review of Global, Regional, and National Coverage." *Lancet* 375 (9719): 1014–28.

MINSA (Ministerio de Salud). 2009. *Análisis de Situación de Salud*. Ministerio de Salud del Peru.

———. 2010. *Perú: Informe nacional sobre los progresos realizados en la aplicación del UNGASS periodo: Enero 2008–Diciembre 2009*. Lima, Peru: MINSA.

Onyango-Ouma, W., H. Birungi, and S. Geibel. 2005. *Understanding the HIV/STI Risks and Prevention Needs of Men Who Have Sex with Men in Nairobi, Kenya*. Horizons Final Report. Washington, DC: Population Council.

Sanders, E. J., S. M. Graham, H. S. Okuku, E. M. van der Elst, A. Muhaari, A. Davies, N. Peshu, M. Price, R. S. McClelland, and A. D. Smith. 2007. "HIV-1 Infection in High Risk Men Who Have Sex with Men in Mombasa, Kenya." *AIDS* 21 (18): 2513–20.

Sergeyev, B., and M. Gorbachev. 2008. *Russia (2008): HIV/AIDS TRaC Study of Risk, Health-Seeking Behaviors, and Their Determinants among Men Who Have Sex with Men in Eight Regions of the Russian Federation. Second Round.* Moscow: PSI.

Sifakis, F., A. Peryskina, B. Sergeev, V. Moguilny, A. Beloglazov, N. Franck-Masenior, S. Baral, and C. Beyrer. 2008. "Rapid Assessment of HIV Infection and Associated Risk Behaviors among Men Who Have Sex with Men in Russia." Presentation at the XVII International AIDS Conference, Mexico City, Mexico, August 3–8.

Stover, J., L. Bollinger, and K. Cooper-Arnold. 2003. "Goals Model: For Estimating the Effects of Resource Allocation Decisions on the Achievement of the Goals of the HIV/AIDS Strategic Plan." Glastonbury, CT: Futures Group International.

Tyusova, O., S. V. Verevochkin, R. Heimer, et al. 2009. "HIV in Population Groups Recruited by Respondent-Driven Sampling in St. Petersburg."

Presentation at the 3rd Eastern Europe and Central Asia AIDS Conference, Moscow, October 28–30.

Ugarte Ubilluz, O., M. Arce Rodriguez, C. Acosta Saal, L. Suarez Ognio, J. L. Sebastián Mesones, and G. Rosell De Almeida. 2010. *Informe nacional sobre los progresos realizados en la aplicación del UNGASS: período: enero 2008–diciembre 2009*. Lima, Peru: Ministerio de Salud, Dirección General de Salud de las Personas.

UNAIDS (Joint United Nations Programme on HIV/AIDS) and Ministry of Health of Ukraine. 2008. *Ukraine: National Report on Monitoring Progress towards the UNGASS Declaration of Commitment on HIV/AIDS. Reporting Period: January 2006–December 2007*. Kyiv: Ministry of Health of Ukraine.

UNAIDS (Joint United Nations Programme on HIV/AIDS) and WHO (World Health Organization). 2008a. "UNAIDS/WHO Epidemiological Fact Sheets on HIV and AIDS, 2008 Update: Kenya." Geneva: UNAIDS/WHO Working Group on Global HIV/AIDS and STI Surveillance.

———. 2008b. "UNAIDS/WHO Epidemiological Fact Sheets on HIV and AIDS, 2008 Update: Peru." Geneva: UNAIDS/WHO Working Group on Global HIV/AIDS and STI Surveillance.

———. 2009. *AIDS Epidemic Update: December 2009*. Geneva: UNAIDS and WHO.

van Griensven, F., S. Thanprasertsuk, R. Jommaroeng, G. Mansergh, S. Naorat, R. A. Jenkins, K. Ungchusak, P. Phanuphak, J. W. Tappero, and Bangkok MSM Study Group. 2005. "Evidence of a Previously Undocumented Epidemic of HIV Infection among Men Who Have Sex with Men in Bangkok, Thailand." *AIDS* 19 (5): 521–26.

van Griensven, F., A. Varangrat, W. Wimonsate, S. Tanpradech, K. Kladsawad, T. Chemnasiri, O. Suksripanich, P. Phanuphak, P. Mock, K. Kanggarnrua, et al. 2009. "Trends in HIV Prevalence, Estimated HIV Incidence, and Risk Behavior among Men Who Have Sex with Men in Bangkok, Thailand, 2003–2007." *Journal of Acquired Immune Deficiency Syndromes* 53 (2): 234–39.

WHO (World Health Organization) Regional Office for Europe. 2007. *HIV Prevalence and Risks among Men Who Have Sex with Men in Moscow and Saint Petersburg*. Copenhagen: WHO.

Wimonsate, W., S. Chaikummao, J. Tongtoyai, C. Kittinunvorakoon, A. Sriporn, A. Varangrat, P. Akarasewi, P. Sirivongrangson, J. McNicholl, and F. van Griensven. 2008. "Successful Start of a Preparatory HIV Cohort Study among Men Who Have Sex With Men (MSM) in Bangkok, Thailand: Preliminary Baseline, Follow-Up and HIV Incidence Data." Presentation at the XVII International AIDS Conference, Mexico City, Mexico, August 3–8.

CHAPTER 10

Modeling Cost and Cost-Effectiveness

Key themes:

- Robust differences exist in HIV intervention costs and intervention effects on HIV infections related to men who have sex with men (MSM).
- To reduce HIV infections among MSM, promotion and distribution of condoms with lubricants is generally the most cost-effective use of resources, followed by community-level behavioral interventions, and then antiretroviral therapy (ART) for prevention.
- ART for prevention may be comparatively less cost-effective than condom and lubricant distribution in reducing overall HIV infections among MSM, though ART is typically already implemented as a strategy with other aims and measures.
- By World Health Organization benchmarks of cost-effectiveness, comparing costs of interventions per disability-adjusted life year averted against per capita gross national income, all of the assessed interventions provide value for money.

This chapter demonstrates the effects and costs of interventions for MSM in selected low- and middle-income countries, modeled with varying coverage levels and combinations of interventions. These modeling and costing exercises were performed to demonstrate the utility of the Goals Model (Stover, Bollinger, and Cooper-Arnold 2001) to inform strategic planning and the variation in results observed across epidemic scenarios and environments.

Methods

Whereas previous chapters have highlighted the impact that interventions targeting MSM can have on the HIV epidemic in selected countries, this chapter uses data available in the literature to assess the costs and cost-effectiveness of these interventions.

Estimating Impact

The impact of the interventions assessed here follows the methods already discussed in chapter 9 of this book. This chapter describes how these methods were adapted to cost-effectiveness analysis.

MSM-specific interventions and coverage scenarios. The impact on the HIV epidemic among MSM can be assessed by varying levels of access to ART among the general population. For this book, the predictions are based on rollout of preventive interventions by estimating the number of HIV infections, assuming all other intervention coverage remains at current levels. The interventions modeled are

- Null, or no MSM-specific interventions
- Community-based behavioral intervention
- Distribution of condoms with lubricant and partner reduction counseling
- Expanding ART coverage

The null intervention scenario is calculated by setting the current coverage of the two MSM interventions at zero, as if all MSM interventions were suddenly removed. Then, the interventions and combinations thereof listed above are tested at current coverage levels (assuming 30 percent coverage from 2008 through 2015 for both community-based behavioral intervention and distribution of condoms with lubricant and partner reduction counseling, given variations between 20 and 40 percent reported for intervention coverage). These combinations are then modeled to observe impacts if 60 percent coverage were reached gradually by 2015. Finally, to estimate the effect of an optimally supportive environment, combinations in which coverage of interventions for MSM and ART reach 100 percent are modeled.

Inputs: Systematic review of HIV prevention interventions for MSM. Using the results of the systematic review of HIV prevention interventions for MSM, meta-analysis was completed to develop summary estimates of the reductions of unprotected anal intercourse or the corollary of increase in condom use rates during anal intercourse. Studies were weighted by their relative sample sizes. See the preceding chapters for more details.

Estimating the Costs of Interventions

The costs of interventions for MSM were estimated by conducting a comprehensive literature review. As far as possible, contextual information concerning the forms and scale of the interventions, the subgroups reached by the interventions, the existence of complementary interventions, and the epidemiological setting were extracted from publications. When possible, data on the location in the country (for example, urban or rural), setting of the intervention (primary health care, hospital, community), target population, numbers in the target population, numbers treated or served, methods used in costing, costing perspective, and items included in the costing were also extracted from the articles. Data relating to the costing methods used and, most important, the cost data reported—converted to 2008 U.S. dollars and international dollars (to reflect differences in purchasing power)—were collected.

Literature search on unit costs. The first literature search was completed in December 2009; the results of this search are shown in table 10.1. Additional searches were conducted for specific interventions based on the findings of other parts of the study. Specifically, searches were conducted for ART, interventions for injecting drug users (needle exchange programs and methadone maintenance therapy), voluntary counseling and testing, and structural interventions (conducted in April 2010). The second search was done in PubMed, with further searches of the reference lists of papers found. The results of this second search are shown in table 10.2.

Papers based on titles totaled 371, and 263 abstracts were read. Overall, 93 studies of relevance were found in the first phase of the literature search, and 74 additional studies of relevance were found in the second phase (total number of studies = 167). Some of these studies

Table 10.1 Search Results for First Phase of Literature Review

	Number of articles			
Search criteria	*PubMed*	*EconLit*	*Google scholar*	*Reference tracking or informant contacts*
1. "economics" OR "costs" OR "cost analysis" OR econom[a] OR "cost" OR "costly" OR "costing" OR "price" OR "prices" OR "pricing" OR pharmacoeconomic[a] OR (expenditure[a] not energy) OR (value and money) OR budget[a]	583,006	800,637	215,000 (limited keywords)	n.a.
2. "HIV" OR "AIDS" OR "STI" OR "sexually transmitted infection"	272,582	20,933	6,530	n.a.
3. ("MSM" OR "men who have sex with men" OR "gay" OR "homosexual" OR "transgender") OR ("CSW" OR "sex worker" OR "prostitute" OR "street women" OR "brothel") OR ("vulnerable population" OR "truck driver" OR "migrant" OR "street kids" OR "homeless")	30,306	3,345	n.a.	n.a.
4. #1 AND #2	17,328	17,641	249	n.a.
5. #3 AND #4	785	707	n.a.	n.a.
Titles selected	72	17	n.a.	65
Abstracts selected	35	5	6	62

Papers for inclusion (unit costs[a])	18[b]	2[c]	2[d]	54[e,f,g]
Papers for inclusion (cost-effectiveness related to MSM)[h]	13[i]	0	0	4[j]

Source: Authors.
Note: n.a. = not applicable.
a. Excluding articles related to MSM.
b. Bollinger et al. 2009; Cohen, Wu, and Farley 2004; Creese et al. 2002; Dandona et al. 2008; Fung et al. 2007; Guinness et al. 2005; Guinness, Kumaranayake, and Hanson 2007; Herida et al. 2006; Hutton, Wyss, and N'Diekhor 2003; Kasymova, Johns, and Sharipova 2009; Kumar et al. 2009; Macauley and Creighton 2009; Price et al. 2006; Sweat et al. 2006; Thomsen et al. 2006; Vickerman, Terris-Prestholt, et al. 2006; Wilson et al. 2010.
c. Revenga et al. 2006; Weaver et al. 2009.
d. Terris-Prestholt, Vyas et al. 2006; Woodhall et al. 2009.
e. Many of these are related to cost of treatment.
f. Aisu et al. 1995; Aracena-Genao et al. 2008; Auvert et al. 2008; Babigumira et al. 2009; Bachmann 2006; Badri, Cleary et al. 2006; Badri, Maartens et al. 2006; Borghi et al. 2005; Boulle et al. 2002; Carrara et al. 2005; Cleary, McIntyre, and Boulle 2006, 2008; Crabbe et al. 1996; Daly et al. 1998; Dandona, Sisodia, Prasad et al. 2005; Dandona, Sisodia, Ramesh et al. 2005; Deghaye, Pawinski, and Desmond 2006; Djajakusumah et al. 1998; Fang et al. 2007; Forsythe et al. 1998, 2002; Freedberg et al. 2001; Gilson et al. 1997; Goldie et al. 2003, 2006; Harrison et al. 2000; Holtgrave and Pinkerton 1997; Holtgrave et al. 1993; Kahn, Marseille, and Auvert 2006; Krieger et al. 2008; Kumaranayake and Watts 2000; La Ruche, Lorougnon, and Digbeu 1995; Leiva et al. 2001; Liu et al. 2003; Long et al. 2006; Losina et al. 2009; Marseille et al. 2001; McConnel et al. 2005; Miners et al. 2001; Moses et al. 1991; Parker et al. 1999; Pinkerton, Holtgrave, and Bloom 1998; Schackman et al. 2005, 2006; Soderlund et al. 1993; Sweat et al. 2000; Terris-Prestholt, Kumaranayake et al. 2006; van der Veen et al. 1994; Vickerman Kumaranayake et al. 2006; Walker et al. 2001; Wang et al. 2003; Wilkinson et al. 1997; Wolf et al. 2007.
g. Includes individual references from systematic searches.
h. Two articles related to developing countries (Peru, India).
i. Aldridge et al. 2009; Desai et al. 2008; Dandona et al. 2009; Goldie et al. 1999, 2000; Kahn et al. 2001; Karnon et al. 2008; Paltiel et al. 2009; Pinkerton, Holtgrave, and Valdiserri 1997; Rieg et al. 2008; Tao and Remafedi 1998; Tuli and Kerndt 2009; Zaric et al. 2008.
j. Heumann et al. 2001; Holtgrave and Kelly 1997; Pinkerton, Holtgrave, DiFranceisco et al. 1998; Pinkerton et al. 2004.

Table 10.2 Search Results for Second Phase of Literature Review

	Third criterion (#3)			
Search criteria	*"ART" OR "HAART" OR "anti-retroviral" OR "treatment" (March 16, 2010)*	*"Replacement therapy" OR "methadone" OR "needle exchange" OR "IDU" OR "harm reduction"*	*"Voluntary counseling and testing" OR "VCT" OR "testing" OR "HIV testing" OR "counseling"*	*"Structural interventions" OR "decriminalization" OR "homophobia" OR "HIV policy" OR "mass media" OR "engagement" OR "community" OR "system strengthening" OR "health sector" OR "new policy"*
1. "economics" OR "costs" OR "cost analysis" OR econom[a] OR "cost" OR "costly" OR "costing" OR "price" OR "prices" OR "pricing" OR pharmacoeconomic[a] OR (expenditure[a] not energy) OR (value and money) OR budget[a]	595,667	595,667	595,667	595,667
2. "HIV" OR "AIDS" OR "STI" OR "sexually transmitted infection"	277,802	277,802	277,802	277,802
4. #1 AND #2	17,693	17,693	17,693	17,693
5. #3 AND #4	4,840	359 (196 new)	2,196 (1,260 new)	2,391 (1,709 new)
Titles selected	128	22	32	40

Abstracts selected	53 (plus 16 found previously) plus 57 from reference search	16 (plus 1 found previously) plus 7 from reference search	13 (plus 2 found previously)	9
Papers for inclusion (unit costs)[a]	30[b] plus 22[c]	10[d] plus 6[e]	3[f]	3[g]

Source: Authors.

Note: a. Not all studies found were necessarily directly related to the search topic; for example, the search for costs on ART found some studies reporting costs for needle exchange programs, and so on.

b. Afriandi et al. 2010; Anis et al. 2000; Bautista-Arredondo et al. 2008; Beck et al. 2004; Bikilla et al. 2009; Binagwaho et al. 2010; Charreau et al. 2008; Cohen, Wu, and Farley 2006; Fieno 2008; Flori and le Vaillant 2004; Freedberg et al. 2007; Hounton et al. 2008; Hubben et al. 2008; Kitajima et al. 2003; Koenig et al. 2008; Lopez-Bastida et al. 2009; Lowy et al. 2005; Martinson et al. 2009; Menzies et al. 2009; Merito et al. 2005; Nachega et al. 2010; Over et al. 2006; Paton et al. 2006; Quentin et al. 2008; Renaud et al. 2009; Rothbard, Lee, and Blank 2009; Thielman et al. 2006; Tornero Estébanez et al. 2004; Tuli et al. 2005; Yazdanpanah et al. 2002.

c. Bedimo et al. 2002; Chaix et al. 2000; Constella Futures et al. 2006; Dijkgraaf et al. 2005; Gardner et al. 2008; Godfrey, Stewart, and Gossop 2004; Goldman et al. 2001; John, Rajagopalan, and Madhuri 2006; Kombe and Smith 2003; Krentz, Auld, and Gill 2003; Krentz and Gill 2008; Kyriopoulos et al. 2001; Masson et al. 2004; Partners for Health Reform*plus*, DELIVER, and POLICY Project 2004; Purdum, Johnson, and Globe 2004; Roberts et al. 2006; Rosen, Long, and Sanne 2008; Tramarin et al. 2004; UN RTF 2009; Velasco et al. 2000, 2007.

d. Bayoumi and Zaric 2008; Cabases and Sanchez 2003; Doran et al. 2003; Gold et al. 1997; Guinness et al. 2010; Harris 2006; Kumaranayake et al. 2004; Moore, Ritter, and Caulkins 2007; Ruger, Ben, and Cottler 2010; Zaric, Barnett, and Brandeau 2000.

e. Barnett 1999; Chandrashekar et al. 2010; Ettner et al. 2006; Healey et al. 2003; Mojtabai and Zivin 2003; Warren et al. 2006.

f. Farnham et al. 1996; Hausler et al. 2006; Shrestha et al. 2009.

g. Negin et al. 2009; Shrestha et al. 2008; Sood and Nambiar 2006.

were not, in the end, used in this analysis because they related to voluntary counseling and testing, treatment of sexually transmitted infections (STIs), and other interventions that were not included in the cost-effectiveness analyses. Table 10.3 gives details of the number of studies, observations, and countries covered for the main interventions: outreach, condom distribution, ART, needle exchange programs, opioid replacement therapy, and structural interventions. The table shows that 114 studies[1] were found that are of relevance for the main interventions examined for this chapter (plus 11 studies related to structural interventions). Of these, 62 reported costs for ART, 19 reported costs for education through peer outreach, 9 reported costs for condom distribution, 9 reported costs for needle exchange programs, and 15 reported costs for opioid replacement therapy.

Analysis of data extracted from the literature: Data extraction, assessment of quality, and analysis. The data from the papers were extracted and entered, in the first instance, into a Microsoft Excel database. The

Table 10.3 Complete Search Results for Selected Interventions

Intervention category	*Specific intervention and target populations*	*Number of studies*	*Number of observations*	*Number of countries*
ART	ART	62	77	26
Condom distribution	Total[a]	9	13	8
	To general population	3	4	4
	To FSWs	4	6	4
	To MSM	3	3	3
Outreach through peer educators	Total[a]	19	40	7
	To vulnerable population (general)	3	3	1
	To IDUs	2	2	1
	To FSWs	7	25	4
	To MSM	9	10	5
Interventions targeting IDUs	Needle exchange programs	9	16	9
	Opioid replacement therapy	15	17	7
Structural interventions	Mass media to general population	8	10	7
	Mass media to vulnerable population	1	1	1
	Changes in laws or policies	2	3	1

Source: Authors.
Note: FSWs = female sex workers; IDUs = injecting drug users.
a. Some studies contain multiple observations, multiple countries, or multiple target populations. Therefore, totals do not represent the sum of the breakdowns below them.

database contains variables related to the type of intervention, target population, number of people served by the intervention, and unit costs and an array of variables to capture what kind of costing was done and to what quality. For example, of the 77 observations obtained for the unit costs of highly active ART, 64 (83 percent) were viewed as being relatively complete in terms of the costs collected (that is, including at least the costs for ART drugs, ART-related laboratory procedures, inpatient and outpatient visits, and treatment of opportunistic infections). However, 35 (45 percent) reported costs explicitly from an economic costing method, whereas others either were not explicit or reported financial costs only. Finally, 26 (34 percent) of the reported costs were based on either models or expert opinion, while the remainder were based on empirical observations and primary data collection.

These types of variables were used in the analysis to control for methodological differences in the data analysis (see next section). Given the nature of the data reported, traditional cost or production function forms were not used because a large proportion of the studies do not report number of people served, target population, or coverage, meaning that these variables cannot be included in the regression.[2] However, gross domestic product (GDP) was used as a proxy for price, along with the variables listed above. The purpose of these regressions is to predict prices where data are missing, which leads to two points. First, in countries where unit costs have been observed in the literature, these unit costs are used for cost-effectiveness analysis, and the regression estimates are used to create plausible ranges around the unit costs. Second, the regressions were modeled using one- and two-knotted splines as well as higher-order terms around the continuous independent variables. The best model is assessed using Akaike's Information Criteria, which is an indication of the balance between fitting the data and overspecification of data to the point where they are not generalizable.

The regressions were used to fill in missing unit costs for both the cost-effectiveness analysis and the global price tag exercises (see appendixes A and B). However, for some interventions—condom distribution, mass media, and changes to legislation or policy—the number of studies found would not support regression analysis. The cost for condom and lubricant distribution ranges from US$0.10 to US$0.40 per condom distributed. Given that the costs of condoms themselves are approximately US$0.02 per condom, the remainder of the cost represents lubrication and distribution. Costs are unlikely to be greater than the high end of the range observed (except in cases of very high levels of inefficiency), so these figures are used for all countries.

Annex 10.A provides details of the data used in each regression and the results of the models. What follows here is a summary of the methods used.

Regression analysis of the ART data. In the case of ART, GDP has an unadjusted correlation of 0.6 with the unit costs (see figure 10.1), indicating that a good amount of the variation can be explained with a regression in a fairly simple specification. However, as shown in the box in the lower left corner of figure 10.1, this relationship is less clear for observations from countries with low GDP, where the correlation between GDP and unit costs appears to be much weaker. This issue proved problematic when determining which regression model best explains the data.

Costs were collected from studies starting in 1992, but the majority of studies were conducted after 2000. A wide range of countries were covered, with GDP per capita ranging from US$125 to US$46,000 and an

Figure 10.1 Initial Exploration of Data for ART Unit Costs
Cost per person per year

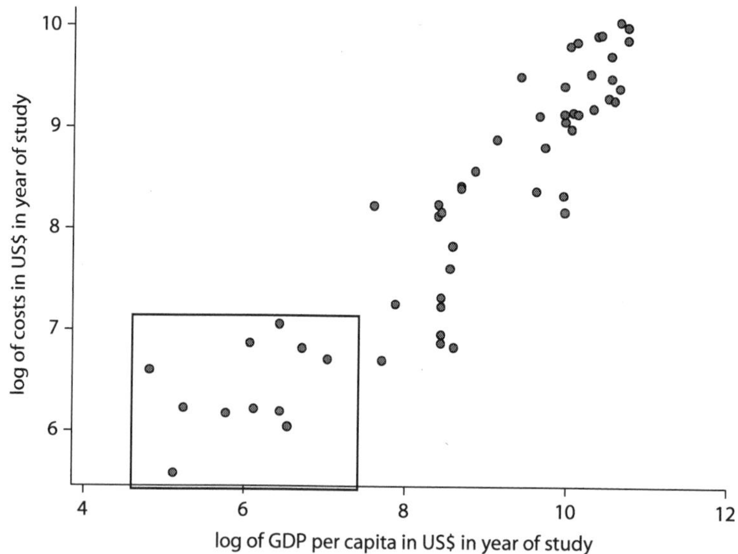

Source: Authors.
Note: Studies reporting average lifetime costs of ART were excluded from the figure. Axes are in natural log scale; in natural units, GDP per capita on the x-axis ranges from US$150 [natural log = 5] to US$60,000 [natural log = 11].

average of about US$14,000. The two countries with the highest number of studies were the United States and South Africa; 43 of the 77 studies were from developed countries. About one-third of the studies were based on models or expert opinion, and most (83 percent) appeared to have captured the major cost categories associated with ART care (see table 10.A.1 of annex 10.A).

This analysis explored using a logarithmic spline and higher-order terms in a log function. In addition, a number of categorizations were tried for year of the study and how the data were collected or estimated. Interaction terms were assessed between all variables, especially because several of the methodological characteristics of the studies seemed to be correlated with each other. Table 10.A.2 of annex 10.A shows the results of the best model from this first analysis. As expected, costs are higher where GDP is higher, although costs seem to increase more rapidly with respect to GDP for $100 to $600 GDP compared with GDP over US$600. Both spline components are highly statistically significant. Longitudinal studies tended to show lower costs when compared with other methods of data collection or estimation, although this difference is not statistically significant when compared with cross-sectional data; modeled and estimated data may overestimate costs because they tend to assume perfect compliance with treatment guidelines, overestimate the costs of opportunistic infections or drug switches, or both. The model shows a decrease in costs after 2003, when many countries were able to negotiate dramatic markdowns in the price of ART drugs.

Several iterations were run to ensure the best fit between costs and GDP and between costs and year. For example, different break points in the spline were tried, different classes for years, and higher-order terms. Additionally, a second set of models was tested on data excluding studies that reported only the lifetime costs of ART because these data must make assumptions about the life expectancy of people on ART and used different discounting rates, which may influence their costs. The results of the best-fit model are reported in table 10.A.3 of annex 10.A. This model results in some findings that are counterintuitive (for example, studies that obviously omitted cost categories are shown to be associated with higher costs, controlling for other factors). A comparison of the predictions up to GDP US$12,000 is shown in figure 10.2. The line for model 1 in this figure shows predictions for the full model with all the data, whereas the line for model 2 shows predictions excluding lifetime costs. The dots represent observed data from the data set for one-year costs, which are not adjusted for the other variables in the models. The

Figure 10.2 Prediction Results from Model 1 and Model 2 for ART Unit Costs
Cost per person per year

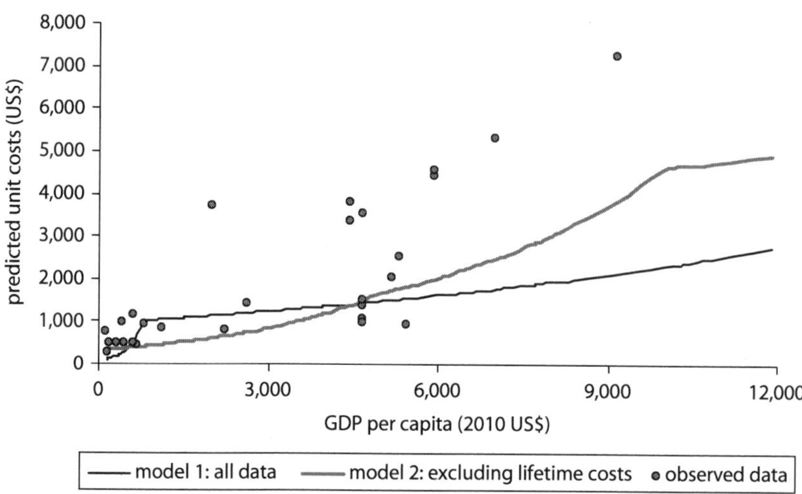

Source: Authors.

first model sharply increases at low-income levels and then has a lower slope than the second model.[3] Both models seem to be underpredicting the observed data for middle-income countries (because of observations from high-income countries that are not shown in the figure). Better overall fit and signs on coefficients consistent with expectations prompted use of the first model to predict costs.

Regression analysis of the outreach data. In the case of the data on the unit costs of outreach, GDP has a less clear relationship with unit costs than it did with the ART model (see figure 10.3), although some relationship does appear to exist. However, it contains a good deal of noise, indicating that other variables are needed to explain the unit costs.

Table 10.A.4 in annex 10.A summarizes the input data collected. The definitions of the variables are the same as those used in the ART analysis.

Costs were collected from studies starting in 1992, but the majority of studies were conducted after 2000. A wide range of countries were covered, with GDP per capita ranging from US$456 to US$40,000, with an average of about US$12,500. The two countries with the highest number of studies were the United States and India; 11 of the 16 studies were from developed countries (32 of 40 cost estimates). The majority (80 percent) of observations are based on empirical data collection; 25 percent of the

Figure 10.3 Initial Exploration of Data for Outreach Unit Costs

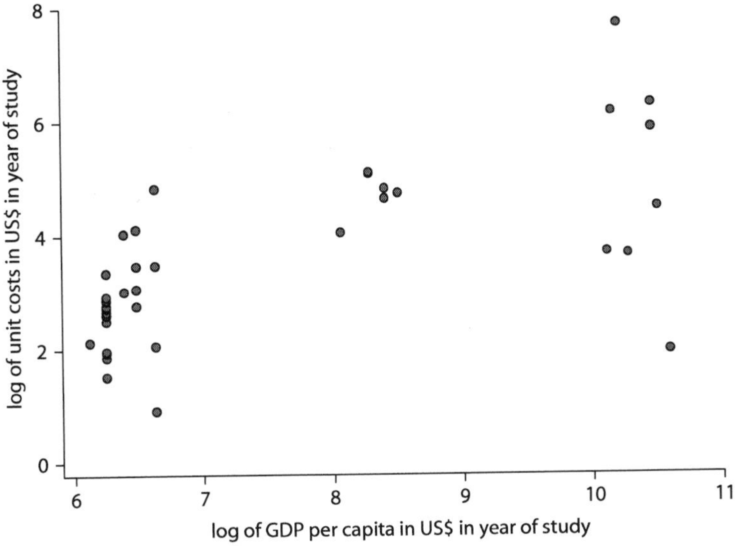

Source: Authors.

observed unit costs were for programs targeting MSM (Aldridge et al. 2009; Constella Futures et al. 2006; Dandona et al. 2009; Holtgrave and Kelly 1997; Kahn et al. 2001; Pinkerton, Holtgrave, DiFranceisco et al. 1998; Pinkerton, Holtgrave, and Valdiserri 1997; Tao and Remafedi 1998), and 27.5 percent were for programs targeting men only.

This analysis explored two models, in each case running a series of different models including splines and higher-order terms on continuous variables to determine the best fit. The first model included all data; in this case, the number of contacts made with clients could not be controlled for because eight observations were missing these data. The second model used the fewer observations but controlled for the number of contacts made with clients. In addition, a number of categorizations were tried for year of the study and how the data were collected or estimated. Interaction terms were assessed between all variables, especially because several of the methodological characteristics of the studies seemed to be correlated with each other. Table 10.A.5 (see annex 10.A) shows the results of the best model for the first model. As expected, costs are higher where GDP is higher; splines and higher-order terms did not improve the fit of the data. Targeting females was shown to have higher costs than targeting men. Several of the coefficients had signs that were in the opposite direction of what was expected. For example, studies that included the costs of treating STIs were shown to have lower costs than those that did not include treatment of STIs; a plausible explanation for this finding does not arise, other than omitted variable bias.

The second model, although based on fewer observations (n = 31 compared with n = 38 for the first model), remains theoretically preferable because it explicitly models potential economies of scale. The results of the best-fit model for these data are shown in table 10.A.6 (see annex 10.A). This table again shows that costs increase with GDP, although at a slower rate over a GDP per capita of $1,000 compared with under $1,000. As expected, the unit cost initially declines with an increase in the number of contacts and then increases. The lowest level of unit costs in this model occurs with about 25,000 client contacts in a year. The signs of most of the coefficients are in the direction expected (for example, treating STIs compared with not treating STIs is associated with a higher unit cost).

A comparison of the predictions up to a GDP of US$12,000 is shown in figure 10.4. The line for model 1 in this figure shows predictions with all the data, whereas the line for model 2 shows predictions including the number of contacts. The black dots represent observed data from the data set for one-year costs—noting that these are not adjusted for the other variables in the models. The first model appears to predict costs at the high end of the observed data, whereas the second model appears to

Figure 10.4 Prediction Results from Model 1 and Model 2 for Outreach Unit Costs

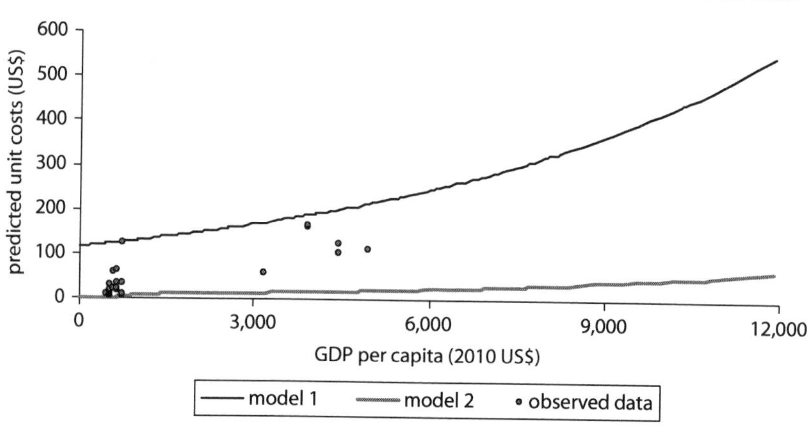

Source: Authors.

predict costs at the low end of the observed data. This low prediction level for the second model is because costs were predicted using the average number of contacts per year from the data available, which is very close to the maximal level of scale efficiency. Thus, most of the observed data are above the predicted values in this model because they represent scale-inefficient observations. The second model is used to predict the unit costs for this study because it is theoretically more correct and because the results are more in line with expectations. The difficulty with using the second model is determining how many contacts will be made per year at different levels of coverage.

Regression analysis of the needle exchange program data. In the case of the data on the unit costs of needle exchange programs, GDP appears to have no clear, unadjusted relationship with unit costs (see figure 10.5); however, a fairly strong relationship appears to exist between the number of contacts at a service delivery center and unit costs (see figure 10.6). Table 10.A.7 (see annex 10.A) summarizes the input data collected. The definitions of the variables are the same as those used in the ART analysis.

Figure 10.5 Initial Exploration of Data for Needle Exchange Program Unit Costs

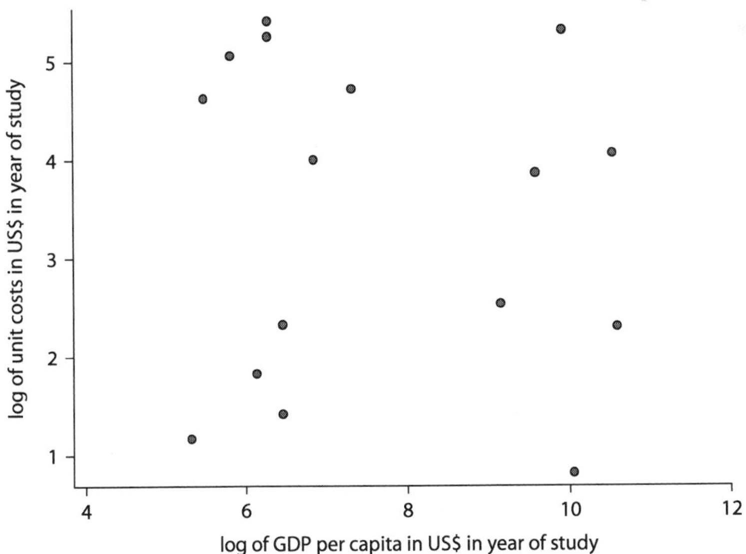

Source: Authors.

Figure 10.6 Initial Exploration of Data for Needle Exchange Program Unit Costs Using Number of Contacts

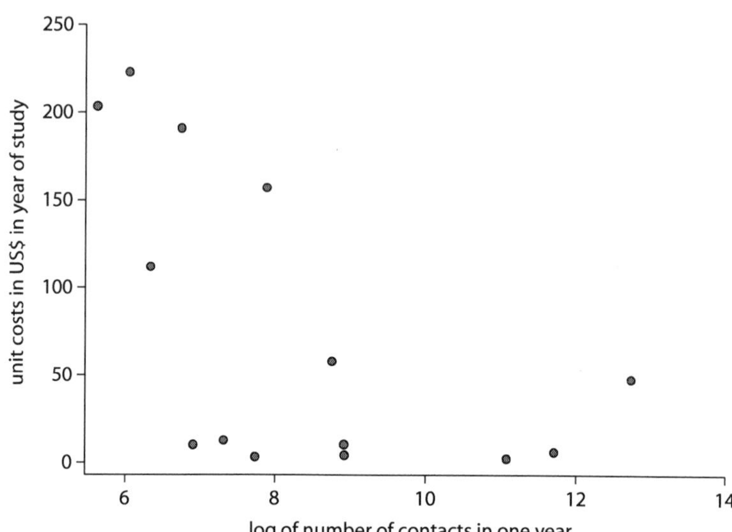

Source: Authors.

Costs were collected from studies starting in 1990, but the majority of studies (9 of 16) were conducted in or after 2000. A wide array of countries was covered, with GDP per capita ranging from US$200 to US$40,000 and an average of about US$9,500. However, few observations were available for middle-income countries (defined as GDP between US$1,000 and US$10,000 per capita), meaning that predictions of unit costs for middle-income countries rely on interpolation between low-income and high-income countries, which limits the ability of the regression model to assess the fit of splines or higher-order terms with respect to GDP per capita. All observations come from Europe, Asia, or developed countries in other areas; South America and Africa are not represented. Most of the studies represented (5 of 9) were from developed countries, but more cost estimates were present for developing countries (11 of 16 cost estimates). The majority (62.5 percent) of observations are based on empirical data collection.

With only 14 observations included in the final model, the limited degrees of freedom for this regression precluded analysis of interactions; simple splines of continuous independent variables did not appear to improve the fit of the model. However, as with the second regression model for outreach, both the number of contacts and the number of contacts squared were statistically significant ($p < 0.05$) and with signs indicating a U-shaped cost curve (see table 10.A.8 in this chapter's annex for the result of the best-fit model). Unit costs were predicted using the modal value of 1,000 contacts per year at a delivery site.

Regression analysis of the methadone replacement therapy data. In the case of the data on the unit costs of methadone replacement therapy programs, GDP appears to have some relationship with unit costs (see figure 10.7), but only two observations for these programs were available from low- or middle-income countries. Thus, deriving unit costs for these data is quite problematic and necessitates making the assumptions that the patterns observed in high-income countries can be extrapolated to low- and middle-income countries (and that the two observations from low- and middle-income countries provide enough data to influence this extrapolation in the correct manner). Obviously, this is a strong assumption, and better data on the costs of this program are needed. Table 10.A.9 (see annex 10.A) summarizes the input data

Figure 10.7 Initial Exploration of Data for Methadone Replacement Therapy Unit Costs

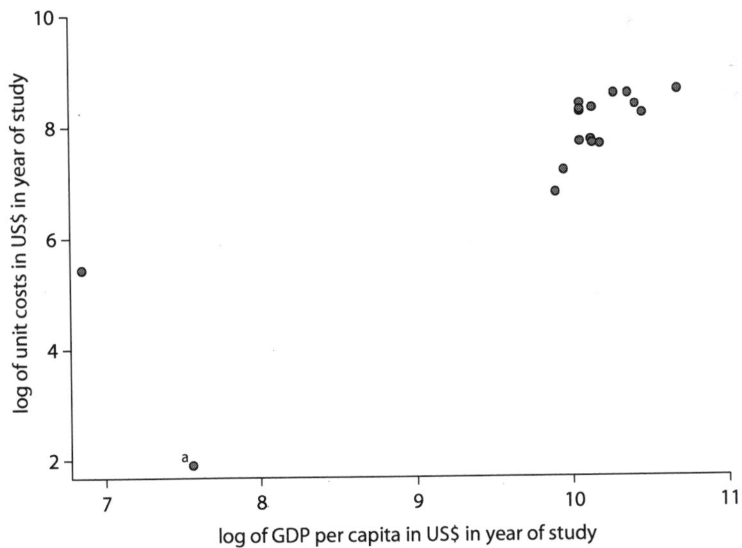

Source: Authors.
a. Cost is per contact; all others are cost per person per year.

collected. The definitions of the variables are the same as those used in the ART analysis. As with the ART analysis, too few of the studies reported the number of patients or the number of contacts to use this variable in the regression analysis.

Costs were collected from studies starting in 1990; about half the studies (9 of 17) were conducted in or after 2000. As noted previously, most observations are from developed countries, and no studies are from countries with a GDP per capita between US$2,000 and US$19,000, which limits the ability of the regression model to assess the fit of splines or higher-order terms with respect to GDP per capita. All observations come from Asia or developed countries; South America, low- and middle-income Europe, and Africa are not represented. The majority (88 percent) of observations are based on empirical data collection; the two unit costs not based on a facility setting did not use empirical data collection.

With 17 observations included in the final model, the limited degrees of freedom for this regression precluded analysis of interactions; simple splines of continuous independent variables did not appear to improve the fit of the model (see table 10.A.10 in this chapter's annex for the result of the best-fit model). The coefficients for full costs compared to incremental costs and complete costs compared to obvious exclusions are not in the expected direction in the final model. This finding is likely caused by the high degree of overlap between these variables and other methodological variables (which were excluded from the final model[4]), making direct interpretation of these coefficients difficult.

Results for Kenya, Peru, Thailand, and Ukraine

Table 10.4 reports the unit costs used in the first analysis of cost-effectiveness in Thailand, Peru, Kenya, and Ukraine. Uncertainty ranges were derived by taking 1,000 draws from a random distribution of the beta coefficients for each variable (using the estimated standard error to draw the random distribution). Results were then summed to determine the mean value and the 95 percent confidence intervals. Data from the literature exist for many of the interventions that are analyzed; for Thailand and Peru, data on the cost of policy change are missing, and for Peru, the cost of condom distribution is missing. For Thailand, the more recent estimate of the costs of ART is used because the older study is from before the sharp decline in the cost of antiretroviral drugs seen in the early part of the 2000s. Although the observations from the individual

Table 10.4 Results for Thailand, Peru, Kenya, and Ukraine

Intervention category	*Specific intervention and target population*	*Number of studies*	*Estimated unit cost (2008 US$)*	*Range*	*Model estimates*	*Model estimate ranges*
Thailand						
ART	n.a.	2[a]	1,235	1,235–4,619	**Model 1: 1,350** Model 2: 1,179	555–2,542 749–1,716
Condom and lubricant distribution	n.a.	1[b,c]	0.10 (per condom distributed)	—	—	—
Outreach through peer educators	n.a.	1[c]	58 (per person reached per year)	—	Model 1: 191 **Model 2[d]: 16.3** (per person reached per year)	18–661 13.7–19.2
Needle exchange program	n.a.	—	—	—	18.7[e] (per person reached per year)	9.6–32.7
Methadone replacement therapy	n.a.	—	—	—	763.0 (cost per person per year)	497.7–1,089.1
Structural interventions	Mass media targeted to vulnerable population	1[b,c]	41,000 (per campaign targeting MSM)	—	—	—
	Changes in laws or policies	—	—	100,000[f]	—	—

(continued next page)

Table 10.4 *(continued)*

Intervention category	*Specific intervention and target population*	*Number of studies*	*Estimated unit cost (2008 US$)*	*Range*	*Model estimates*	*Model estimate ranges*
Peru						
ART	n.a.	1[g]	3,788	—	**Model 1: 1,377** Model 2: 1,271	567–2,592 818–1,838
Condom and lubricant distribution	n.a.	—	—	0.1–0.4[h]	—	—
Outreach through peer educators	n.a.	1[b,g]	103[i] (per person reached per year)	—	Model 1: 196 **Model 2[d]: 17.0** (per person reached per year)	18–675 14.2–19.9
Structural interventions	Mass media targeted to vulnerable population	1[g]	0.40 (per person per year)	—	—	—
	Changes in laws or policies	—	—	100,000[f]	—	—
Kenya						
ART	n.a.	—	—	—	**Model 1: 1,018** Model 2: 418	411–1,918 178–796
Condom and lubricant distribution	n.a.	—	—	0.1–0.4[h]	—	—
Outreach through peer educators	n.a.	—	—	—	Model 1: 128 **Model 2[d]: 4.1** (per person reached per year)	9–473 2.8–5.7
Structural interventions	Mass media targeted to vulnerable population	—	—		—	—
	Changes in laws or policies	—	—	100,000[f]	—	—

Ukraine						
ART	n.a.	—	—	—	**Model 1: 1,183** Model 2: 718	482–2,230 384–1,145
Condom and lubricant distribution	n.a.	—	—	0.1–0.4[h]	—	—
Outreach through peer educators	n.a.	—	—	—	Model 1: 158 **Model 2[d]: 12.6** (per person reached per year)	13–573 10.6–14.8
Needle exchange program	n.a.	1[j]	10.21	—	17.9[e] (per person reached per year)	9.2–31.2
Methadone replacement therapy	n.a.	—	—	—	707.3 (cost per person per year)	454.0–1,023.1
Structural interventions	Mass media targeted to vulnerable population	—	—		—	—
	Changes in laws or policies	—	—	100,000[f]	—	—

Source: Authors.
Note: n.a. = not applicable; — not available. Highlighted models were used for the analysis.
a. Kitajima et al. 2003; Revenga et al. 2006.
b. MSM-specific unit cost.
c. Constella Futures et al. 2006.
d. Predicted for the average number of contacts in one year observed in data collected.
e. Predicted for the modal number of contacts in one year observed in the data collected.
f. Cohen, Wu, and Farley 2004.
g. Aldridge et al. 2009.
h. Bedimo et al. 2002; Constella Futures et al. 2006; Soderlund et al. 1993; Terris-Prestholt, Kumaranayake et al. 2006.
i. Includes condoms and lubricant.
j. Vickerman et al. 2006.

countries may have less than ideal methodologies behind them, they likely more closely represent the situation in an individual country than the results from the models prepared for this analysis (given the weaknesses of the models). In cases for which data from a country are available, they are used for the base case assessment, and the model is used for uncertainty ranges.

In many cases, the uncertainty ranges from the models include the base case estimate using literature from a particular country. The model for outreach through peer educators is the exception, likely because the model has been used to predict costs for an efficient level of contacts. The models also seem to do worse for Peru than for Thailand or Ukraine, which is likely because the models from the Latin American regions have few observations (one country in the peer outreach model and three countries in the ART model) and because injecting drug users in Peru are few in number and typically use cocaine, which is not amenable to substitution therapy with methadone.

Total costs are calculated as the linear sum of *target population * coverage * unit costs* for all interventions except for the distribution of condoms and lubricants. For the distribution of condoms and lubricants, costs were calculated as *target population * number of partners per year * number of sex acts per partner * adjustment for wastage rate by users * coverage * unit costs*. Wastage rate by users is assumed to be 5 percent. For the two MSM-specific interventions, the target population is all MSM. However, for ART, the target population is MSM in need. The prevalence of HIV is estimated in other parts of this book and is duplicated here.

Estimating the Impacts

Tables 10.5 to 10.8 provide the total infections averted and average cost-effectiveness of various single interventions to control HIV/AIDS among MSM in Peru, Thailand, Ukraine, and Kenya for the period 2007–15, compared to no intervention. In all countries, the largest number of HIV infections is averted through ART for MSM, apart from the scenarios where the interventions are set at 30 percent coverage. In that case, community-level behavioral interventions avert more infections. However, ART is consistently the most costly of the three interventions examined.

Tables 10.9 to 10.12 report on the incremental cost-effectiveness ratios for interventions, listed in the order they would be added with increasing budgets if cost-effectiveness were the only consideration. Figures 10.8 to 10.11 show the expansion paths graphically, with the slope of the line joining any two points indicating the incremental

Table 10.5 Total Costs, Total Infections Averted, and Average Cost-Effectiveness of Various Single Interventions to Control HIV/AIDS among MSM in Peru, for the Period 2007–15, Compared to No Intervention

Intervention	*Coverage level (%)*	*Total costs (2008 US$)*	*Total infections averted*	*Average cost per HIV infection averted (2008 US$)*
Promotion and distribution of condoms with lubricants	30	33,676,446	16,465	2,045
Promotion and distribution of condoms with lubricants	30–60	49,764,315	25,252	1,971
Promotion and distribution of condoms with lubricants	100	111,621,982	53,276	2,095
Community level	30	131,857,534	30,068	4,385
Community level	30–60	194,567,912	45,455	4,280
Community level	100	435,288,819	92,307	4,716
ART	30	472,701,927	26,274	186,245
ART	60	950,443,131	59,781	164,583
ART	100	1,598,770,873	120,704	137,116

Source: Authors.

Table 10.6 Total Costs, Total Infections Averted, and Average Cost-Effectiveness of Various Single Interventions to Control HIV/AIDS among MSM in Thailand, for the Period 2007–15, Compared to No Intervention

Intervention	*Coverage level (%)*	*Total costs (2008 US$)*	*Total infections averted*	*Average cost per HIV infection averted (2008 US$)*
Promotion and distribution of condoms with lubricants	30	9,497,691	6,137	1,548
Promotion and distribution of condoms with lubricants	30–60	13,918,866	9,300	1,497
Promotion and distribution of condoms with lubricants	100	31,593,714	19,841	1,592
Community level	30	72,777,368	14,172	5,135
Community level	30–60	106,605,856	20,946	5,090
Community level	100	241,597,698	41,527	5,818
ART	30	1,556,225,324	12,905	120,591
ART	60	3,120,886,234	28,753	108,541
ART	100	5,229,571,611	54,831	95,376

Source: Authors.

cost-effectiveness ratio for the more costly option. The expansion paths for all four countries are similar, indicating that the promotion and distribution of condoms with lubricants is generally the most cost-effective approach to controlling the HIV epidemic among MSM (except in Kenya and Ukraine where community interventions are

Table 10.7 Total Costs, Total Infections Averted, and Average Cost-Effectiveness of Various Single Interventions to Control HIV/AIDS among MSM in Ukraine, for the Period 2007–15, Compared to No Intervention

Intervention	*Coverage level (%)*	*Total costs (2008 US$)*	*Total infections averted*	*Average cost per HIV infection averted (2008 US$)*
Promotion and distribution of condoms with lubricants	30	17,013,040	948	17,946
Promotion and distribution of condoms with lubricants	30–60	24,446,988	1,490	16,407
Promotion and distribution of condoms with lubricants	100	56,689,932	3,524	16,087
Community level	30	8,164,590	2,455	3,326
Community level	30–60	11,731,364	3,889	3,017
Community level	100	27,180,427	9,748	2,788
ART	30	57,883,388	2,681	21,590
ART	60	116,745,369	5,287	22,082
ART	100	205,034,342	11,996	17,236

Source: Authors.

Table 10.8 Total Costs, Total Infections Averted, and Average Cost-Effectiveness of Various Single Interventions to Control HIV/AIDS among MSM in Kenya, for the Period 2007–15, Compared to No Intervention

Intervention	*Coverage level (%)*	*Total costs (2008 US$)*	*Total infections averted*	*Average cost per HIV infection averted (2008 US$)*
Promotion and distribution of condoms with lubricants	30	2,913,723	2,344	1,243
Promotion and distribution of condoms with lubricants	30–60	4,325,468	3,949	1,095
Promotion and distribution of condoms with lubricants	100	9,692,852	8,594	1,128
Community level	30	1,893,499	6,460	293
Community level	30–60	2,808,014	10,385	270
Community level	100	6,275,058	23,049	272
ART	30	51,407,009	5,448	9,436
ART	60	106,201,281	14,574	7,287
ART	100	187,640,039	38,272	4,903

Source: Authors.

more cost-effective, which seems to be driven by the low unit cost of that intervention in that setting). Adding community-level behavioral interventions is the next most cost-effective option (except in Kenya and Ukraine), and adding ART is the relatively least cost-effective option across three of the four countries.

Table 10.9 Total Costs, Total Infections Averted, and Incremental Cost-Effectiveness of Nondominated[a] Intervention Combinations to Control HIV/AIDS among MSM in Peru for the Period 2007–15

Intervention package number	*Description*	*Total costs (2008 US$)*	*Total infections averted*	*Incremental cost-effectiveness ratio (2008 US$)*
P1	Promotion and distribution of condoms with lubricants, 30–60% coverage	49,764,315	25,252	1,971
P2	Promotion and distribution of condoms with lubricants, 100% coverage	111,621,982	53,276	2,207
P3	Promotion and distribution of condoms with lubricants, 100% coverage + community-level MSM, 60% coverage	306,189,894	98,731	4,280
P4	Promotion and distribution of condoms with lubricants + community-level MSM, both 100% coverage	546,910,801	145,583	5,138
P5	Promotion and distribution of condoms with lubricants + community-level MSM, + ART, all 100% coverage	2,145,681,674	266,287	13,245

Source: Authors.
a. Excludes interventions that were more costly but less effective than others (dominated interventions) and those with higher incremental cost-effectiveness ratios than more effective options (weakly dominated interventions).

Table 10.10 Total Costs, Total Infections Averted, and Incremental Cost-Effectiveness of Nondominated[a] Intervention Combinations to Control HIV/AIDS among MSM in Thailand for the Period 2007–15

Intervention package number	*Description*	*Total costs (2008 US$)*	*Total infections averted*	*Incremental cost-effectiveness ratio (2008 US$)*
T1	Promotion and distribution of condoms with lubricants, 30–60% coverage	13,918,866	9,300	1,497
T2	Promotion and distribution of condoms with lubricants, 100% coverage	31,593,714	19,841	1,677

(continued next page)

Table 10.10 *(continued)*

Intervention package number	*Description*	*Total costs (2008 US$)*	*Total infections averted*	*Incremental cost-effectiveness ratio (2008 US$)*
T3	Promotion and distribution of condoms with lubricants, 100% coverage + community-level MSM 60% coverage	138,199,570	40,787	5,090
T4	Promotion and distribution of condoms with lubricants + community-level MSM, both 100% coverage	273,191,413	61,368	6,559
T5	Promotion and distribution of condoms with lubricants + community-level MSM + ART, all 100% coverage	5,502,763,023	116,199	95,376

Source: Authors.
a. Excludes interventions that were more costly but less effective than others (dominated interventions) and those with higher incremental cost-effectiveness ratios than more effective options (weakly dominated interventions).

Table 10.11 Total Costs, Total Infections Averted, and Incremental Cost-Effectiveness of Nondominated[a] Intervention Combinations to Control HIV/AIDS among MSM in Ukraine for the Period 2007–15

Intervention package number	*Description*	*Total costs (2008 US$)*	*Total infections averted*	*Incremental cost-effectiveness ratio (2008 US$)*
U1	Community-level MSM, 100% coverage	27,180,427	9,748	2,788
U2	Community-level MSM + promotion and distribution of condoms with lubricants, both 100% coverage	83,870,359	13,272	16,087
U3	Community-level MSM + promotion and distribution of condoms with lubricants + ART, all 100% coverage	288,904,701	25,168	17,236

Source: Authors.
a. Excludes interventions that were more costly but less effective than others (dominated interventions) and those with higher incremental cost-effectiveness ratios than more effective options (weakly dominated interventions).

Table 10.12 Total Costs, Total Infections Averted, and Incremental Cost-Effectiveness of Nondominated[a] Intervention Combinations to Control HIV/AIDS among MSM in Kenya for the Period 2007–15

Intervention package number	*Description*	*Total costs (2008 US$)*	*Total infections averted*	*Incremental cost-effectiveness ratio (2008 US$)*
K1	Community-level MSM, 60% coverage	2,808,014	10,385	270
K2	Community-level MSM, 100% coverage	6,275,058	23,049	274
K3	Community-level MSM, 100% coverage + promotion and distribution of condoms with lubricants, 60% coverage	7,133,482	26,998	217
K4	Community-level MSM + promotion and distribution of condoms with lubricants, both 100% coverage	15,967,909	31,643	1,902
K5	Community-level MSM + promotion and distribution of condoms with lubricants + ART, all 100% coverage	203,607,948	69,915	4,903

Source: Authors.
a. Excludes interventions that were more costly but less effective than others (dominated interventions) and those with higher incremental cost-effectiveness ratios than more effective options (weakly dominated interventions).

Figure 10.8 Expansion Path for Incremental Addition of Interventions in Peru

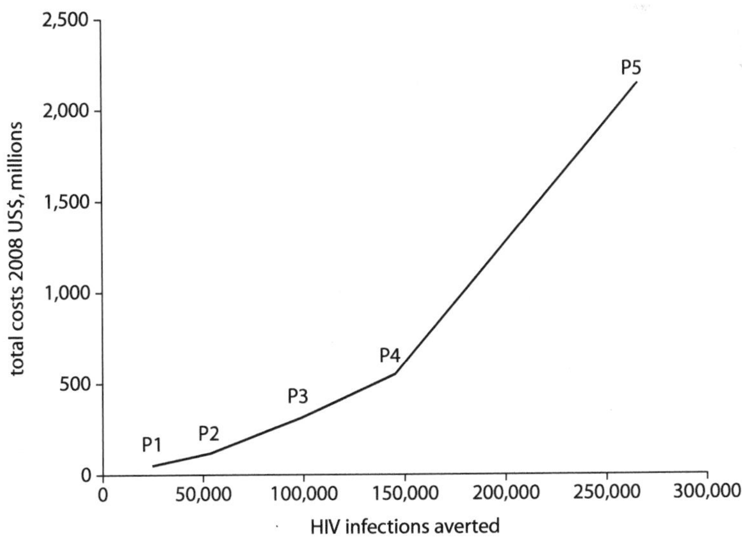

Source: Authors.
Note: See table 10.9 for description of combinations P1–P5.

Figure 10.9 Expansion Path for Incremental Addition of Interventions in Thailand

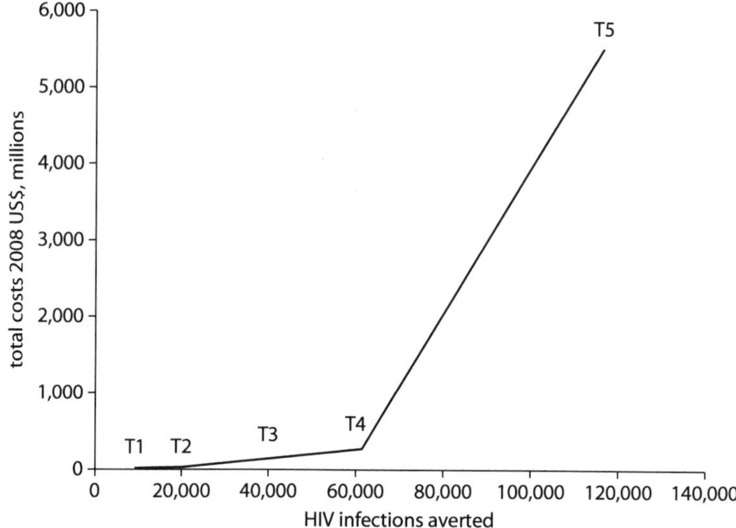

Source: Authors.
Note: See table 10.10 for description of combinations T1–T5.

Figure 10.10 Expansion Path for Incremental Addition of Interventions in Ukraine

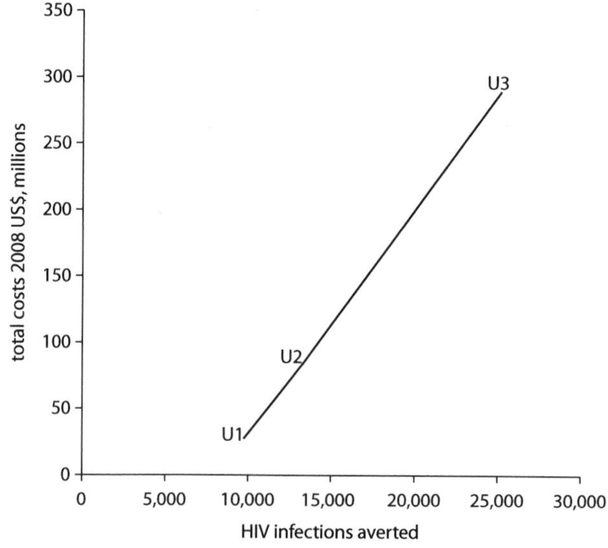

Source: Authors.
Note: See table 10.11 for description of combinations U1–U3.

Figure 10.11 Expansion Path for Incremental Addition of Interventions in Kenya

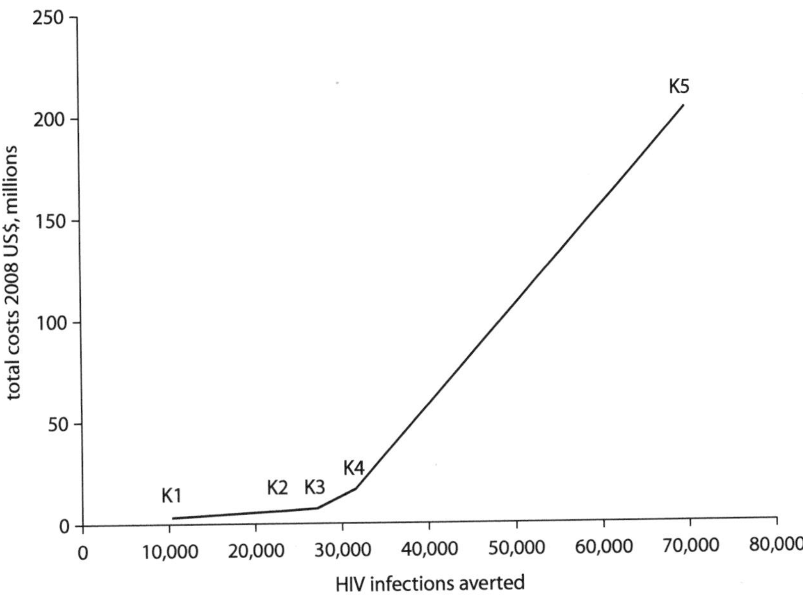

Source: Authors.
Note: See table 10.12 for description of combinations K1–K5.

Discussion

The results of these analyses have implications for costs and costing exercises, cost-effectiveness, and decision making, which are discussed in turn below.

Costs. In general, the main finding from this literature search and analysis is that few data are reported in the public literature on the costs of providing HIV/AIDS interventions to MSM. The literature search revealed only 18 studies specific for MSM. Thus, without additional primary data collection, assessing the costs or the cost-effectiveness of interventions targeting MSM will remain uncertain. For this book, data for interventions targeting other groups that may be somewhat similar to MSM-targeted programs have been relied on, but the results should be interpreted as tentative, order-of-magnitude unit costs. The uncertainty ranges tend to reflect this conclusion.

Second, the data used in these analyses are often collected in different ways, illustrating different perspectives, and using different methodologies;

this problem has been noted previously for cost data in general (Adam, Koopmanschap, and Evans 2003). It makes comparing these studies problematic at best. Clearly, many of these studies were answering different questions from the one posed here; this book tried to accommodate such differences by explicitly including variables in its models to account for these methodological differences. However, these differences do not always lend themselves to perfect classification or quantification, and therefore some measurement error will be present in the regressions. The purpose of the regressions was not to test if these methodological differences have a statistically significant impact on the cost estimates, but to predict as well as possible what unit costs might be in different countries; therefore this measurement error, while not ideal, might be tolerable.

Furthermore, the purpose of the regression models is not to interpret the coefficients; variables were included or excluded based on their ability to explain available data (and therefore to serve as predictors for areas where data are not currently available) and only secondarily because of theoretical considerations. The beta coefficients in the models may not reflect the isolated effects of the variables they are associated with, but may be subject to confounding, and the like. Nevertheless, the signs of the beta coefficients for most of the main variables were in the directions expected. Most notably, increased GDP is associated with higher unit costs in all models, and in the models where such data are available, costs have a U-shaped relationship with number of contacts.[5]

Another potential problem with these models is using localized, program- or facility-specific data to estimate average costs for an entire nation. This problem is most clearly highlighted in the models where number of contacts has been included as a variable. What the average of "the number of annual contacts at a facility/program" will be for all facilities or programs in a nation is unknown, as is how this average might change with different national coverage levels. For the models where this variable is not available, this problem remains, although it cannot be modeled explicitly. Moreover, national-level variables that may have an influence on unit costs have not been included, such as the extent of donor participation or length of time since starting service provision (Over 2010), in part because these variables may not apply to a particular setting and in part because data are not available for many years or countries. Again, this omission may bias the results when predicting for a particular country.

As noted previously, the results presented here are far from conclusive, and interpreting the beta coefficients in the models is problematic. However, the models for the outreach intervention do show that different target populations (for example, male only vs. female only, or male only vs. both sexes) do have a significant ($p < 0.05$) effect on unit costs. This finding does not mean that the differences in the unit costs are important: the magnitude of the differences that is important depends on the question that is being asked (for example, is it important when determining a budget vs. does it make a difference in a cost-effectiveness analysis). However, this finding does reinforce the notion that further research into the costs of interventions and programs for MSM is needed to define not only the extent to which these programs have different costs than other types of programs, but also why they have different costs. Such research could help make results more generalizable (initial hypotheses may include the following, which could all influence the unit costs: the outreach techniques needed for different programs, the number of contacts that peer outreach workers can establish in one location, and the need for lubricants).

Furthermore, as has been noted previously (Guinness et al. 2005; Guinness, Kumaranayake, and Hanson 2007; Kumaranayake 2008), the size of a particular site does seem to influence unit costs. The difficulty is translating that difference into different unit costs at varying levels of national coverage. More work is needed in this area to fully assess the cost-effectiveness of interventions.

Other methods than those used here are available for estimating unit costs, primarily ingredients-based methods in which individual inputs to the unit costs are estimated separately (see, for example, Over 2010). These ingredients-based methods are highly driven by assumptions about quantities of resources used to deliver services (and tend to assume a rather close adherence to either guidelines or a few limited studies) as well as the prices of the inputs used. They are also subject to bias because of the omission of certain cost categories. This chapter's results, in contrast, are driven by assumptions about the external validity of existing data and the ability of regression analysis to adequately capture or control for differences in the data to produce predictions for where data are missing. Lacking data on what is needed for most of the interventions for MSM (except possibly the more clinical-based interventions such as ART and methadone replacement therapy), this chapter has adapted the latter approach, but all results should be interpreted with the limitations of the methods used borne in mind.

Impact and cost-effectiveness. Because of uncertainty in many of this book's data and assumptions, the results presented here should be viewed by broad bands of incremental cost-effectiveness ratios. However, in this respect, the results suggest that robust differences exist in the value for money of the three interventions examined, with the promotion and distribution of condoms with lubricants generally being the most cost-effective use of resources, followed by community-level behavioral interventions, and finally ART.

A previous study of the cost-effectiveness of strategies to control HIV/AIDS in Peru (Aldridge et al. 2009) found that "interventions targeted at MSM consistently performed well in terms of total infections averted, [. . .] however it did not perform well in terms of cost-effectiveness." The analysis here is not strictly comparable with that analysis because a different version of Goals and different coverage levels for the three interventions were used and also because modifications were made to the model to allow exploration of different risk group among MSM. The earlier version of Goals classified MSM as a single, homogeneous at-risk group, which ignores the reality of varying behavioral and risk characteristics. Despite these differences, a brief comparison is informative. The cost-effectiveness of an intervention for MSM was estimated to be approximately US$6,700 per HIV infection averted (authors' calculations based on data reported by Aldridge et al. 2009). The intervention for MSM examined by Aldridge and colleagues (2009) is described as peer counseling and treatment of STIs, with condoms provided during counseling sessions. This package is similar to the community-level behavioral intervention modeled for this chapter and for cost-effectiveness was found to be about US$4,500 per HIV infection averted.

Aldridge and colleagues (2009) also remark that "if interventions were targeted more specifically at these groups [MSM risk groups] then numbers of participants included would be smaller and the interventions would likely to improve significantly in the cost-effectiveness rankings." Currently, options are being explored to take advantage of the risk classification of MSM performed for this book and incorporated into the Goals Model to compare the cost-effectiveness of targeted versus universal MSM interventions.

Also of note is that the earlier version of Goals that Aldridge and colleagues (2009) used did not include the ability of ART to affect sexual behavior and transmissibility. The current version did allow exploration of the impact and cost-effectiveness of ART, and it resulted in the largest impact in terms of HIV infections averted. However, because

ART is substantially more costly than the other two options evaluated, it was still considered the least cost-effective way to manage the epidemic among MSM in Kenya, Peru, and Thailand among the three interventions assessed. Nevertheless, a cost per HIV infection averted of US$137,000 roughly equates to a cost per disability-adjusted life year averted of US$5,300, which is between one and three times the gross national income of Peru (US$3,990) in 2008; hence, using the normative benchmark of cost-effectiveness set forth by the World Health Organization (Commission on Macroeconomics and Health 2001), ART would be considered good value for money.

One must emphasize that decisions are never, nor should they be, made only on the basis of cost-effectiveness data. Many other factors influence priority setting, including ethical criteria and human rights (which is addressed in chapter 11 of this report). Therefore, policy makers should interpret this chapter's results in the context of these other important considerations.

See appendix A, where the price tag is estimated to launch a comprehensive prevention and treatment program for MSM in these four countries, plus Brazil, India, the Russian Federation, and Senegal. The analysis is extended to an additional 47 countries in appendix B.

Annex 10.A

Tables 10.A.1 to 10.A.10 provide details of the data used in each regression and the results of the models.

Table 10.A.1 Input Data into ART Regression Model

Variable	*Number*	*Mean*	*Standard deviation*	*Minimum*	*Maximum*
Year of observation	77	2002.90	3.42	1992	2008
Percentage of studies reporting lifetime costs vs. cost per patient year	77	29	0.45	0	1
Unit cost in year of study (US$)	77	18,095	50,100	265	385,200
GDP per capita in year of study (US$)	77	13,951	14,065	125	46,040
Unit cost inflated to 2008 (US$)	77	22,303	58,011	441.16	431.82
GDP per capita in 2008 (US$)	77	20,904	20,310	138	68,433
Percentage of studies reporting economic costs vs. financial costs	77	45	.50	0	1

(continued next page)

Table 10.A.1 *(continued)*

Variable	*Number*	*Mean*	*Standard deviation*	*Minimum*	*Maximum*
Percentage of studies reporting full costs vs. incremental costs	77	90	.31	0	1
Percentage of studies collecting longitudinal data	77	27	n.a.	n.a.	n.a.
Percentage of studies collecting data in a cross section	77	39	n.a.	n.a.	n.a.
Percentage of studies using a model to estimate costs	77	29	n.a.	n.a.	n.a.
Percentage of studies reporting data based on expert opinion	77	5	n.a.	n.a.	n.a.
Percentage of studies reporting costs from a societal perspective vs. health system perspective	77	1	.11	0	1
Percentage of studies that omitted obvious cost categories vs. all cost categories	77	17	.38	0	1
Percentage of studies reporting costs for patients in their first year of treatment vs. patients in multiple years of treatment	77	3	.16	0	1
Percentage of costing taking place in a hospital setting vs. primary health care	77	95	.22	0	1

Source: Authors.
Note: n.a. = not applicable.

Table 10.A.2 Results of the Best Model from Preliminary Analysis of the ART Data

Unit costs in the year of the study (US$)	*Beta*	*Robust standard error*	*z*	*P > z*
Spline for GDP below US$600	.0035554	.0004616	7.70	0.000
Spline for GDP above US$600	.0000895	4.29e-06	20.85	0.000
Lifetime costs vs. cost per patient year	2.183962	.764403	2.86	0.004
Economic costs vs. financial costs	−.9674951	.5977861	−1.62	0.106
Cross-sectional vs. longitudinal data collection	.1614562	.4658455	0.35	0.729
Modeled costs vs. longitudinal data collection	1.085035	.4697007	2.31	0.021
Expert opinion vs. longitudinal data collection	1.675547	.2018708	8.30	0.000

(continued next page)

Table 10.A.2 *(continued)*

Unit costs in the year of the study (US$)	*Beta*	*Robust standard error*	*z*	*P > z*
Societal perspective vs. health system perspective	.784839	.1919791	4.09	0.000
Omitted obvious cost categories vs. all cost categories	−.2978026	.1320604	−2.26	0.024
After year 2003 vs. before year 2003	−.3952051	.2143303	−1.84	0.065
Interaction: Economic costs * omitted cost categories	−.9927247	.6232381	−1.59	0.111
Interaction: Economic costs * after year 2003	.8264552	.2256439	3.66	0.000
Interaction: Cross-sectional data collection * omitted cost categories	.730016	.3423907	2.13	0.033
Interaction: Modeled data * omitted cost categories	.022589	.6098211	0.04	0.970
Constant	4.481715	.362199	12.37	0.000

Source: Authors.
Note: Regression run using the glm command in Stata using a log link function; coefficients are presented as log transformed.

Table 10.A.3 Results of the Best Model from Analysis of the ART Data Excluding Studies Reporting Lifetime Costs

Unit costs in the year of the study (US$)	*Beta*	*Robust standard error*	*z*	*P > z*
Spline for GDP below US$5,000	.0003459	.0000931	3.71	0.000
Spline for GDP between US$5,000 and 10,000	.0001966	.0000711	2.77	0.006
Spline for GDP above US$10,000	.0000318	9.99e-06	3.18	0.001
Spline for year before 2000	.0456218	.0793634	0.57	0.565
Spline for year after 2000	−.081442	.0271555	−3.00	0.003
Economic costs vs. financial costs	.1701934	.1613888	1.05	0.292
Full costs vs. incremental costs	.8984096	.2169095	4.14	0.000
Modeled costs vs. observed costs	1.818832	.4110894	4.42	0.000
Interaction = 1 if full costs and modeled costs	−1.453123	.3777715	−3.85	0.000
Omitted obvious cost categories vs. all cost categories	.1850366	.1031737	1.79	0.073

(continued next page)

Table 10.A.3 *(continued)*

Unit costs in the year of the study (US$)	*Beta*	*Robust standard error*	*z*	*P > z*
Cost for patients only in first year of treatment vs. cost for patients in multiple years	−.8192254	.2570806	−3.19	0.001
Constant	−85.84465	158.8378	−0.54	0.589

Source: Authors.
Note: Regression run using the glm command in Stata using a log link function; coefficients are presented as log transformed.

Table 10.A.4 Input Data into Outreach Model

Variable	*Number*	*Mean*	*Standard deviation*	*Minimum*	*Maximum*
Target population: MSM only	40	25%	n.a.	n.a.	n.a.
Target population: Female sex workers only	40	62.5%	n.a.	n.a.	n.a.
Target population: Other vulnerable populations	40	12.5%	n.a.	n.a.	n.a.
Target population: Men only	40	27.5%	n.a.	n.a.	n.a.
Target population: Female only	40	67.5%	n.a.	n.a.	n.a.
Target population: Both male and female	40	5%	n.a.	n.a.	n.a.
Location: Entire country vs. urban only	40	60%	.50	0	1
Number of contacts made with client population in one year	33	22,763	38,134	168	150,000
Year of study	40	2002.5	3.72	1992	2009
Unit costs in year of study (US$)	40	126	359	2.5	2,211.4
GDP per capita in year of study (US$)	40	7,297	12,547	456	39,852
Economic costs vs. financial costs	40	80%	.41	0	1
Full costing vs. incremental costing	40	82.5%	.38	0	1
Cost reported as cost per person per year	40	45%	n.a.	n.a.	n.a.

(continued next page)

Table 10.A.4 *(continued)*

Variable	*Number*	*Mean*	*Standard deviation*	*Minimum*	*Maximum*
Cost reported as cost per person reached per year	40	20%	n.a.	n.a.	n.a.
Cost reported per person (unclear)	40	5%	n.a.	n.a.	n.a.
Method of cost estimation: Expert opinion	40	12.5%	n.a.	n.a.	n.a.
Method of cost estimation: Model based	40	7.5%	n.a.	n.a.	n.a.
Method of cost estimation: Empirical data collection in cross section	40	72.5%	n.a.	n.a.	n.a.
Method of cost estimation: Empirical data collection in longitudinal study	40	7.5%	n.a.	n.a.	n.a.
Societal costs vs. health system or program costs	40	10%	.30	0	1
Complete costs vs. obvious exclusions	40	85%	.36	0	1
Program implemented as outreach from fixed facility vs. community based	40	70%	.46	0	1
Unit costs include treatment of STIs vs. do not include treatment of STIs	40	60%	.50	0	1

Source: Authors.
Note: n.a. = not applicable.

Table 10.A.5 Results of the Best Model from Analysis of the Community Outreach Data

Unit costs in the year of the study (US$)	*Beta*	*Robust standard error*	*z*	*P > z*
GDP per capita in year of study (US$)	.0001646	.0000367	4.48	0.000
Year	.3491947	.0368174	9.48	0.000
Female-only target population vs. male-only target population	.3063353	.1548912	1.98	0.048
Target population of both sexes vs. male-only target population	−2.781628	.1128904	−24.64	0.000
Economic vs. financial costing method	.4327514	.012152	35.61	0.000

(continued next page)

Table 10.A.5 *(continued)*

Unit costs in the year of the study (US$)	*Beta*	*Robust standard error*	*z*	*P>z*
Per target population per year vs. per person reached per year	.6395169	1.026502	0.62	0.533
Observed data collection method vs. model or expert opinion	−14.28275	3.559005	−4.01	0.000
Full list of items included in cost vs. partial list of items included in cost	12.81632	2.536801	5.05	0.000
Outreach from health facility vs. community-based program	−7.917872	1.200025	−6.60	0.000
Costs include treatment of STIs vs. not treating STIs	−5.467877	1.305512	−4.19	0.000
Interaction of economic costs and outreach	11.73527	1.631382	7.19	0.000
Interaction of female-only target population and empirical observation	1.819096	1.164981	1.56	0.118
Constant[a]	−696.7883	73.90562	−9.43	0.000

Source: Authors.
Note: Regression run using the glm command in Stata using a log link function; coefficients are presented as log transformed.
a. Constant is negative because year is a continuous variable that was not centered (so constant is for year AD 0).

Table 10.A.6 Results of the Best Model from Analysis of the Community Outreach Data Including Number of Contacts as an Independent Variable

Unit costs in the year of the study (US$)	*Beta*	*Robust standard error*	*z*	*P>z*
Spline for GDP per capita in year of study if GDP is under US$1,000	.0050895	.0007242	7.03	0.000
Spline for GDP per capita in year of study if GDP Z > US$1,000	.0001739	1.00e-06	173.28	0.000
Year	.3986516	.0036	110.74	0.000
Number of contacts made with client population in one year	−.0001301	.000012	−10.80	0.000
Number of contacts made with client population in one year squared	1.91e-09	1.75e-10	10.91	0.000
Location: Entire country vs. urban only	−.1874547	.1115483	−1.68	0.093

(continued next page)

Table 10.A.6 *(continued)*

Unit costs in the year of the study (US$)	*Beta*	*Robust standard error*	*z*	*P > z*
Target population: Female only vs. male only	15.43797	1.913283	8.07	0.000
Target population: Both male and female vs. male only	−2.312948	.0532263	−43.46	0.000
Economic costs vs. financial costs	.4385633	.0059705	73.46	0.000
Cost per target population vs. cost per person reached	.5843889	.026618	21.95	0.000
Complete costs vs. obvious exclusions	10.7241	1.783908	6.01	0.000
Program implemented as outreach from fixed facility vs. community based	−34.33245	2.570988	−13.35	0.000
Unit costs include treatment of STIs vs. not treating STIs	23.09818	.9130612	25.30	0.000
Constant	−813.1135	7.640423	−106.42	0.000

Source: Authors.

Table 10.A.7 Input Data into Needle Exchange Model

Variable	*Number*	*Mean*	*Standard deviation*	*Minimum*	*Maximum*
Female-only target population vs. both sexes	16	6.25%	.25	0	1
Location: Entire country vs. urban setting	16	37.5%	.5	0	1
Number of contacts in one year	14	39,864	93,038	275	339,714
Year	16	1998.4	4.94	1990	2007
Cost per person reached per year vs. cost per contact	16	75%	.45	0	1
Unit costs in year of study (US$)	16	74.80	79.40	2.25	223
GDP per capita in year of study (US$)	16	9431	13,750.50	203	39,852
Economic costs vs. financial costs	16	43.75%	.51	0	1
Method of cost estimation: Expert opinion	16	37.5%	n.a.	n.a.	n.a.
Method of cost estimation: Empirical data collection in cross section	16	56.25%	n.a.	n.a.	n.a.

(continued next page)

Table 10.A.7 *(continued)*

Variable	*Number*	*Mean*	*Standard deviation*	*Minimum*	*Maximum*
Method of cost estimation:					
Empirical data collection in longitudinal study	16	6.25%	n.a.	n.a.	n.a.
Societal costs vs. health system or program costs	16	6.25%	.25	0	1
Complete costs vs. obvious exclusions	16	62.5%	.5	0	1
Setting: Community based	16	18.75%	n.a.	n.a.	n.a.
Setting: Outreach from a fixed facility	16	56.25%	n.a.	n.a.	n.a.
Setting: Services provided at a fixed facility	16	25%	n.a.	n.a.	n.a.

Source: Authors.
Note: n.a. = not applicable.

Table 10.A.8 Results of the Best Model from Analysis of the Needle Exchange Program Data

Unit costs in the year of the study (US$)	*Beta*	*Robust standard errror*	*z*	*P > z*
GDP per capita in year of study	.0000286	2.87e-06	9.96	0.000
Year category: After 2000 vs. up to and including 2000	−3.242729	1.061944	−3.05	0.002
Number of contacts made with client population in one year	−.0001242	.0000552	−2.25	0.024
Number of contacts made with client population in one year squared	3.54e-10	1.62e-10	2.18	0.029
Data collected from empirical study vs. model or expert opinion	−2.523697	.337902	−7.47	0.000
Setting: Outreach from fixed facility vs. community based	.6482994	.3117629	2.08	0.038
Setting: Services at a fixed facility vs. community based	2.554566	.1209329	21.12	0.000
Constant	4.740716	.2445634	19.38	0.000

Source: Authors.

Table 10.A.9 Input Data into Methadone Replacement Therapy Model

Variable	*Number*	*Mean*	*Standard deviation*	*Minimum*	*Maximum*
Location: Entire country vs. urban setting	17	18%	.39	0	1
Number of contacts in one year	7	2,595	6,062	88	16,335
Year	17	1998.2	5.5	1990	2007
Cost per person reached per year vs. cost per contact	17	94%	.24	0	1
Unit costs in year of the study (US$)	17	3,016	1,765	6.70	5,611
GDP per capita in year of the study (US$)	17	24,157	10,394	946	43,674
Economic costs vs. financial costs	17	29%	.47	0	1
Full costs vs. incremental costs	17	82%	.39	0	1
Method of cost estimation: Expert opinion	17	11.76%	n.a.	n.a.	n.a.
Method of cost estimation: Empirical data collection in cross section	17	88.24%	n.a.	n.a.	n.a.
Societal costs vs. health system or program costs	17	23.5%	.44	0	1
Complete costs vs. obvious exclusions	17	88%	.33	0	1
Setting: Community based	16	5.88%	n.a.	n.a.	n.a.
Setting: Outreach from a fixed facility	16	5.88%	n.a.	n.a.	n.a.
Setting: Services provided at a fixed facility	16	88.24%	n.a.	n.a.	n.a.

Source: Authors.
Note: n.a. = not applicable.

Table 10.A.10 Results of the Best Model from Analysis of the Methadone Replacement Therapy Data

Unit costs in the year of the study (US$)	*Beta*	*Robust standard error*	*z*	*P>z*
GDP per capita in the year of the study	.0000529	6.26e-06	8.44	0.000
Year category: After 1995 vs. up to and including 1995	–.6708178	.1584232	–4.23	0.000

(continued next page)

Table 10.A.10 *(continued)*

Unit costs in the year of the study (US$)	*Beta*	*Robust standard error*	*z*	*P > z*
Cost per person per year vs. cost per contact	4.568949	.2631472	17.36	0.000
Economic costs vs. financial costs	.106346	.1243488	0.86	0.392
Full costs vs. incremental costs	−.678927	.0818811	−8.29	0.000
Complete costs vs. obvious exclusions	−.0042361	.0668161	−0.06	0.949
Constant	3.064128	.2180517	14.05	0.000

Source: Authors.

Notes

1. Some of these studies may overlap; for example, a study reporting costs for condom distribution and mass media would be counted twice here.
2. For this reason, factors such as economies of scale cannot be assessed; therefore, these factors are dealt with in uncertainty analysis.
3. Note that a second spline node for GDP was tried in the first model's specifications but was not found to improve the performance of the model.
4. The coefficient for "complete costs vs. obvious exclusions" is not statistically significant based on the p-value reported, but was the best among the available variables when using Akaike's Information Criteria and therefore was included in the final model.
5. Additionally, in the ART model, any model where year was included as a continuous variable showed a negative sign for year. Because this variable is controlled for GDP (that is, a later year compared to an earlier year, assuming GDP is the same), this outcome conforms with expectations about decreases over time in the prices of drugs and lab tests needed for ART.

References

Adam, T., M. A. Koopmanschap, and D. B. Evans. 2003. "Cost-Effectiveness Analysis: Can We Reduce Variability in Costing Methods?" *International Journal of Technology Assessment in Health Care* 19 (2): 407–20.

Afriandi, I., A. Y. Siregar, F. Meheus, T. Hidayat, A. van der Ven, R. van Crevel, and R. Baltussen. 2010. "Costs of Hospital-Based Methadone Maintenance Treatment in HIV/AIDS Control among Injecting Drug Users in Indonesia." *Health Policy* 95 (1): 69–73.

Aisu, T., M. C. Raviglione, E. van Praag, P. Eriki, J. P. Narain, L. Barugahare, G. Tembo, D. McFarland, and F. A. Engwau. 1995. "Preventive Chemotherapy for HIV-Associated Tuberculosis in Uganda: An Operational Assessment at a Voluntary Counselling and Testing Centre." *AIDS* 9 (3): 267–73.

Aldridge, R. W., D. Iglesias, C. F. Cáceres, and J. J. Miranda. 2009. "Determining a Cost Effective Intervention Response to HIV/AIDS in Peru." *BMC Public Health* 9: 352.

Anis, A. H., D. Guh, R. S. Hogg, X. H. Wang, B. Yip, K. J. Craib, M. V. O'Shaughnessy, M. T. Schechter, and J. S. Montaner. 2000. "The Cost Effectiveness of Antiretroviral Regimens for the Treatment of HIV/AIDS." *Pharmacoeconomics* 18 (4): 393–404.

Aracena-Genao, B., J. O. Navarro, H. Lamadrid-Figueroa, S. Forsythe, and B. Trejo-Valdivia. 2008. "Costs and Benefits of HAART for Patients with HIV in a Public Hospital in Mexico." *AIDS* (Suppl. 1): S141–48.

Auvert, B., E. Marseille, E. L. Korenromp, J. Lloyd-Smith, R. Sitta, D. Taljaard, C. Pretorius, B. Williams, and J. G. Kahn. 2008. "Estimating the Resources Needed and Savings Anticipated from Roll-Out of Adult Male Circumcision in Sub-Saharan Africa." *PLoS One* 3 (8): 2679.

Babigumira, J. B., A. K. Sethi, K. A. Smyth, and M. E. Singer. 2009. "Cost Effectiveness of Facility-Based Care, Home-Based Care and Mobile Clinics for Provision of Antiretroviral Therapy in Uganda." *Pharmacoeconomics* 27 (11): 963–73.

Bachmann, M. O. 2006. "Effectiveness and Cost Effectiveness of Early and Late Prevention of HIV/AIDS Progression with Antiretrovirals or Antibiotics in Southern African Adults." *AIDS Care* 18 (2): 109–20.

Badri, M., S. Cleary, G. Maartens, J. Pitt, L. G. Bekker, C. Orrell, and R. Wood. 2006. "When to Initiate Highly Active Antiretroviral Therapy in Sub-Saharan Africa? A South African Cost-Effectiveness Study." *Antiviral Therapy* 11 (1): 63–72.

Badri, M., G. Maartens, S. Mandalia, L. G. Bekker, J. R. Penrod, R. W. Platt, R. Wood, and E. J. Beck. 2006. "Cost-Effectiveness of Highly Active Antiretroviral Therapy in South Africa." *PLoS Med* 23 (1): e4.

Barnett, P. G. 1999. "The Cost-Effectiveness of Methadone Maintenance as a Health Care Intervention." *Addiction* 94 (4): 479–88.

Bautista-Arredondo, S., T. Dmytraczenko, G. Kombe, and S. M. Bertozzi. 2008. "Costing of Scaling Up HIV/AIDS Treatment in Mexico." *Salud Pública de México* 50 (Suppl. 4): S437–44.

Bayoumi, A. M., and G. S. Zaric. 2008. "The Cost-Effectiveness of Vancouver's Supervised Injection Facility." *Canadian Medical Association Journal* 179 (11): 1143–51.

Beck, E. J., S. Mandalia, M. Gaudreault, C. Brewer, H. Zowall, N. Gilmore, M. B. Klein, R. Lalonde, A. Piché, and C. A. Hankins. 2004. "The Cost-Effectiveness of Highly Active Antiretroviral Therapy, Canada 1991–2001." *AIDS* 18 (18): 2411–18.

Bedimo, A. L., S. D. Pinkerton, D. A. Cohen, B. Gray, and T. A. Farley. 2002. "Condom Distribution: A Cost-Utility Analysis." *International Journal of STD and AIDS* 13 (6): 384–92.

Bikilla, A. D., D. Jerene, B. Robberstad, and B. Lindtjorn. 2009. "Cost-Effectiveness of Anti-retroviral Therapy at a District Hospital in Southern Ethiopia." *Cost Effectiveness and Resource Allocation* 7: 13.

Binagwaho, A., E. Pegurri, J. Muita, and S. Bertozzi. 2010. "Male Circumcision at Different Ages in Rwanda: A Cost-Effectiveness Study." *PLoS Med* 7 (1): e1000211.

Bollinger, L. A., J. Stover, G. Musuka, B. Fidzani, T. Moeti, and L. Busang. 2009. "The Cost and Impact of Male Circumcision on HIV/AIDS in Botswana." *Journal of the International AIDS Society* 12 (1): 7.

Borghi, J., A. Gorter, P. Sandiford, and Z. Segura. 2005. "The Cost-Effectiveness of a Competitive Voucher Scheme to Reduce Sexually Transmitted Infections in High-Risk Groups in Nicaragua." *Health Policy and Planning* 20 (4): 222–31.

Boulle, A., C. Kenyon, J. Skordis, and R. Wood. 2002. "Exploring the Costs of a Limited Public Sector Antiretroviral Treatment Programme in South Africa." *South African Medical Journal* 92 (10): 811–17.

Cabases, J. M., and E. Sanchez. 2003. "Costs and Effectiveness of a Syringe Distribution and Needle Exchange Program for HIV Prevention in a Regional Setting." *European Journal of Health Economics* 4 (3): 203–208.

Carrara, V., F. Terris-Prestholt, L. Kumaranayake, and P. Mayaud. 2005. "Operational and Economic Evaluation of an NGO-Led Sexually Transmitted Infections Intervention: North-Western Cambodia." *Bulletin of the World Health Organization* 83 (6): 434–42.

Chaix, C., C. Grenier-Sennelier, P. Clevenbergh, J. Durant, J. M. Schapiro, P. Dellamonica, and I. Durand-Zaleski. 2000. "Economic Evaluation of Drug Resistance Genotyping for the Adaptation of Treatment in HIV-Infected Patients in the VIRADAPT Study." *Journal of Acquired Immune Deficiency Syndromes* 24 (3): 227–31.

Chandrashekar, S., L. Guinness, L. Kumaranayake, B. Reddy, Y. Govindraj, P. Vickerman, and M. Alary. 2010. "The Effects of Scale on the Costs of Targeted HIV Prevention Interventions among Female and Male Sex Workers, Men Who Have Sex with Men and Transgenders in India." *Sexually Transmitted Infections* 86 (Suppl. 1): i89–94.

Charreau, I., G. Jeanblanc, P. Tangre, L. Boyer, M. Saouzanet, B. Marchou, J. M. Molina, J. P. Aboulke, and I. Durand-Zaleski. 2008. "Costs of Intermittent

Versus Continuous Antiretroviral Therapy in Patients with Controlled HIV Infection: A Substudy of the ANRS 106 Window Trial." *Journal of Acquired Immune Deficiency Syndromes* 49 (4): 416–21.

Cleary, S. M., D. McIntyre, and A. M. Boulle. 2006. "The Cost-Effectiveness of Antiretroviral Treatment in Khayelitsha, South Africa—a Primary Data Analysis." *Cost Effectiveness and Resource Allocation* 4: 20.

———. 2008. "Assessing Efficiency and Costs of Scaling Up HIV Treatment." *AIDS* 22 (Suppl. 1): S35–42.

Cohen, D. A., S. Y. Wu, and T. A. Farley. 2004. "Comparing the Cost-Effectiveness of HIV Prevention Interventions." *Journal of Acquired Immune Deficiency Syndromes* 37 (3): 1404–14.

———. 2006. "Structural Interventions to Prevent HIV/Sexually Transmitted Disease: Are They Cost-Effective for Women in the Southern United States?" *Sexually Transmitted Diseases* 33 (7 Suppl.): S46–49.

Commission on Macroeconomics and Health. 2001. *Macroeconomics and Health: Investing in Health for Economic Development. Report of the Commission on Macroeconomics and Health.* Geneva: World Health Organization.

Constella Futures, Centre for Development and Population Activities, White Ribbon Alliance for Safe Motherhood, and World Conference of Religions for Peace. 2006. "HIV Expenditure on MSM Programming in the Asia-Pacific Region." Background paper produced for the International Consultation on Male Sexual Health and HIV in Asia and the Pacific titled "Risks and Responsibilities" held in New Delhi, India, September 22–26. U.S. Agency for International Development, Health Policy Initiative, Task Order 1, Washington, DC.

Crabbe, F., H. Carsauw, A. Buve, M. Laga, J. P. Tchupo, and A. Trebucq. 1996. "Why Do Men with Urethritis in Cameroon Prefer to Seek Care in the Informal Health Sector?" *Genitourinary Medicine* 72 (3): 220–22.

Creese, A., K. Floyd, A. Alban, and L. Guinness. 2002. "Cost-Effectiveness of HIV/AIDS Interventions in Africa: A Systematic Review of the Evidence." *Lancet* 359 (9318): 1635–43.

Daly, C. C., L. Franco, D. A. Chilongozi, and G. Dallabetta. 1998. "A Cost Comparison of Approaches to Sexually Transmitted Disease Treatment in Malawi." *Health Policy and Planning* 13 (1): 87–93.

Dandona, L., S. G. Kumar, G. A. Kumar, and R. Dandona. 2009. "Economic Analysis of HIV Prevention Interventions in Andhra Pradesh State of India to Inform Resource Allocation." *AIDS* 23 (2): 233–42.

Dandona, L., S. G. Kumar, Y. Ramesh, M. C. Rao, A. A. Kumar, E. Marseille, J. G. Kahn, and R. Dandona. 2008. "Changing Cost of HIV Interventions in the Context of Scaling-Up in India." *AIDS* 22 (Suppl. 1): S43–49.

Dandona, L., P. Sisodia, S. G. Kumar, Y. K. Ramesh, A. A. Kumar, M. C. Rao, E. Marseille, M. Someshwar, N. Marshall, and J. G. Kahn. 2005. "HIV

Prevention Programmes for Female Sex Workers in Andhra Pradesh, India: Outputs, Cost and Efficiency." *BMC Public Health* 5: 98.

Dandona, L., P. Sisodia, T. L. Prasad, E. Marseille, R. M. Chalapathi, A. A. Kumar, S. G. Kumar, Y. K. Ramesh, M. Over, M. Someshwar, and J. G. Kahn. 2005. "Cost and Efficiency of Public Sector Sexually Transmitted Infection Clinics in Andhra Pradesh, India." *BMC Health Services Research* 5: 69.

Dandona, L., P. Sisodia, Y. K. Ramesh, S. G. Kumar, A. A. Kumar, M. C. Rao, M. Someshwar, B. Hansl, N. Marshall, E. Marseille, and J. G. Kahn. 2005. "Cost and Efficiency of HIV Voluntary Counselling and Testing Centres in Andhra Pradesh, India." *National Medical Journal of India* 18 (1): 26–31.

Deghaye, N., R. A. Pawinski, and C. Desmond. 2006. "Financial and Economic Costs of Scaling Up the Provision of HAART to HIV-Infected Health Care Workers in KwaZulu-Natal." *South African Medical Journal* 96 (2): 140–43.

Desai, K., S. L. Sansom, M. L. Ackers, S. R. Stewart, H. I. Hall, D. J. Hu, R. Sanders, C. R. Scotton, S. Soorapanth, M. C. Boily, et al. 2008. "Modeling the Impact of HIV Chemoprophylaxis Strategies among Men Who Have Sex with Men in the United States: HIV Infections Prevented and Cost-Effectiveness." *AIDS* 22 (14): 1829–39.

Dijkgraaf, M. G., B. P. van der Zanden, C. A. de Borgie, P. Blanken, J. M. van Ree, and W. van den Brink. 2005. "Cost Utility Analysis of Co-prescribed Heroin Compared with Methadone Maintenance Treatment in Heroin Addicts in Two Randomised Trials." *BMJ* 330 (7503): 1297.

Djajakusumah, T., S. Sudigdoadi, K. Keersmaekers, and A. Meheus. 1998. "Evaluation of Syndromic Patient Management Algorithm for Urethral Discharge." *Sexually Transmitted Infections* 74 (Suppl. 1): S29–33.

Doran, C. M., M. Shanahan, R. P. Mattick, R. Ali, J. White, and J. Bell. 2003. "Buprenorphine versus Methadone Maintenance: A Cost-Effectiveness Analysis." *Drug and Alcohol Dependence* 71 (3): 295–302.

Dowdy, D. W., M. D. Sweat, and D. R. Holtgrave. 2006. "Country-Wide Distribution of the Nitrile Female Condom (FC2) in Brazil and South Africa: A Cost-Effectiveness Analysis." *AIDS* 20 (16): 2091–98.

Ettner, S. L., D. Huang, E. Evans, D. R. Ash, M. Hardy, M. Jourabchi, and Y. I. Hser. 2006. "Benefit-Cost in the California Treatment Outcome Project: Does Substance Abuse Treatment 'Pay for Itself'?" *Health Services Research* 41 (1): 192–213.

Fang, C. T., Y. Y. Chang, H. M. Hsu, S. J. Twu, K. T. Chen, M. Y. Chen, L. Y. L. Huang, J-S. Hwang, J-D. Wang. 2007. "Cost-Effectiveness of Highly Active Antiretroviral Therapy for HIV Infection in Taiwan." *Journal of the Formosan Medical Association* 106 (8): 631–40.

Farnham, P. G., R. D. Gorsky, D. R. Holtgrave, W. K. Jones, and M. E. Guinan. 1996. "Counseling and Testing for HIV Prevention: Costs, Effects, and

Cost-Effectiveness of More Rapid Screening Tests." *Public Health Reports* 111 (1): 44–53.

Fieno, J. V. 2008. "Costing Adult Male Circumcision in High HIV Prevalence, Low Circumcision Rate Countries." *AIDS Care* 20 (5): 515–20.

Flori, Y. A., and M. le Vaillant. 2004. "Use and Cost of Antiretrovirals in France 1995–2000: An Analysis Based on the Medical Dossier on Human Immunodeficiency (Release 2) Database." *Pharmacoeconomics* 22 (16): 1061–70.

Forsythe, S., G. Arthur, G. Ngatia, R. Mutemi, J. Odhiambo, and C. Gilks. 2002. "Assessing the Cost and Willingness to Pay for Voluntary HIV Counselling and Testing in Kenya." *Health Policy and Planning* 17 (2): 187–95.

Forsythe, S., C. Mangkalopakorn, A. Chitwarakorn, and N. Masvichian. 1998. "Cost of Providing Sexually Transmitted Disease Services in Bangkok." *AIDS* 12 (Suppl. 2): S73–80.

Freedberg, K. A., N. Kumarasamy, E. Losina, A. J. Cecelia, C. A. Scott, N. Divi, T. P. Flanigan, Z. Lu, M. C. Weinstein, B. Wang, et al. 2007. "Clinical Impact and Cost-Effectiveness of Antiretroviral Therapy in India: Starting Criteria and Second-Line Therapy." *AIDS* 21 (Suppl. 4): S117–28.

Freedberg, K. A., E. Losina, M. C. Weinstein, A. D. Paltiel, C. J. Cohen, G. R. Seage, D. E. Craven, H. Zhang, A. D. Kimmel, and S. J. Goldie. 2001. "The Cost Effectiveness of Combination Antiretroviral Therapy for HIV Disease." *New England Journal of Medicine* 344 (11): 824–31.

Fung, I. C., L. Guinness, P. Vickerman, C. Watts, G. Vannela, J. Vadhvana, A. M. Foss, L. Malodia, M. Gandhi, and G. Jani. 2007. "Modelling the Impact and Cost-Effectiveness of the HIV Intervention Programme amongst Commercial Sex Workers in Ahmedabad, Gujarat, India." *BMC Public Health* 7: 195.

Gardner, E. M., M. E. Maravi, C. Rietmeijer, A. J. Davidson, and W. J. Burman. 2008. "The Association of Adherence to Antiretroviral Therapy with Healthcare Utilization and Costs for Medical Care." *Applied Health Economics and Health Policy* 6 (2–3): 145–55.

Gilson, L., R. Mkanje, H. Grosskurth, F. Mosha, J. Picard, A. Gavyole, J. Todd, P. Mayaud, R. Swai, L. Fransen, et al. 1997. "Cost-Effectiveness of Improved Treatment Services for Sexually Transmitted Diseases in Preventing HIV-1 Infection in Mwanza Region, Tanzania." *Lancet* 350 (9094): 1805–9.

Godfrey, C., D. Stewart, and M. Gossop. 2004. "Economic Analysis of Costs and Consequences of the Treatment of Drug Misuse: 2-Year Outcome Data from the National Treatment Outcome Research Study (NTORS)." *Addiction* 99 (6): 697–707.

Gold, M., A. Gafni, P. Nelligan, and P. Millson. 1997. "Needle Exchange Programs: An Economic Evaluation of a Local Experience." *Canadian Medical Association Journal* 157 (3): 255–62.

Goldie, S. J., K. M. Kuntz, M. C. Weinstein, K. A. Freedberg, and J. M. Palefsky. 2000. "Cost-Effectiveness of Screening for Anal Squamous Intraepithelial Lesions and Anal Cancer in Human Immunodeficiency Virus-Negative Homosexual and Bisexual Men." *American Journal of Medicine* 108 (8): 634–41.

Goldie, S. J., K. M. Kuntz, M. C. Weinstein, K. A. Freedberg, M. L. Welton, and J. M. Palefsky. 1999. "The Clinical Effectiveness and Cost-Effectiveness of Screening for Anal Squamous Intraepithelial Lesions in Homosexual and Bisexual HIV-Positive Men." *JAMA* 281 (19): 1822–29.

Goldie, S. J., A. D. Paltiel, M. C. Weinstein, E. Losina, G. R. Seage III, A. D. Kimmel, R. P. Walensky, P. E. Sax, and K. A. Freedberg. 2003. "Projecting the Cost-Effectiveness of Adherence Interventions in Persons with Human Immunodeficiency Virus Infection." *American Journal of Medicine* 115 (8): 632–41.

Goldie, S. J., Y. Yazdanpanah, E. Losina, M. C. Weinstein, X. Anglaret, R. P. Walensky, H. E. Hsu, A. Kimmel, C. Holmes, J. E. Kaplan, and K. A. Freedberg. 2006. "Cost-Effectiveness of HIV Treatment in Resource-Poor Settings—the Case of Côte d'Ivoire." *New England Journal of Medicine* 355 (11): 1141–53.

Goldman, D. P., J. Bhattacharya, A. A. Leibowitz, G. F. Joyce, M. F. Shapiro, and S. A. Bozzette. 2001. "The Impact of State Policy on the Costs of HIV Infection." *Medical Care Research and Review* 58 (1): 31–53.

Guinness, L., L. Kumaranayake, and K. Hanson. 2007. "A Cost Function for HIV Prevention Services: Is There a 'U'-Shape?" *Cost Effectiveness and Resource Allocation* 5: 13.

Guinness, L., L. Kumaranayake, B. Rajaraman, G. Sankaranarayanan, G. Vannela, P. Raghupathi, and A. George. 2005. "Does Scale Matter? The Costs of HIV-Prevention Interventions for Commercial Sex Workers in India." *Bulletin of the World Health Organization* 83 (10): 747–55.

Guinness, L., P. Vickerman, Z. Quayyum, A. Foss, C. Watts, A. Rodericks, T. Azim, S. Jana, and L. Kumaranayake. 2010. "The Cost-Effectiveness of Consistent and Early Intervention of Harm Reduction for Injecting Drug Users in Bangladesh." *Addiction* 105 (2): 319–28.

Harris, Z. K. 2006. "Efficient Allocation of Resources to Prevent HIV Infection among Injection Drug Users: The Prevention Point Philadelphia (PPP) Needle Exchange Program." *Health Economics* 15 (2): 147–58.

Harrison, A., S. A. Karim, K. Floyd, C. Lombard, M. Lurie, N. Ntuli, and D. Wilkinson. 2000. "Syndrome Packets and Health Worker Training Improve Sexually Transmitted Disease Case Management in Rural South Africa: Randomized Controlled Trial." *AIDS* 14 (17): 2769–79.

Hausler, H. P., E. Sinanovic, L. Kumaranayake, P. Naidoo, H. Schoeman, B. Karpakis, and P. Godfrey-Faussett. 2006. "Costs of Measures to Control

Tuberculosis/HIV in Public Primary Care Facilities in Cape Town, South Africa." *Bulletin of the World Health Organization* 84 (7): 528–36.

Healey, A., M. Knapp, J. Marsden, M. Gossop, and D. Stewart. 2003. "Criminal Outcomes and Costs of Treatment Services for Injecting and Non-Injecting Heroin Users: Evidence from a National Prospective Cohort Survey." *Journal of Health Services Research and Policy* 8 (3): 134–41.

Herida, M., C. Larsen, F. Lot, A. Laporte, J. C. Desenclos, and F. F. Hamers. 2006. "Cost-Effectiveness of HIV Post-Exposure Prophylaxis in France." *AIDS* 20 (13): 1753–61.

Heumann, K. S., R. Marx, S. J. Lawrence, D. L. Stump, D. P. Carroll, A. M. Hirozawa, M. H. Katz, and J. G. Kahn. 2001. "Cost-Effectiveness of Prevention Referrals for High-Risk HIV-Negatives in San Francisco." *AIDS Care* 13 (5): 637–42.

Holtgrave, D. R., and J. A. Kelly. 1997. "Cost-Effectiveness of an HIV/AIDS Prevention Intervention for Gay Men." *AIDS and Behavior* 1 (3): 173–80.

Holtgrave, D. R., and S. D. Pinkerton. 1997. "Updates of Cost of Illness and Quality of Life Estimates for Use in Economic Evaluations of HIV Prevention Programs." *Journal of Acquired Immune Deficiency Syndromes and Human Retrovirology* 16 (1): 54–62.

Holtgrave, D. R., R. O. Valdiserri, A. R. Gerber, and A. R. Hinman. 1993. "Human Immunodeficiency Virus Counseling, Testing, Referral, and Partner Notification Services: A Cost-Benefit Analysis." *Archives of Internal Medicine* 153 (10): 1225–30.

Hounton, S. H., A. Akonde, D. M. Zannou, J. Bashi, N. Meda, and D. Newlands. 2008. "Costing Universal Access of Highly Active Antiretroviral Therapy in Benin." *AIDS Care* 20 (5): 582–87.

Hubben, G. A., D. Bishai, P. Pechlivanoglou, A. M. Cattelan, R. Grisetti, C. Facchin, F. A. Compostella, J. M. Bos, M. J. Postma, and A. Tramarin. 2008. "The Societal Burden of HIV/AIDS in Northern Italy: An Analysis of Costs and Quality of Life." *AIDS Care* 20 (4): 449–55.

Hutton, G., K. Wyss, and Y. N'Diekhor. 2003. "Prioritization of Prevention Activities to Combat the Spread of HIV/AIDS in Resource Constrained Settings: A Cost-Effectiveness Analysis from Chad, Central Africa." *International Journal of Health Planning and Management* 18 (2): 117–36.

John, K. R., N. Rajagopalan, and K. V. Madhuri. 2006. "Brief Communication: Economic Comparison of Opportunistic Infection Management with Antiretroviral Treatment in People Living with HIV/AIDS Presenting at an NGO Clinic in Bangalore, India." *Medscape General Medicine* 8 (4): 24.

Kahn, J. G., S. M. Kegeles, R. Hays, and N. Beltzer. 2001. "Cost-Effectiveness of the Mpowerment Project, a Community-Level Intervention for Young Gay Men." *Journal of Acquired Immune Deficiency Syndromes* 27 (5): 482–91.

Kahn, J. G., E. Marseille, and B. Auvert. 2006. "Cost-Effectiveness of Male Circumcision for HIV Prevention in a South African Setting." *PLoS Med* 3 (12): e517.

Karnon, J., R. Jones, C. Czoski-Murray, and K. J. Smith. 2008. "Cost-Utility Analysis of Screening High-Risk Groups for Anal Cancer." *Journal of Public Health* (Oxford, U.K.) 30 (3): 293–304.

Kasymova, N., B. Johns, and B. Sharipova. 2009. "The Costs of a Sexually Transmitted Infection Outreach and Treatment Programme Targeting Most At Risk Youth in Tajikistan." *Cost Effectiveness and Resource Allocation* 7: 19.

Kitajima, T., Y. Kobayashi, W. Chaipah, H. Sato, W. Chadbunchachai, and R. Thuennadee. 2003. "Costs of Medical Services for Patients with HIV/AIDS in Khon Kaen, Thailand." *AIDS* 17 (16): 2375–81.

Koenig, S. P., C. Riviere, P. Leger, P. Severe, S. Atwood, D. W. Fitzgerald, J. W. Pape, and B. R. Schackman. 2008. "The Cost of Antiretroviral Therapy in Haiti." *Cost Effectiveness and Resource Allocation* 6: 3.

Kombe, G., and O. Smith. 2003. *The Costs of Anti-Retroviral Treatment in Zambia.* Technical Report No. 029. Bethesda, MD: The Partners for Health Reform*plus* Project, Abt Associates Inc.

Krentz, H. B., M. C. Auld, and M. J. Gill. 2003. "The Changing Direct Costs of Medical Care for Patients with HIV/AIDS, 1995–2001." *Canadian Medical Association Journal* 169 (2): 106–10.

Krentz, H. B., and M. J. Gill. 2008. "Cost of Medical Care for HIV-Infected Patients within a Regional Population from 1997 to 2006." *HIV Medicine* 9 (9): 721–30.

Krieger, J. N., S. D. Mehta, R. C. Bailey, K. Agot, J. O. Ndinya-Achola, C. Parker, et al. 2008. "Adult Male Circumcision: Effects on Sexual Function and Sexual Satisfaction in Kisumu, Kenya." *Journal of Sexual Medicine* 5 (11): 2610–22.

Kumar, S. G., R. Dandona, J. A. Schneider, Y. K. Ramesh, and L. Dandona. 2009. "Outputs and Cost of HIV Prevention Programmes for Truck Drivers in Andhra Pradesh, India." *BMC Health Services Research* 9: 82.

Kumaranayake, L. 2008. "The Economics of Scaling Up: Cost Estimation for HIV/AIDS Interventions." *AIDS* 22 (Suppl. 1): S23–33.

Kumaranayake, L., P. Vickerman, D. Walker, S. Samoshkin, V. Romantzov, Z. Emelyanova, V. Zviagin, and C. Watts. 2004. "The Cost-Effectiveness of HIV Preventive Measures among Injecting Drug Users in Svetlogorsk, Belarus." *Addiction* 99 (12): 1565–76.

Kumaranayake, L., and C. Watts. 2000. "Economic Costs of HIV/AIDS Prevention Activities in Sub-Saharan Africa." *AIDS* 14 (Suppl. 3): S239–52.

Kyriopoulos, J. E., M. A. Geitona, V. A. Paparizos, K. K. Kyriakis, C. A. Botsi, and N. G. Stavrianeas. 2001. "The Impact of New Antiretroic Therapeutic

Schemes on the Cost for AIDS Treatment in Greece." *Journal of Medical Systems* 25 (1): 73–80.

La Ruche, G., F. Lorougnon, and N. Digbeu. 1995. "Therapeutic Algorithms for the Management of Sexually Transmitted Diseases at the Peripheral Level in Côte d'Ivoire: Assessment of Efficacy and Cost." *Bulletin of the World Health Organization* 73 (3): 305–13.

Leiva, A., M. Shaw, K. Paine, K. Manneh, K. McAdam, and P. Mayaud. 2001. "Management of Sexually Transmitted Diseases in Urban Pharmacies in The Gambia." *International Journal of STD and AIDS* 12 (7): 444–52.

Liu, H., D. Jamison, X. Li, E. Ma, Y. Yin, and R. Detels. 2003. "Is Syndromic Management Better Than the Current Approach for Treatment of STDs in China? Evaluation of the Cost-Effectiveness of Syndromic Management for Male STD Patients." *Sexually Transmitted Diseases* 30 (4): 327–30.

Long, E. F., M. L. Brandeau, C. M. Galvin, T. Vinichenko, S. P. Tole, A. Schwartz, G. D. Sanders, and D. K. Owens. 2006. "Effectiveness and Cost-Effectiveness of Strategies to Expand Antiretroviral Therapy in St. Petersburg, Russia." *AIDS* 20 (17): 2207–15.

Lopez-Bastida, J., J. Oliva-Moreno, L. Perestelo-Perez, and P. Serrano-Aguilar. 2009. "The Economic Costs and Health-Related Quality of Life of People with HIV/AIDS in the Canary Islands, Spain." *BMC Health Services Research* 9: 55.

Losina, E., H. Toure, L. M. Uhler, X. Anglaret, A. D. Paltiel, E. Balestre, R. P. Walensky, E. Messou, M. C. Weinstein, F. Dabis, et al. 2009. "Cost-Effectiveness of Preventing Loss to Follow-up in HIV Treatment Programs: A Côte d'Ivoire Appraisal." *PLoS Med* 6 (10): e1000173.

Lowy, A., J. Page, R. Jaccard, B. Ledergerber, B. Somaini, R. Weber, and T. Szucs. 2005. "Costs of Treatment of Swiss Patients with HIV on Antiretroviral Therapy in Hospital-Based and General Practice-Based Care: A Prospective Cohort Study." *AIDS Care* 17 (6): 698–710.

Macauley, S., and S. Creighton. 2009. "Testing Commercial Sex Workers for Chlamydia and Gonorrhoea on Outreach." *Sexually Transmitted Infections* 85 (3): 231–32.

Marseille, E., J. G. Kahn, K. Billinghurst, and J. Saba. 2001. "Cost-Effectiveness of the Female Condom in Preventing HIV and STDs in Commercial Sex Workers in Rural South Africa." *Social Science and Medicine* 52 (1): 135–48.

Martinson, N., L. Mohapi, D. Bakos, G. E. Gray, J. A. McIntyre, and C. B. Holmes. 2009. "Costs of Providing Care for HIV-Infected Adults in an Urban HIV Clinic in Soweto, South Africa." *Journal of Acquired Immune Deficiency Syndromes* 50 (3): 327–30.

Masson, C. L., P. G. Barnett, K. L. Sees, K. L. Delucchi, A. Rosen, W. Wong, and S. M. Hall. 2004. "Cost and Cost-Effectiveness of Standard Methadone

Maintenance Treatment Compared to Enriched 180-Day Methadone Detoxification." *Addiction* 99 (6): 718–26.

McConnel, C. E., N. Stanley, J. A. Du Plessis, C. S. Pitter, F. Abdulla, H. M. Coovadia, E. Marseille, and J. G. Kahn. 2005. "The Cost of a Rapid-Test VCT Clinic in South Africa." *South African Medical Journal* 95 (12): 968–71.

Menzies, N., B. Abang, R. Wanyenze, F. Nuwaha, B. Mugisha, A. Coutinho, R. Bunnell, J. Mermin, and J. M. Blandford. 2009. "The Costs and Effectiveness of Four HIV Counseling and Testing Strategies in Uganda." *AIDS* 23 (3): 395–401.

Merito, M., A. Bonaccorsi, F. Pammolli, M. Riccaboni, G. Baio, C. Arici, A. D. Monforte, P. Pezzotti, D. Corsini, A. Tramarin, et al. 2005. "Economic Evaluation of HIV Treatments: The I.CO.N.A. Cohort Study." *Health Policy* (Amsterdam, Netherlands) 74 (3): 304–13.

Miners, A. H., C. A. Sabin, P. Trueman, M. Youle, A. Mocroft, M. Johnson, and E. J. Beck. 2001. "Assessing the Cost-Effectiveness of HAART for Adults with HIV in England." *HIV Medicine* 2 (1): 52–58.

Mojtabai, R., and J. G. Zivin. 2003. "Effectiveness and Cost-Effectiveness of Four Treatment Modalities for Substance Disorders: A Propensity Score Analysis." *Health Services Research* 38 (1 Pt 1): 233–59.

Moore, T. J., A. Ritter, and J. P. Caulkins. 2007. "The Costs and Consequences of Three Policy Options for Reducing Heroin Dependency." *Drug and Alcohol Review* 26 (4): 369–78.

Moses, S., F. A. Plummer, E. N. Ngugi, N. J. Nagelkerke, A. O. Anzala, and J. O. Ndinya-Achola. 1991. "Controlling HIV in Africa: Effectiveness and Cost of an Intervention in a High-Frequency STD Transmitter Core Group." *AIDS* 5 (4): 407–11.

Nachega, J. B., R. Leisegang, D. Bishai, H. Nguyen, M. Hislop, S. Cleary, L. Regensberg, and G. Maartens. 2010. "Association of Antiretroviral Therapy Adherence and Health Care Costs." *Annals of Internal Medicine* 152 (1): 18–25.

Negin, J., J. Wariero, P. Mutuo, S. Jan, and P. Pronyk. 2009. "Feasibility, Acceptability and Cost of Home-Based HIV Testing in Rural Kenya." *Tropical Medicine and International Health* 14 (8): 849–55.

Over, M. 2010. *Sustaining and Leveraging AIDS Treatment.* Washington, DC: Center for Global Development.

Over, M., E. Marseille, K. Sudhakar, J. Gold, I. Gupta, A. Indrayan, S. Hira, N. Nagelkerke, A. S. Rao, and P. Heywood. 2006. "Antiretroviral Therapy and HIV Prevention in India: Modeling Costs and Consequences of Policy Options." *Sexually Transmitted Diseases* 33 (10 Suppl.): S145–52.

Paltiel, A. D., K. A. Freedberg, C. A. Scott, B. R. Schackman, E. Losina, B. Wang, G. R. Seage 3rd, C. E. Sloan, P. E. Sax, and R. P. Walensky. 2009. "HIV

Preexposure Prophylaxis in the United States: Impact on Lifetime Infection Risk, Clinical Outcomes, and Cost-Effectiveness." *Clinical Infectious Diseases* 48 (6): 806–15.

Parker, K. A., E. H. Koumans, R. V. Hawkins, M. Massanga, P. Somse, K. Barker, and J. Moran. 1999. "Providing Low-Cost Sexually Transmitted Diseases Services in Two Semi-Urban Health Centers in Central African Republic (CAR): Characteristics of Patients and Patterns of Health Care-Seeking Behavior." *Sexually Transmitted Diseases* 26 (9): 508–16.

Partners for Health Reform*plus*, DELIVER, and POLICY Project. 2004. *Nigeria: Rapid Assessment of HIV/AIDS Care in the Public and Private Sectors.* Bethesda, MD: The Partners for Health Reform*plus* Project, Abt Associates Inc.

Paton, N. I., C. A. Chapman, S. Sangeetha, S. Mandalia, R. Bellamy, and E. J. Beck. 2006. "Cost and Cost-Effectiveness of Antiretroviral Therapy for HIV Infection in Singapore." *International Journal of STD and AIDS* 17 (10): 699–705.

Pinkerton, S. D., D. R. Holtgrave, and F. R. Bloom. 1998. "Cost-Effectiveness of Post-Exposure Prophylaxis Following Sexual Exposure to HIV." *AIDS* 12 (9): 1067–78.

Pinkerton, S. D., D. R. Holtgrave, W. J. DiFranceisco, L. Y. Stevenson, and J. A. Kelly. 1998. "Cost-Effectiveness of a Community-Level HIV Risk Reduction Intervention." *American Journal of Public Health* 88 (8): 1239–42.

Pinkerton, S. D., D. R. Holtgrave, and R. O. Valdiserri. 1997. "Cost-Effectiveness of HIV-Prevention Skills Training for Men Who Have Sex with Men." *AIDS* 11 (3): 347–57.

Pinkerton, S. D., J. N. Martin, M. E. Roland, M. H. Katz, T. J. Coates, and J. O. Kahn. 2004. "Cost-Effectiveness of HIV Postexposure Prophylaxis Following Sexual or Injection Drug Exposure in 96 Metropolitan Areas in the United States." *AIDS* 18 (15): 2065–73.

Price, M. A., S. R. Stewart, W. C. Miller, F. Behets, W.H. Dow, F. E. Martinson, D. Chilongozi, and M. S. Cohen. 2006. "The Cost-Effectiveness of Treating Male Trichomoniasis to Avert HIV Transmission in Men Seeking Sexually Transmitted Disease Care in Malawi." *Journal of Acquired Immune Deficiency Syndromes* 43 (2): 202–209.

Purdum, A.G., K. A. Johnson, and D. R. Globe. 2004. "Comparing Total Health Care Costs and Treatment Patterns of HIV Patients in a Managed Care Setting." *AIDS Care* 16 (6): 767–80.

Quentin, W., H. H. Konig, J. O. Schmidt, and A. Kalk. 2008. "Recurrent Costs of HIV/AIDS-Related Health Services in Rwanda: Implications for Financing." *Tropical Medicine and International Health* 13 (10): 1245–56.

Renaud, A., O. Basenya, N. de Borman, I. Greindl, and G. Meyer-Rath. 2009. "The Cost Effectiveness of Integrated Care for People Living with HIV Including

Antiretroviral Treatment in a Primary Health Care Centre in Bujumbura, Burundi." *AIDS Care* 21 (11): 1388–94.

Revenga, A., M. Over, E. Masaki, W. Peerapatanapokin, J. Gold, V. Tangcharoensathien, and S. Thanprasertsuk. 2006. *The Economics of Effective AIDS Treatment: Evaluating Policy Options for Thailand*. Washington, DC: World Bank.

Rieg, G., R. J. Lewis, L. G. Miller, M. D. Witt, M. Guerrero, and E. S. Daar. 2008. "Asymptomatic Sexually Transmitted Infections in HIV-Infected Men Who Have Sex with Men: Prevalence, Incidence, Predictors, and Screening Strategies." *AIDS Patient Care and STDS* 22 (12): 947–54.

Roberts, R. R., L. M. Kampe, M. Hammerman, R. D. Scott, T. Soto, G. G. Ciavarella, R. J. Rydman, K. Gorosh, and R. A. Weinstein. 2006. "The Cost of Care for Patients with HIV from the Provider Economic Perspective." *AIDS Patient Care and STDS* 20 (12): 876–86.

Rosen, S., L. Long, and I. Sanne. 2008. "The Outcomes and Outpatient Costs of Different Models of Antiretroviral Treatment Delivery in South Africa." *Tropical Medicine and International Health* 13 (8): 1005–15.

Rothbard, A. B., S. Lee, and M. B. Blank. 2009. "Cost of Treating Seriously Mentally Ill Persons with HIV Following Highly Active Retroviral Therapy (HAART)." *Journal of Mental Health Policy and Economics* 12 (4): 187–94.

Ruger, J. P., A. A. Ben, and L. Cottler. 2010. "Costs of HIV Prevention among Out-of-Treatment Drug-Using Women: Results of a Randomized Controlled Trial." *Public Health Reports* 125 (Suppl. 1): 83–94.

Schackman, B. R., R. Finkelstein, C. P. Neukermans, L. Lewis, and L. Eldred. 2005. "The Cost of HIV Medication Adherence Support Interventions: Results of a Cross-Site Evaluation." *AIDS Care* 17 (8): 927–37.

Schackman, B. R., K. A. Gebo, R. P. Walensky, E. Losina, T. Muccio, P. E. Sax, M. C. Weinstein, G. R. Seage 3rd, R. D. Moore, and K. A. Freedberg. 2006. "The Lifetime Cost of Current Human Immunodeficiency Virus Care in the United States." *Medical Care* 44 (11): 990–97.

Shrestha, R. K., H. A. Clark, S. L. Sansom, B. Song, H. Buckendahl, C. B. Calhoun, A. B. Hutchinson, and J. D. Heffelfinger. 2008. "Cost-Effectiveness of Finding New HIV Diagnoses Using Rapid HIV Testing in Community-Based Organizations." *Public Health Reports* 123 (Suppl. 3): 94–100.

Shrestha, R. K., S. L. Sansom, A. Richardson-Moore, P. T. French, B. Scalco, M. Lalota, M. Llanas, J. Stodola, R. Macgowan, and A. Margolis. 2009. "Costs of Voluntary Rapid HIV Testing and Counseling in Jails in 4 States—Advancing HIV Prevention Demonstration Project, 2003–2006." *Sexually Transmitted Diseases* 36 (2 Suppl.): S5–8.

Soderlund, N., J. Lavis, J. Broomberg, and A. Mills. 1993. "The Costs of HIV Prevention Strategies in Developing Countries." *Bulletin of the World Health Organization* 71 (5): 595–604.

Sood, S., and D. Nambiar. 2006. "Comparative Cost-Effectiveness of the Components of a Behavior Change Communication Campaign on HIV/AIDS in North India." *Journal of Health Communication* 11 (Suppl. 2): 143–62.

Stover, J., L. Bollinger, and K. Cooper-Arnold. 2001. *Goals Model: For Estimating the Effects of Resource Allocation Decisions on the Achievement of Goals of the HIV/AIDS Strategic Plan.* Glastonbury, CT: Futures Group International.

Sweat, M., S. Gregorich, G. Sangiwa, C. Furlonge, D. Balmer, C. Kamenga, O. Grinstead, and T. Coates. 2000. "Cost-Effectiveness of Voluntary HIV-1 Counselling and Testing in Reducing Sexual Transmission of HIV-1 in Kenya and Tanzania." *Lancet* 356 (9224): 113–21.

Sweat, M., D. Kerrigan, L. Moreno, S. Rosario, B. Gomez, H. Jerez, E. Weiss, and C. Barrington. 2006. "Cost-Effectiveness of Environmental-Structural Communication Interventions for HIV Prevention in the Female Sex Industry in the Dominican Republic." *Journal of Health Communication* 11 (Suppl. 2): 123–42.

Tao, G., and G. Remafedi. 1998. "Economic Evaluation of an HIV Prevention Intervention for Gay and Bisexual Male Adolescents." *Journal of Acquired Immune Deficiency Syndromes and Human Retrovirology* 17 (1): 83–90.

Terris-Prestholt, F., L. Kumaranayake, S. Foster, A. Kamali, J. Kinsman, V. Basajja, N. Nalweyso, M. Quigley, J. Kengeya-Kayondo, and J. Whitworth. 2006. "The Role of Community Acceptance over Time for Costs of HIV and STI Prevention Interventions: Analysis of the Masaka Intervention Trial, Uganda, 1996–1999." *Sexually Transmitted Diseases* 33 (10 Suppl.): S111–16.

Terris-Prestholt, F., S. Vyas, L. Kumaranayake, P. Mayaud, and C. Watts. 2006. "The Costs of Treating Curable Sexually Transmitted Infections in Low- and Middle-Income Countries: A Systematic Review." *Sexually Transmitted Diseases* 33 (10 Suppl.): S153–66.

Thielman, N. M., H. Y. Chu, J. Ostermann, D. K. Itemba, A. Mgonja, S. Mtweve, J. A. Bartlett, J. F. Shao, and J. A. Crump. 2006. "Cost-Effectiveness of Free HIV Voluntary Counseling and Testing through a Community-Based AIDS Service Organization in Northern Tanzania." *American Journal of Public Health* 96 (1): 114–19.

Thomsen, S. C., W. Ombidi, C. Toroitich-Ruto, E. L. Wong, H. O. Tucker, R. Homan, N. Kingola, and S. Luchters. 2006. "A Prospective Study Assessing the Effects of Introducing the Female Condom in a Sex Worker Population in Mombasa, Kenya." *Sexually Transmitted Infections* 82 (5): 397–402.

Tornero Estébanez, C., A. Cuenca Soria, A. Santamaría Martín, E. Gil Tomás, E. Soler Company, and S. Rull Segura. 2004. "Distribución del gasto farmacéutico en medicación antirretoviral." *Anales de Medicina Interna* 21 (6): 269–71.

Tramarin, A., S. Campostrini, M. J. Postma, G. Calleri, K. Tolley, N. Parise, F. de Lalla, and Palladio Study Group. 2004. "A Multicentre Study of Patient Survival, Disability, Quality of Life and Cost of Care: Among Patients with AIDS in Northern Italy." *Pharmacoeconomics* 22 (1): 43–53.

Tuli, K., and P. R. Kerndt. 2009. "Preventing Sexually Transmitted Infections among Incarcerated Men Who Have Sex with Men: A Cost-Effectiveness Analysis." *Sexually Transmitted Diseases* 36 (2 Suppl.): S41–48.

Tuli, K., S. Sansom, D. W. Purcell, L. R. Metsch, C. A. Latkin, M. N. Gourevitch, C. A. Gómez, and INSPIRE Team. 2005. "Economic Evaluation of an HIV Prevention Intervention for Seropositive Injection Drug Users." *Journal of Public Health Management and Practice* 11 (6): 508–15.

UN RTF (United Nations Regional Task Force on Injecting Drug Use and HIV/AIDS for Asia and the Pacific). 2009. "Estimation of Resource Needs and Availability for HIV Prevention and Care among People Who Inject Drugs in Asia." Manila: United Nations Regional Task Force on Injecting Drug Use and HIV/AIDS for Asia and the Pacific.

van der Veen, F. H., I. Ndoye, S. Guindo, I. Deschampheleire, and L. Fransen. 1994. "Management of STDs and Cost of Treatment in Primary Health Care Centres in Pikine, Senegal." *International Journal of STD and AIDS* 5 (4): 262–67.

Velasco, M., A. Gómez, C. Fernández, E. Pérez-Cecilia, M. J. Téllez, V. Roca, and A. Fernández-Cruz. 2000. "Economic Impact of HIV Protease Inhibitor Therapy in the Global Use of Health-Care Resources." *HIV Medicine* 1 (4): 246–51.

Velasco, M., J. E. Losa, A. Espinosa, J. Sanz, G. Gaspar, M. Cervero, R. Torres, E. Condes, C. Barros, and V. Castilla. 2007. "Economic Evaluation of Assistance to HIV Patients in a Spanish Hospital." *European Journal of Internal Medicine* 18 (5): 400–404.

Vickerman, P., L. Kumaranayake, O. Balakireva, L. Guinness, O. Artyukh, T. Semikop, O. Yaremenko, and C. Watts. 2006. "The Cost-Effectiveness of Expanding Harm Reduction Activities for Injecting Drug Users in Odessa, Ukraine." *Sexually Transmitted Diseases* 33 (10 Suppl.): S89–102.

Vickerman, P., F. Terris-Prestholt, S. Delany, L. Kumaranayake, H. Rees, and C. Watts. 2006. "Are Targeted HIV Prevention Activities Cost-Effective in High Prevalence Settings? Results from a Sexually Transmitted Infection Treatment Project for Sex Workers in Johannesburg, South Africa." *Sexually Transmitted Diseases* 33 (10 Suppl.): S122–32.

Walker, D., H. Muyinda, S. Foster, J. Kengeya-Kayondo, and J. Whitworth. 2001. "The Quality of Care by Private Practitioners for Sexually Transmitted Diseases in Uganda." *Health Policy and Planning* 16 (1): 35–40.

Wang, Q., P. Yang, M. Zhong, and G. Wang. 2003. "Validation of Diagnostic Algorithms for Syndromic Management of Sexually Transmitted Diseases." *Chinese Medical Journal* 116 (2): 181–86.

Warren, E., R. Viney, J. Shearer, M. Shanahan, A. Wodak, and K. Dolan. 2006. "Value for Money in Drug Treatment: Economic Evaluation of Prison Methadone." *Drug and Alcohol Dependence* 84 (2): 160–66.

Weaver, M. R., C. J. Conover, R. J. Proescholdbell, P. S. Arno, A. Ang, K. K. Uldall, and S. L. Ettner. 2009. "Cost-Effectiveness Analysis of Integrated Care for People with HIV, Chronic Mental Illness and Substance Abuse Disorders." *Journal of Mental Health Policy and Economics* 12 (1): 33–46.

Wilkinson, D., N. Wilkinson, C. Lombard, D. Martin, A. Smith, K. Floyd, and R. Ballard. 1997. "On-Site HIV Testing in Resource-Poor Settings: Is One Rapid Test Enough?" *AIDS* 11 (3): 377–81.

Wilson, D. P., K. J. Heymer, J. Anderson, J. O'Connor, C. Harcourt, and B. Donovan. 2010. "Sex Workers Can Be Screened Too Often: A Cost-Effectiveness Analysis in Victoria, Australia." *Sexually Transmitted Infections* 86 (2): 117–25.

Wolf, L. L., P. Ricketts, K. A. Freedberg, H. Williams-Roberts, L. R. Hirschhorn, K. Allen-Ferdinand, W. R. Rodriguez, N. Divi, M. T. Wong, and E. Losina. 2007. "The Cost-Effectiveness of Antiretroviral Therapy for Treating HIV Disease in the Caribbean." *Journal of Acquired Immune Deficiency Syndromes* 46 (4): 463–71.

Woodhall, S. C., M. Jit, C. Cai, T. Ramsey, S. Zia, S. Crouch, Y. Birks, R. Newton, W. J. Edmunds, and C. J. Lacey. 2009. "Cost of Treatment and QALYs Lost Due to Genital Warts: Data for the Economic Evaluation of HPV Vaccines in the United Kingdom." *Sexually Transmitted Diseases* 36 (8): 515–21.

Yazdanpanah, Y., S. J. Goldie, E. Losina, M. C. Weinstein, T. Lebrun, A. D. Paltiel, G. R. Seage 3rd, G. Leblanc, F. Ajana, A. D. Kimmel, et al. 2002. "Lifetime Cost of HIV Care in France during the Era of Highly Active Antiretroviral Therapy." *Antiviral Therapy* 7 (4): 257–66.

Zaric, G. S., P. G. Barnett, and M. L. Brandeau. 2000. "HIV Transmission and the Cost-Effectiveness of Methadone Maintenance." *American Journal of Public Health* 90 (7): 1100–11.

Zaric, G. S., A. M. Bayoumi, M. L. Brandeau, and D. K. Owens. 2008. "The Cost-Effectiveness of Counseling Strategies to Improve Adherence to Highly Active Antiretroviral Therapy among Men Who Have Sex with Men." *Medical Decision Making* 28 (3): 359–76.

PART IV

A Broader Policy Perspective

CHAPTER 11

Policy and Human Rights

Key themes:

- Criminalization of same-sex behavior has profound implications across the spectrum of policies, issues, and programs relating to men who have sex with men (MSM): criminalization matters.
- Responses to HIV epidemics among MSM in these highly disparate political and human rights environments have to be context specific: one size will not fit all.
- Mainstreaming of programs and services for MSM into public sector health systems may improve rights contexts in some settings but may be harmful in others, making HIV programs targets of public attack: mainstreaming must be carefully evaluated and cannot be assumed to be an improvement in rights or care.
- Community participation in every step of program development and implementation for MSM is crucial: the community is *the* key partner for this population.
- Laws and policies that promote universal access and gender equality in principle may fail for MSM in practice where homophobic cultural, religious, or political forces are active: good policies for HIV do not guarantee good outcomes for MSM and other sexual minorities.

(continued)

- Epidemiologic and cost-effectiveness findings are consistent with the rights argument, not counter to it: responding to MSM with high rates of coverage has positive effects for overall HIV trajectories in all four scenarios studied.
- Although quantification of the impact of structural interventions is important, action is mandated to decrease human rights abuses against MSM on social justice and human dignity grounds alone. Enough evidence exists to act now.

The international community is at a critical period in the HIV response. HIV infections continue to rise in a number of subpopulations, resources for continuing the response are threatened, and the human rights and social and political standing of MSM are the subject of intense public, media, political, and public health debate. Major advances in the legal standing of sexual minorities, most notably the repeal of India's sodomy laws and the end of criminalization of same-sex relations and diverse gender identities in Nepal, have been tempered by sharp rises in homophobic attacks and discriminatory legislative efforts in a number of countries, including Kenya, Malawi, and Uganda in Africa and the Russian Federation and Uzbekistan in Europe and Asia. Yet, as this report has demonstrated, the epidemics among MSM in many low- and middle-income countries (LMICs) are a severe, expanding, and underappreciated component of global HIV. For more than 80 LMICs, data on HIV among MSM are still unavailable. Essential services for these men remain grossly limited in resources, challenging to access, and insufficient in scale and scope to address these expanding epidemics and to provide services for the growing number of MSM in need.

The results of a recent preexposure prophylaxis study of oral daily Truvada to reduce acquisition risk for HIV infection among MSM and transgendered women, which demonstrated a 42 percent reduction in risk, bring these resource and access issues for MSM to the fore. Although the preexposure prophylaxis result was encouraging, and upcoming trials may confirm the utility of this approach for other at-risk populations, MSM who might benefit from this new approach still lack access to much more basic components of services, such as condoms and safe clinical contexts, access to quality HIV testing with counseling relevant to risks for MSM, and basic care for other sexually transmitted infections. New advances in

AIDS science will still face the human rights barriers confronting MSM and will only heighten the importance of rights-based responses.

The struggle to expand services for MSM in LMICs is now clearly under way, and the United Nations (UN) family of agencies has emerged as a leader in calling for human rights for sexual and gender minorities as part of the HIV response. On World AIDS Day, December 1, 2009, UN Secretary-General Ban Ki-moon said the world must

> shine the full light of human rights on HIV. I urge all countries to remove punitive laws, policies, and practices that hamper the AIDS response. In many countries, legal frameworks institutionalize discrimination against groups most at risk. Yet discrimination against sex workers, drug users, and men who have sex with men only fuels the epidemic and prevents cost-effective interventions. We must ensure that AIDS responses are based on evidence, not ideology, and reach those most in need and most affected. (UN 2009)

More recently, in September 2010, Secretary-General Ban stressed the importance of decriminalization of lesbian, gay, bisexual, and transgendered (LGBT) populations globally in saying,

> I therefore repeat the appeal I made in May: for all countries that criminalize people on the basis of their sexual orientation or gender identity to take the steps necessary to remove such offences from the statute books and to encourage greater respect for all people, irrespective of their sexuality or gender identity. (UN 2010)

The UN recently established an Independent Commission on HIV and the Law, led by the United Nations Development Programme and the Joint United Nations Programme on HIV/AIDS (UNAIDS), which has agreed to address the issue of decriminalization of same-sex behavior and its impact on improving HIV services for MSM, among other legal issues with bearing on the pandemic.

What are the human rights issues of most relevance to MSM and the HIV response? First and most important, those laws, policies, and practices that lead to reduced access to health care services are limitations of the right to health care.

Discrimination based on sexual orientation or gender identity is a violation of Article 26 of the International Covenant on Civil and Political Rights, which prohibits "discrimination . . . on any ground such as race, colour, sex, language, religion, political or other opinion, national or social origin, property, birth or other status." In the 1994 UN Human Rights Committee decision of *Toonen v. Australia*, the committee ruled that "sex" includes sexual orientation. This decision was the first recognition of gay and lesbian rights within the UN human rights system. *Toonen* was also argued on privacy rights, because Article 17 of the International Covenant on Civil and Political Rights bars "arbitrary or unlawful interference" with privacy.

Because denial of HIV care to this high-prevalence population is life-threatening, laws, policies, and practices that limit access to prevention, treatment, and care of MSM may also be violations of the most fundamental right of all—that to life itself.

Stigma and discrimination in markedly homophobic contexts may go beyond those rights protected in international human rights law to affect MSM in intensely personal ways. In a recent study by Baral and colleagues (2009) in Botswana, Malawi, and Namibia, MSM reported a range of rights-related abuses. They included being afraid to seek health care services (18.5 percent of men), being afraid to walk in their own communities (19.0 percent), and having been blackmailed because of their sexuality (21.2 percent) (table 11.1). Overall, some 42 percent of MSM reported at least one abuse (Baral et al. 2009).

More detailed analysis showed that MSM who reported having been blackmailed were also more likely to have disclosed sexual orientation to a family member, were less likely to have had an HIV test in the last six months, and were more likely to be afraid to seek health care. Having disclosed sexual orientation to a health care worker was highly associated with being denied health care and with being much less likely to have had an HIV test in the last six months. These findings demonstrate the very direct impact that stigma and discrimination can have on important prevention and treatment-related activities such as HIV testing, disclosure of actual risks to health care providers, and seeking health care in general.

Table 11.1 Prevalence of Human Rights Concerns for MSM in Botswana, Malawi, and Namibia, 2009
percent

Characteristic	*Botswana*	*Malawi*	*Namibia*	*Pooled*
Denied health care based on sexuality	0.9	4.0	8.3	5.1 (27/533)
Afraid to seek health services	20.5	17.6	18.3	18.5 (99/535)
Afraid to walk in community	29.1	15.5	16.7	19.0 (101/532)
Blackmailed because of sexuality	26.5	18.0	21.3	21.2 (113/533)
Yes to any of the above related to sexuality	56.9	34.3	41.5	42.1 (222/527)

Source: Baral et al. 2009.

The UN Family, PEPFAR, and Rights and Policies Relating to MSM

The Global Fund to Fight AIDS, Tuberculosis and Malaria (GFATM) put forward a Sexual Orientation and Gender Identities Strategy in May 2009 that encourages all partners, concentrating on governments, to strengthen their focus on those marginalized because of sexual orientation, gender identity, or consensual sexual behaviors. The GFATM includes in this strategy MSM; men, women, and transgendered persons who sell sex; and transgendered persons more broadly. The GFATM also asserts that "These groups exist in all countries" (GFATM 2010, 1). Although this point seems basic, it has been contentious for a number of states that deny or minimize the existence of their sexual minorities for cultural or political reasons.

The GFATM is one of the largest funders of HIV programs globally, with a considerably wider number of country programs than the U.S. President's Emergency Plan for AIDS Relief (PEPFAR), which targets U.S. strategic priorities. Hence, the funding policies of the GFATM can play key roles in incentivizing rights-based approaches to sexual minorities, including MSM, in country funding proposals. The GFATM mandates the participation of affected and infected communities in its Country Coordinating Mechanisms (CCMs) and makes funding available to build such participation and outreach. This goal is explicit in the 2010 Funding Policy of the GFATM and should serve as a further incentive for the inclusion of MSM in country-level programs.

The GFATM also funds non-CCM proposals when the evidence is clear that governments are unwilling or unable to address a key activity area. The GFATM funded a US$18.6 million award through a non-CCM mechanism for South Asian MSM (Afghanistan, Bangladesh, Bhutan, India, Nepal, Pakistan, and Sri Lanka) in round 9, with the Naz Foundation International, a long-standing community-based organization for MSM. This program includes a substantial human rights component with a plan to adapt rights advocacy and efforts to local contexts with in-country nongovernmental organization partners.

In 2009, UNAIDS also put forward a policy guidance on MSM that includes a central human rights and nondiscrimination component. The *UNAIDS Action Framework: Universal Access for Men Who Have Sex with Men and Transgender People* urges that a conducive legal, policy, and social environment to support programming address HIV-related issues among MSM and transgendered people and that this can be strengthened through the promotion and guarantee of human rights (UNAIDS 2009).

The U.S. Office of the Global AIDS Coordinator and its PEPFAR program have also been developing a guidance on HIV prevention, treatment, and care for MSM. This guidance has informed the work presented in this report, among other sources. The guidance is likely to strongly endorse human rights and nondiscrimination in access to health care, given the recent policy shift of the U.S. government in supporting the UN call for decriminalization worldwide and the recent statement of U.S. Secretary of State Clinton on the occasion of National LGBT Pride day in June 2010: "Just as I was very proud to say the obvious more than 15 years ago in Beijing that human rights are women's rights—and women's rights are human rights—let me say today that human rights are gay rights and gay rights are human rights" (U.S. Department of State 2010).

On the U.S. domestic front, the Obama administration released the first *National HIV/AIDS Strategy for the United States* in July 2010 and the plan for implementation of the policy in February 2011. (White House 2010, 2011). The strategy is of critical import for the U.S. HIV response overall, because it affirms the principles of being evidence based, recognizes that gay and other MSM are the majority of U.S. men living with HIV infection and that African American MSM are disproportionally burdened with HIV, and calls for an end to stigma and discrimination in access to services. Although not a document with direct relevance to the United States as a donor nation for LMICs, the national strategy nevertheless affirms the Obama administration's commitment to evidence-based policy in HIV/AIDS. In this context, again, the evidence strongly supports an expanded focus on the underserved MSM component of global HIV/AIDS.

Current Legal Status of MSM in LMICs

Table 11.2 shows HIV prevalence rates of MSM and the general population for the LMICs where data were available for this book. The legal status of male homosexuality (sexual behavior between consenting adult men) is categorized by the scenarios developed through the epidemic algorithm.

The legal environment for MSM is best in scenario 1 (Latin America) and scenario 2 (Eastern Europe) and remains most problematic in scenario 3 (largely Africa), scenario 4 (parts of Asia), and the low-data settings of the Middle East and North Africa. Although legal status does not ensure rights protections or enabling environments, it is a key parameter for understanding social tolerance and the space for rights advocacy at country levels.

Table 11.2 MSM and General Population HIV Prevalence Rates for 54 LMICs Categorized by Epidemic Scenario

Country	*Aggregate HIV prevalence among MSM*		*Law against male-to-male relationships and punishments*
	Percent	*95% C.I.*	
Scenario 1. Risks among MSM are the predominant exposure mode for HIV infection in the population			
Argentina	12.10	(10.8–13.4)	No law
Bolivia	21.20	(17.6–24.7)	No law
Brazil	8.20	(6.9–9.4)	No law
Colombia	19.40	(17.2–21.6)	No law
Ecuador	15.10	(12.8–17.4)	No law
El Salvador	7.90	(4.8–10.9)	No law
Guatemala	11.50	(6.7–16.4)	No law
Honduras	9.80	(8.1–11.5)	No law
Mexico	25.60	(24.8–26.5)	No law
Nicaragua	9.30	(4.8–13.7)	No law
Panama	10.60	(6.7–14.6)	No law
Paraguay	13.00	(6.2–19.9)	No law
Peru[a]	13.80	(13.4–14.3)	No law
Uruguay	18.90	(16.1–21.7)	No law
Jamaica	31.80	(25.4–38.3)	Imprisonment less than 10 years
Scenario 2. Risks among MSM occur within established HIV epidemics driven by injecting drug use			
Armenia	0.90	(0.0–2.7)	No law
Georgia	5.30	(1.2–9.4)	No law
Moldova	1.70	(0.0–4.0)	No law
Poland	5.40	(3.3–7.6)	No law
Russian Federation	3.40	(2.6–4.2)	No law
Serbia	8.70	(5.4–12.0)	No law
Timor-Leste	1.00	(0.0–2.6)	No law
Ukraine[a]	10.60	(7.8–14.2)	No law
Scenario 3. Risks among MSM occur in the context of mature and widespread HIV epidemics among heterosexuals			
South Africa	15.30	(12.4–18.3)	Legal protection
Namibia	12.40	(8.1–16.8)	Not legal; no data on punishment
Botswana	19.70	(12.5–26.9)	Imprisonment less than 10 years
Senegal[b]	24.30	(21.9–26.7)	Imprisonment less than 10 years
Ghana[b]	25.00	(20.5–29.5)	Imprisonment 10 years or more
Kenya[a]	15.20	(13.3–17.2)	Imprisonment more than 10 years
Malawi	21.40	(15.7–27.1)	Imprisonment more than 10 years
Tanzania	12.40	(9.5–15.2)	Imprisonment more than 10 years
Zambia	32.90	(29.3–36.6)	Imprisonment more than 10 years
Nigeria	13.50	(12.0–15.5)	Death penalty
Sudan	8.80	(7.1–10.4)	Death penalty

(continued next page)

Table 11.2 *(continued)*

Country	*Aggregate HIV prevalence among MSM* *Percent*	*95% C. I.*	*Law against male-to-male relationships and punishments*
Scenario 4. MSM, injecting drug users, and heterosexual transmissions all contribute significantly to the HIV epidemic			
Cambodia	7.80	(5.9–9.7)	No law
China	4.30	(4.0–4.7)	No law
Lao PDR	5.40	(3.5–7.2)	No law
Thailand[a]	23.00	(20.1–25.4)	No law
Vietnam	6.20	(5.1–7.3)	No law
India	14.50	(13.3–15.6)	Decriminalization
Indonesia	9.00	(6.9–11.0)	Legal in some areas; imprisonment less than 10 years
Nepal	4.80	(2.6–7.0)	Legal protection
Egypt, Arab Rep.	5.30	(2.9–7.7)	Imprisonment less than 10 years
Pakistan	1.80	(1.1–2.6)	Imprisonment less than 10 years
Countries with unavailable or incomplete data			
Azerbaijan	42.90	(6.2–79.5)	No law
Belarus	0	(0.0–0.0)	No law
Kazakhstan	0	(0.0–0.0)	No law
Kyrgyz Republic	0	(0.0–0.0)	No law
Angola	—	—	Fines or restrictions
Lebanon	—	—	Imprisonment less than 10 years
Turkmenistan	—	—	Imprisonment less than 10 years
Zimbabwe	—	—	Imprisonment less than 10 years
Iran, Islamic Rep.	—	—	Death
Yemen, Rep.	—	—	Death

Source: ILGA 2010.
Note: — No data available. High-income countries excluded from analysis: Andorra; Antigua and Barbuda; Aruba; Australia; Austria; The Bahamas; Bahrain; Barbados; Belgium; Bermuda; Brunei Darussalam; Canada; Cayman Islands; Channel Islands; Croatia; Cyprus; Czech Republic; Denmark; Equatorial Guinea; Estonia; Faeroe Islands; Finland; France; French Polynesia; Germany; Greece; Greenland; Guam; Hong Kong SAR, China; Hungary; Iceland; Ireland; Isle of Man; Israel; Italy; Japan; Republic of Korea; Kuwait; Liechtenstein; Luxembourg; Macao SAR, China; Malta; Monaco; Netherlands; Netherlands Antilles; New Caledonia; New Zealand; Northern Mariana Islands; Norway; Oman; Portugal; Puerto Rico; Qatar; San Marino; Saudi Arabia; Singapore; Slovak Republic; Slovenia; Spain; Sweden; Switzerland; Trinidad and Tobago; United Arab Emirates; United Kingdom; United States; Virgin Islands (U.S.).
a. Example countries used to describe each scenario.
b. Following the algorithm and based on available data, Senegal would also be assigned to scenario 4 and Ghana to scenario 1; both are somewhat outliers in these categories, and both have some uncertainties in risks and prevalence of HIV for female sex workers, IDU, and MSM, which make characterization difficult.

Focus Countries

The four countries selected for in-depth analysis in this report represent a range of human rights contexts for MSM. Peru has removed punitive laws and policies and implemented policies of access to care for sexual minorities and active outreach to communities of MSM. Nevertheless, cultural attitudes continue to stigmatize behavior of MSM, effeminacy in men, and being the receptive partner in sex between men. Peru's high HIV prevalence in MSM and low prevalence in virtually every other risk group ensure that MSM predominate among HIV patients and make the potential for HIV stigma significant among open MSM.

Thailand has never had laws penalizing same-sex behavior, largely because of its unique history in having avoided European colonization. A long-standing cultural tradition of tolerance of traditional transgendered persons (*Katoey*, biological males who take on the cultural role and appearance of women) has led to a relatively tolerant, if not accepting, society. MSM are not formally discriminated against in health care settings. During the 2003 law-and-order campaign, gay-identified venues including bars, saunas, and other clubs were targeted for harassment by the police. During these crackdowns, condoms were seen as evidence of the "promotion" of homosexual behavior, and venues were forced to remove all visible condom displays—a reversal of Thailand's previously successful 100 percent condom campaign targeting heterosexual sex venues.

Ukraine decriminalized homosexuality after independence from the former Soviet Union. Social stigma and fear of disclosure of sexual orientation and MSM status, however, remain prevalent in society, and services for MSM are extremely limited.

Kenya has colonial-era sodomy laws that remain in force, making same-sex behavior between consenting adults a crime punishable by up to 14 years' imprisonment. Behavior of MSM is highly stigmatized and therefore hidden, although an open community is emerging. Clinical services for MSM were beginning to emerge in 2010, and data from several studies suggested Kenyan MSM were at substantial risk for infection. In February 2010, in Mtwapa town in the coastal Kilifi District (near Mombasa), rumors of a purported gay wedding sparked attacks against individuals suspected of being gay and soon led to organized vigilante attacks on the Kenya Medical Research Institute (KEMRI). KEMRI had been providing services to MSM and had a policy of inclusion in services on its website. These attacks on KEMRI may have been organized by religious leaders in Kenya, including leaders of the Council of Imams and Preachers of Kenya and of the National Council of Churches of Kenya (Human Rights Watch 2010). They held a press conference on February 11, 2010, in which they called for investigation of KEMRI and criticized the government of Kenya for "providing counseling services for criminals" (Human Rights Watch 2010). The mob attached KEMRI on

February 13, immediately affecting the clinic's activities and LGBT persons in the community and in Kenya more broadly; mob attacks lasted for some days and eventually spread to Mombasa. A climate of fear and the very real threat of violence have driven many MSM underground and interrupted provision of services.

Modeling the Effect of Enabling Policy Environments

The current Goals Model, which has been adapted with the collaboration of the Goals development team of John Stover and Lori Bollinger of the Futures Institute (Glastonbury, Connecticut), had limited capacity to include structural interventions such as decriminalization in projections. The Goals Model has been expanded for MSM by using this book's scenario-based approach, including more intervention parameters, expanding the risk categorization for MSM, and exploring a situation of enabling policy environments and full resources that would allow intervention coverage to reach 100 percent. This approach assumes that attention to human rights issues—such as addressing discrimination in health care access, ensuring protection and not harassment as policing policy, and decriminalizing same-sex behavior—would have an overall enabling effect on uptake and use of services for MSM. This potentiating impact would act indirectly, through maximizing uptake and use of services, on HIV risks and hence on HIV incidence. This indirect positive impact on services can be called *theta* (θ). A challenge to this approach is the lack of empirical data on the impact size of θ for MSM in different contexts.

Although little work has been done on estimating the effect of structural interventions on HIV in other populations, one recent report from Strathdee and colleagues (2010) attempted to quantify θ among drug users in Ukraine. Using prospective data on injecting drug users in the cities of Kyiv, Makeevka, Odessa, and Strathdee and colleagues modeled the effect of declines in police brutality on transmission of new HIV infections. They found that elimination of police beatings would reduce new infections in Odessa, the city with the highest rates of police brutality, by 4 to 19 percent over five years. A conservative midrange assumption would yield a θ of 11.5 percent over five years. They argued that police brutality affected HIV incidence indirectly, by discouraging attendance at needle and syringe exchanges, reducing drug users' willingness to seek treatment, and otherwise limiting uptake and use of services.

Reducing police brutality, a structural intervention, would also act indirectly on HIV infections by increasing use of services and enabling drug users to access treatment and care.

Adapting the approach used by Strathdee and colleagues to MSM, and assuming a low estimate of the potential θ for structural interventions of 10 percent reduction in new infections over five years, one finds such interventions could have a substantial impact on HIV infections in settings where structural risks continue to decrease access to services by MSM. Empirical data are urgently needed to assess θs in epidemic contexts among MSM.

This book's use of the Goals Model, in which the best-case scenario assumption was set at 100 percent coverage of MSM in a given population and enough antiretroviral therapy to cover all HIV-positive MSM in a given population, implicitly assumes no systematic barriers to access. Thus, it actually models an "ideal" context for MSM. Without empirical data on θs, however, one cannot assess how much human rights advances for MSM may actually contribute to this kind of best-case scenario. All who are interested in taking this work further must recognize and address the reality that HIV epidemics among MSM continue—and some continue to expand—in settings as different from LMICs as France and the Netherlands, where most would agree human rights and social justice concerns for MSM play little role in structural risks for HIV.

For MSM in most of the world, however, the contexts of their lives and their need for services are far indeed from these tolerant and inclusive environments. Moreover, police brutality, as in the Ukraine case of injecting drug users, continues to play a role in denial of services for MSM. The decriminalization of homosexuality in India, for example, was argued for by the National AIDS Control Organisation on the grounds that the criminal statute was a barrier to HIV prevention services—it allowed police to harass MSM and transgendered outreach workers with impunity for promoting "illegal acts" and so limited condom distribution at venues for MSM (parks and other "beats") in India. This history suggests that, at least in some settings, police brutality would be an appropriate target for structural intervention and that, as in Ukraine for drug users, this intervention effect should be measurable.

Although quantification of the impact of structural interventions is important, action is mandated to decrease human rights abuses against MSM on social justice and human dignity grounds alone.

Policy Findings

The eight countries investigated in this book broadly cover the spectrum of legal and policy environments for MSM in LMICs:

- Countries that have long-standing legal protection for MSM (Brazil and Peru)
- Countries that have recently decriminalized such practices (most recently, India and, in the early 1990s, Russia and Ukraine)
- Countries that demonstrate acceptance, if not tolerance, with no prior history of criminalization (Thailand)
- Countries that actively discriminate against MSM and have laws against homosexuality (Kenya and Senegal)

Several fundamental policy recommendations are drawn from these reviews:

- Criminalization of same-sex behavior has profound implications across the spectrum of policies, issues, and programs relating to MSM: criminalization matters.
- Responses to HIV epidemics among MSM in these highly disparate political and human rights environments have to be context specific: one size will not fit all.
- Mainstreaming of MSM programs and services into public sector health systems may improve rights contexts in some settings but may be harmful in others, making HIV programs targets of public attack: mainstreaming must be carefully evaluated and cannot be assumed to be an improvement in rights or care.
- Community participation in every step of program development and implementation for MSM is crucial: the community is *the* key partner for this population.
- Laws and policies that promote universal access and gender equality in principle may fail for MSM in practice where homophobic cultural, religious, or political forces are active: good policies for HIV do not guarantee good outcomes for MSM and other sexual minorities.
- Epidemiologic and cost-effectiveness findings are consistent with the rights argument, not counter to it: responding to MSM with high rates of coverage has positive impacts for overall HIV trajectories in all four scenarios studied.

- Although quantification of the impact of structural interventions is important, action is mandated to decrease human rights abuses against MSM on social justice and human dignity grounds alone.

Policy Contexts and Programming

Brazil and Peru are relatively tolerant societies with a strong LGBT civil society; a long history of decriminalization of homosexuality; and a national commitment to inclusion of MSM in HIV prevention, treatment, and care. Brazil has engaged in interventions to address social exclusion and homophobia—such as the "Brazil without Homophobia" campaign—*as an HIV preventive intervention.* A marked policy parallel exists here to India's recent repeal of its colonial-era sodomy laws, which were overturned by a court ruling based on the argument put forward by India's National AIDS Control Organisation. These are examples of structural interventions at national levels aimed at enhancing the environment for MSM to come forward for HIV and other health services.

In marked contrast are the policy environments and legal restrictions in Kenya and Senegal. The national Senegalese AIDS strategy for 2007–11 identified MSM as a key target population for prevention, and the Senegalese Ministry of Health has implemented some outreach programs from MSM. Senegalese LGBT organizations have been partners in prevention programs run by the ministry. In December 2008, the International Conference on AIDS and STIs in Africa was held in Dakar. There, Senegalese government officials publicly pledged their support to reducing HIV among sexual minorities.

The willingness of the Ministry of Health to address HIV among MSM appears to have led to a political backlash. Within weeks of the conference, police arrested nine male HIV prevention workers in Dakar on suspicion of engaging in homosexual conduct. Article 319.3 of the Senegalese penal code states that "whoever commits an improper or unnatural act with a person of the same sex" will be punished by imprisonment of between one and five years and a fine of CFAF 100,000 to 1,500,000 (US$200 to US$3,000). In January 2009, these men were sentenced to eight years in prison and a CFAF 500,000 fine. The arrest and sentencing were widely publicized locally and garnered international attention. All of the men were subsequently released on appeal, because no evidence existed of actual homosexual acts—the men were at a meeting in a private apartment at the time of their arrest—but the social and religious (in this case Islamic leadership) pressure has been intense, and these men remain in hiding or have left the country. The Center for Public Health and Human Rights at Johns Hopkins University has recently conducted an investigation into health-seeking behavior among MSM in Senegal in the wake of these events, and preliminary data suggest that use of services has dramatically declined among MSM in Senegal.

The Senegal situation starkly portrays a reality for MSM in many settings and in much of Africa: policy reform may be difficult or impossible in some political contexts, and enabling environments may simply not exist. For these settings, stand-alone LGBT-friendly health services or MSM clinic services may be both unfeasible and unwise if they generate the kinds of backlash that have marked the Senegal experience. In these settings, quiet work with sympathetic providers and reform efforts within HIV services may be more realistic policy goals. Engagement and support with community partners will be even more essential in these settings than in environments less hostile to MSM.

The Human Rights Framework and MSM Programming

Homosexuality remains criminalized in more than 80 UN member states, with punishments ranging from jail time to the death penalty. Repressive legal contexts and pervasive social stigma can limit access for these men to appropriate services for sexually transmitted infections and HIV, including prevention and treatment, and can even be life-threatening—as is the case for ongoing executions of gay men in the Islamic Republic of Iran and Iraq or the current Ugandan legislative process to sharply increase legal punishments for homosexuality, including the death penalty for "aggravated homosexuality." In these environments, even if funding were available for state-of-the-art comprehensive HIV prevention and care packages for MSM, such assistance would likely be of limited value because men in such settings are quite justified in not seeking care. Therefore, growing HIV epidemics among MSM in many LMICs are in part attributable to inappropriate governance responses on multiple levels. Moreover, criminalization of same-sex practices could be posited as an extreme case of misguided governance in the development of a comprehensive HIV/AIDS response.

The role of governance in the AIDS response is relevant because for HIV the social drivers of risk are much more predictive of disease burden than endogenous susceptibility, which is the case in very few other diseases. To effectively respond to social drivers of risk, governments should adopt evidence-based interventions mitigating the effects of the risk environment. In the context of MSM, many governments have done the opposite and have potentiated the risk environment by limiting the availability of service provision and preventing the uptake of whatever services are available. Although the majority of the laws criminalizing same-sex practices in these settings are national, they are implemented and enforced by municipal and regional tiers of government. This fact is relevant to the international community because all of the countries that criminalize same-sex practices are UN member states and signatories to a number of conventions that include legislated protections for sexual minorities. Separate from the issue of governance decisions related to politicians is the concept of public health governance. Whereas public health is global in that infectious diseases know no boundaries, and global institutions, including UN agencies, provide technical support and guidance to all UN member states, the public health prevention activities are still implemented at a local or regional level. It is the mandate of the public health practitioner to develop comprehensive programming for health protection and promotion for all populations at risk for a disease. For HIV, that population includes MSM in the vast majority of the settings where the disease has been studied. The criminalization of same-sex practices limits the development of a comprehensive HIV/AIDS response, including prevention, treatment, and care.

References

Baral, S., G. Trapence, F. Motimedi, E. Umar, S. Iipinge, F. Dausab, and C. Beyrer. 2009. "HIV Prevalence, Risks for HIV Infection, and Human Rights among Men Who Have Sex with Men (MSM) in Malawi, Namibia, and Botswana." *PLoS One* 4 (3): e4997.

GFATM (Global Fund to Fight AIDS, Tuberculosis and Malaria). 2009. *The Global Fund Strategy in Relation to Sexual Orientation and Gender Identities*. Geneva: GFATM.

———. 2010. "Global Fund Information Note: Sexual Orientation and Gender Identities." GFATM, Geneva.

Human Rights Watch. 2010. "Kenya: Halt Anti-Gay Campaign." News, New York City, NY, February 17. http://www.hrw.org/en/news/2010/02/17/kenya-halt-anti-gay-campaign.

ILGA (International Lesbian, Gay, Bisexual, Trans and Intersex Association). 2010. "Punishments for Male to Male Relationships" (map). http://ilga.org/ilga/en/index.html. Accessed June 20, 2010.

Strathdee, S., T. Hallett, N. Bobrova, T. Rhodes, R. Booth, R. Abdool, and C. A. Hankins. 2010. "HIV and Risk Environment for Injecting Drug Users: The Past, Present, and Future." *Lancet* 376 (9737): 268–84.

UN (United Nations). 2009. "The Secretary-General, Message on World Aids Day, 1 December 2009." Press Release. http://data.unaids.org/pub/PressStatement/2009/20091201_SG_WAD09_message_en.pdf.

———. 2010. "The Secretary-General, Message to Event on Ending Violence and Criminal Sanctions Based on Sexual Orientation and Gender Identity, Geneva, 17 September 2010." http://geneva.usmission.gov/wp-content/uploads/2010/09/SYG.pdf.

UNAIDS (Joint United Nations Programme on HIV/AIDS). 2009. *UNAIDS Action Framework: Universal Access for Men Who Have Sex with Men and Transgender People.* UNAIDS/09.22E/JC1720E. Geneva: UNAIDS.

U.S. Department of State. 2010. "Remarks by Secretary of State Hillary Rodham Clinton at an Event Celebrating Lesbian, Gay, Bisexual and Transgender (LGBT) Month." Washington, DC, June 22. http://www.state.gov/secretary/rm/2010/06/143517.htm.

White House. 2010. *National HIV/AIDS Strategy for the United States.* Washington, DC: White House Office of National AIDS Policy.

———. 2011. Implementation of the *National HIV/AIDS Strategy for the United States.* White House Office of National AIDS Policy, Washington, DC.

APPENDIX A

Price Tag for a Comprehensive Prevention and Treatment Program for MSM

A comprehensive response to address the findings in this report requires that resources be mobilized to meet the HIV prevention and treatment needs of populations of men who have sex with men (MSM) throughout the world. This appendix provides an estimate of the amount of resources, at different levels of implementation coverage, that will be needed in the eight countries highlighted in this report to launch a comprehensive prevention and treatment program for MSM.

Methods

The estimates presented here are based on a cross-sectional analysis of current population numbers and needs. (Appendix B presents the results for and discusses the problems with this analysis for a select set of additional countries.) The estimation of costs for the focal countries is repeated here, using abridged methods, to demonstrate how well these costs reflect the more detailed costing presented in chapter 10.

Items Included

Costs include the resources needed for the direct implementation of programs for MSM. Specifically, they include the costs for distributing condoms and lubricant, implementing community-based peer outreach interventions, and providing antiretroviral therapy (ART). In four countries, the costs of needle exchange programs and opioid substitution therapy programs are also included because these interventions are seen as critical in responding to HIV among MSM as well as injecting drug users (IDUs).

A comprehensive response to the HIV pandemic requires efforts on multiple levels. Specifically for MSM, efforts are needed to advocate for structural reforms to create an enabling environment conducive to reaching, communicating, and mobilizing the community of MSM. The costs of these advocacy, legislative, and organizational efforts are difficult to quantify. The costs of these essential activities cannot be determined from a thorough review of the literature in part because of a lack of scholarly interest in the topic of costing successful advocacy campaigns and the uncertain relationship between advocacy and successful advocacy (which depends in part on existing awareness of the problems of HIV and attitudes in general about MSM). Thus, a great deal of money and effort could be expended in a particular country or region with no guarantee of success.

A second area not included in these costs are other structural interventions, such as mass media messages targeting MSM and sensitizing health (and other) staff on issues related to MSM. These areas are not included because of a lack of data. For example, although media messages may form an important component of an overall HIV response, no data were available on the cost of media messages that target high-risk groups (in general) and MSM (in particular). Only one study in this area specific to MSM was found (Constella Futures et al. 2006); it did not provide details of how the media campaign was carried out.

A third area not included here is the costs of counseling and testing (VCT) and treatment for sexually transmitted infections. These activities are often included in peer outreach interventions, but they have been excluded here. This is not to argue that these costs are unimportant, but to suggest that these costs are often subsumed in general HIV or health sector programming. In countries where a high degree of stigma is associated with MSM, stand-alone clinics may not be advisable because they may become targets for closure or other discriminatory activities. In many cases, MSM will access general clinics without need to disclose their sexual activities. In other settings, such as those outlined in scenario 1 in this book where risks among MSM are the predominant exposure mode for HIV infection, VCT services may de facto cater largely to the populations of MSM, and general VCT costs are applicable to MSM. However, other settings may exist where a strong policy and social environment would allow VCT and clinics for sexually transmitted infections targeted to MSM to operate in conjunction with, for example, peer outreach programs. Identifying these settings is difficult. Even in such settings, however, an indeterminate proportion of MSM may still access general services, making estimation of the MSM-specific resources difficult without more in-depth knowledge of the appropriate programs. Nevertheless, the costs of ART for MSM have been included in these estimates to highlight the importance of treatment as part of the overall response and as an important component of HIV prevention in its own right (that is, treatment as prevention).

A final area not included in this analysis is the cost of program management, including such areas as logistic management, monitoring and evaluation, and supervision. This omission is in part because these costs are theoretically included in the unit cost estimates, although many studies are not clear about the extent to which these costs are captured. Thus, the unit cost might underestimate the extent of resources needed to fully operate these programs.

Demographic Data

Table A.1 provides the demographic data used for this analysis. The number of MSM in 2010 is used. Numbers were based on the models developed for the cost-effectiveness analysis, or from United Nations Population Division figures (UN Population Division 2010). The assumption was that 3 percent of adult men were MSM, which is unlikely to be universally true (Adam et al. 2009) but represents a first estimate that needs further revision at the country level. This analysis was done for the population present in 2010, but population growth (or, in the case of the Russian Federation and Ukraine, population decline) through 2015 will mean that greater (or fewer) resources are needed in the future. The prevalence of HIV is estimated in other parts of the book and is duplicated here. It is assumed that about 70 percent of HIV-positive people will need ART; this figure reflects a mature epidemic and will overestimate the need in areas where incidence is high relative to current prevalence (that is, in areas that have a larger percentage of persons with HIV in the early years of infection). The number of IDUs, where applicable, is based on previous literature (Mathers et al. 2010).

Table A.1 Demographic Variables Used for Estimation of Resources Needed

Country	*Estimated number of MSM, 2010*	*Estimated number of MSM, 2015*[a]	*Estimated HIV prevalence among MSM (%)*	*Estimated HIV prevalence among MSM, low (%)*	*Estimated HIV prevalence among MSM, high (%)*	*Estimated number of HIV-positive MSM, 2010*	*Estimated number of MSM needing ART*[b]	*Estimated number of IDUs*[c]
Brazil	618,335	640,040	8.2	6.9	9.4	50,703	35,492	n.a.
India	3,898,337	4,088,050	14.5	13.3	15.6	565,259	395,681	175,641
Kenya	118,000	130,000	15.2	13.3	17.2	17,936	12,555	n.a.
Peru[d]	312,630	340,470	13.8	13.4	14.3	43,143	30,200	n.a.
Russian Federation[d]	1,449,360	1,380,000	3.4	2.6	4.2	49,278	34,495	1,757,100
Senegal[d]	102,570	119,040	24.3	19.4	29.2	24,925	17,447	n.a.
Thailand	164,978	164,010	23.0	20.1	25.4	37,945	26,561	147,433
Ukraine	362,024	332,206	10.6	7.8	14.2	38,375	26,862	290,954

Sources: Number of MSM drawn from authors' projections except as otherwise indicated, assuming 3 percent of adult men are MSM. HIV prevalence is based on data in other sections of this book. Estimated number of IDUs is drawn from Mathers et al 2010.

Note: n.a. = not applicable.

a. These estimates are included to present an indication of how costs might change in the future, but the data are not used in this analysis.

b. Seventy percent of HIV-positive MSM are assumed to require ART.

c. These numbers represent all IDUs, not just MSM who are IDUs.

d. Numbers are drawn from UN Population Division 2010.

Unit Costs

The unit cost methodology has been described in chapter 10 of this book. Table A.2 provides the unit costs used for the four countries not included in chapter 10.

Coverage

As noted previously, rather than projecting costs into future years, which requires modeling the effects of current preventive activities on future

Table A.2 Unit Cost Estimates for Brazil, India, Russian Federation, and Senegal

Intervention category	*Number of studies*	*Estimated unit cost (2008 US$)*	*Range (2008 US$)*	*Model estimates (2008 US$)*	*Model estimate ranges (2008 US$)*
Brazil					
ART	n.a.	n.a.	—	Model 1: 1,689	702–3,175
Condom and lubricant distribution	2[a]	0.71	—		0.1–0.4[b]
Outreach through peer educators	n.a.	n.a.	—	Model 2[c]: 25.3 (per person reached per year)	21.3–29.7
India					
ART	4[d]	672 (paper judged to have best methodology)	496–6,573	Model 1: 1,032	417–1,945
Condom and lubricant distribution	n.a.	n.a.	—	—	0.1–0.4[b]
Outreach through peer educators	4[e]	18 (per person reached per year)	8.4–125	Model 2[c]: 8.8 (per person reached per year)	7.3–10.6
Needle exchange program	n.a.	n.a.	—	17.1[f] (per person reached per year)	8.8–29.6
Methadone replacement therapy	n.a.	n.a.	—	653.8 (per person per year)	411.6–958.8

(continued next page)

Table A.2 *(continued)*

Intervention category	*Number of studies*	*Estimated unit cost (2008 US$)*	*Range (2008 US$)*	*Model estimates (2008 US$)*	*Model estimate ranges (2008 US$)*
Russian Federation					
ART	1[g]	3,949	—	Model 1: 1,965	815–3,687
Condom and lubricant distribution	n.a.	n.a.	—	—	0.1–0.4[b]
Outreach through peer educators	n.a.	n.a.	—	Model 2[d]: 34.0 (per person reached per year)	28.6–39.9
Needle exchange program	n.a.	n.a.	—	21.2[f] (per person reached per year)	10.6–37.6
Methadone replacement therapy	n.a.	n.a.	—	947.4 (per person per year)	447.6–1,312.5
Senegal					
ART	n.a.	n.a.	—	Model 1: 1,032	417–1,943
Condom and lubricant distribution	n.a.	n.a.	—	—	0.1–0.4[b]
Outreach through peer educators	n.a.	n.a.	—	Model 2[c]: 8.6 (per person reached per year)	7.0–10.4

Source: Authors.
Note: n.a. = not applicable; — not available.
a. Dowdy, Sweat, and Holtgrave 2006 (for female condoms); Soderlund et al. 1993 (cost per contact).
b. Bedimo et al. 2002; Constella Futures et al. 2006; Soderlund et al. 1993; Terris-Prestholt et al. 2006.
c. Predicted for the average number of contacts in one year observed in data collected.
d. Bender et al. 2010; Freedberg et al. 2007; John, Rajagopalan, and Madhuri 2006; Over et al. 2006.
e. Chandrashekar et al. 2010; Dandona et al. 2005; Dandona et al. 2009; Fung et al. 2007; Guinness, Kumaranayake, and Hanson 2007.
f. Predicted for the modal number of contacts in one year observed in the data collected.
g. Long et al. 2006.

HIV infections, this book focuses on the costs for the 2010 population. Furthermore, projecting costs into the future requires knowledge about what rates of coverage expansion are possible, which requires knowledge about the current organization and capacity of communities of MSM, health care providers, and the overall HIV program. Describing coverage scale-up rates is thus not feasible. Costs are therefore presented in three scenarios: 30 percent coverage, 60 percent coverage (as the Joint United Nations Committee on HIV/AIDS [UNAIDS] target for 2015), and full coverage (100 percent coverage for HIV prevention activities targeting MSM and ART, and 60 percent coverage of programs targeting IDUs). Thus, for example, 30 percent coverage represents the cost of covering 30 percent of the 2010 population. Costs were calculated as the total needed for that coverage—gap analysis between current coverage and the target coverage was not done. In many cases, adequate coverage of interventions is very low (Adam et al. 2009), so the difference between a gap analysis and the total costs presented here will be small. The exceptions may be for the distribution of condoms and lubricant (although coverage for lubricants is often lower than that for use of condoms) and for the countries in Latin America, where higher levels of coverage may already be in place (Adam et al. 2009).

Coverage for IDUs represents coverage for all IDUs, not just MSM who are IDUs.

Formulas

Total costs are calculated as the linear sum of *target population * coverage * unit costs* for all interventions except for the distribution of condoms and lubricant. For the distribution of condoms and lubricant, costs were calculated as *target population * number of partners per year * number of sex acts per partner * adjustment for wastage rate by users * coverage * unit costs*. Wastage rate by users is assumed to be 5 percent; the number of partners per year and the number of sex acts per partner were based on the modeling exercise performed for chapter 10 in this book. In cases where these latter data were not available, numbers were used from a country in the same epidemic scenario.

Sensitivity Analysis

The data included in this exercise are fraught with uncertainty; two areas were subjected to explicit sensitivity analysis in this exercise. First, the prevalence of HIV among MSM was used to estimate high and low levels of need for ART. Second, the range of unit costs was used to estimate overall uncertainty in the costs. Thus, uncertainties about the size of the population of MSM were not dealt with in this exercise.

Results

The total cost of each intervention, by coverage level, is reported in table A.3 along with the uncertainty ranges for each. Total costs vary substantially as a result of four factors: number of MSM, HIV prevalence among MSM, inclusion of IDU interventions, and differences in unit costs. Kenya is estimated to need the least resources, at about US$8.9 million to achieve 60 percent coverage, whereas the Russian Federation will need the most, at about US$739 million to achieve 60 percent coverage. In Russia and Ukraine, interventions targeting IDUs represent over two-thirds of the total costs, even if other interventions reach 100 percent coverage, whereas in Thailand, interventions targeting IDUs represent about half the resources needed. In India, Kenya, Peru, and Senegal, ART represents over half of the costs (and over 85 percent of total costs in Kenya and Senegal), whereas in Brazil, preventive interventions targeting MSM are just over half of total costs. In all cases, the plausible range of resources needed is very broad. For example, in Russia, for the full-costs scenario, the sensitivity analysis shows the total costs changing by more than US$1 billion.

Table A.4 shows the costs of the interventions per individual for MSM. In Russia, Peru, and Thailand, full coverage will cost about US$500 per individual; whereas in Brazil, costs are much lower (about US$200 per individual) because of the lower prevalence of HIV among MSM. Full coverage of all interventions is shown to cost over US$100 per individual for MSM in all countries included in this analysis.

Discussion

This analysis has shown that considerable resources are likely to be needed to provide a comprehensive response to HIV among MSM, with over US$100 per individual for MSM needed to reach full coverage in each of the countries analyzed. However, this cost should be countered with the large effects that can be gained (as shown in part III of this book). Prevention activities specifically targeting MSM represent less than 10 percent of these costs in Russia and Ukraine; between 10 and 15 percent of these costs in Kenya, Senegal, and Thailand; and between 30 and 50 percent of these costs in Brazil, India, and Peru.

Considerable uncertainty exists in these results, and the findings should be taken only as first, indicative estimates of the amount of resources needed. Likely, these figures underrepresent the true need for resources for HIV prevention among MSM for numerous reasons. First,

Table A.3 Results of Cost Estimation for Eight Focus Countries

Intervention	Coverage (%)	Brazil	India	Kenya	Peru	Russian Federation	Senegal	Thailand	Ukraine
		Cost in 2010 US$, millions (uncertainty range)							
Condom and lubricant distribution	30	13.9 (2–13.9)	19.7 (9.8–39.4)	0.4 (0.2–0.9)	2 (1–3.9)	7.3 (3.7–14.6)	0.4 (0.2–0.8)	0.4 (0.4–0.4)	1.8 (0.9–3.7)
	60	27.7 (3.9–27.7)	39.4 (19.7–78.8)	0.9 (0.4–1.8)	3.9 (2–7.9)	14.6 (7.3–29.3)	0.8 (0.4–1.6)	0.8 (0.8–0.8)	3.7 (1.8–7.3)
	100	46.2 (6.5–46.2)	65.7 (32.8–131.3)	1.5 (0.7–3)	6.6 (3.3–13.2)	24.4 (12.2–48.8)	1.3 (0.6–2.6)	1.3 (1.3–1.3)	6.1 (3–12.2)
Outreach through peer educators	30	4.7 (4–5.5)	21.1 (8.5–12.4)	0.1 (0.1–0.2)	9.7 (1.3–9.7)	14.8 (12.4–17.3)	0.3 (0.2–0.3)	2.9 (0.7–2.9)	1.4 (1.2–1.6)
	60	9.4 (7.9–11)	42.1 (17.1–24.8)	0.3 (0.2–0.4)	19.3 (2.7–19.3)	29.6 (24.9–34.7)	0.5 (0.4–0.6)	5.7 (1.4–5.7)	2.7 (2.3–3.2)
	100	15.6 (13.2–18.4)	70.2 (28.5–41.3)	0.5 (0.3–0.7)	32.2 (4.4–32.2)	49.3 (41.5–57.8)	0.9 (0.7–1.1)	9.6 (2.3–9.6)	4.6 (3.8–5.4)
ART	30	18 (6.3–38.8)	79.8 (45.4–839.4)	3.8 (1.4–8.2)	34.3 (5–35.6)	40.9 (6.4–50.5)	5.4 (1.7–12.2)	9.8 (3.9–40.6)	9.5 (2.9–24.1)
	60	36 (12.6–77.5)	159.5 (90.8–1,678.9)	7.7 (2.7–16.3)	68.6 (10–71.1)	81.7 (12.9–101)	10.8 (3.5–24.4)	19.7 (7.7–81.3)	19.1 (5.7–48.1)
	100	59.9 (21–129.2)	265.9 (151.3–2,798.1)	12.8 (4.5–27.2)	114.4 (16.6–118.5)	136.2 (21.5–168.3)	18 (5.8–40.7)	32.8 (12.9–135.5)	31.8 (9.5–80.2)
Needle exchange program	30	n.a.	0.5 (0.3–0.9)	n.a.	n.a.	6.7 (3.4–11.9)	n.a.	0.5 (0.3–0.9)	0.5 (0.5–1.6)
	60	n.a.	1.1 (0.6–1.9)	n.a.	n.a.	13.4 (6.7–23.8)	n.a.	1 (0.5–1.7)	1.1 (1–3.3)

(continued next page)

Table A.3 *(continued)*

Intervention	*Coverage (%)*	*Cost in 2010 US$, millions (uncertainty range)*							
		Brazil	*India*	*Kenya*	*Peru*	*Russian Federation*	*Senegal*	*Thailand*	*Ukraine*
Opioid substitution therapy	30	n.a.	20.7 (13–30.3)	n.a.	n.a.	299.6 (141.6–415.1)	n.a.	20.2 (13.2–28.9)	37 (23.8–53.6)
	60	n.a.	41.3 (26–60.6)	n.a.	n.a.	599.3 (283.1–830.2)	n.a.	40.5 (26.4–57.8)	74.1 (47.6–107.2)
Total	30	36.5 (12.2–58.1)	141.7 (77.1–922.5)	4.4 (1.7–9.3)	46 (7.3–49.2)	369.3 (167.5–509.5)	6.1 (2.2–13.3)	33.8 (18.4–73.7)	50.3 (29.2–84.6)
	60	73.1 (24.4–116.3)	283.5 (154.2–1,844.9)	8.9 (3.4–18.5)	91.9 (14.6–98.3)	738.6 (334.9–1,019)	12.1 (4.3–26.6)	67.7 (36.8–147.3)	100.6 (58.4–169.1)
	100	121.8 (40.6–193.8)	472.4 (256.9–3,074.9)	14.8 (5.6–30.9)	153.2 (24.4–163.9)	1,231.1 (558.2–1,698.3)	20.2 (7.2–44.4)	112.8 (61.3–245.5)	167.7 (97.3–281.9)

Source: Authors.
Note: n.a. = not applicable.

Table A.4 Cost per Individual for MSM
Cost in 2010 US$

	60% coverage			*Full coverage*		
Country	*Two prevention interventions*	*Prevention + ART*	*Full package[a]*	*Two prevention interventions*	*Prevention + ART*	*Full package[a]*
Brazil	60.0	118.2	n.a.	100.0	197.0	n.a.
India	20.9	61.8	72.7	34.8	103.1	113.9
Kenya	10.0	75.0	n.a.	16.7	125.0	n.a.
Peru	74.4	294.0	n.a.	124.1	490.0	n.a.
Russian Federation	30.5	86.9	509.6	50.8	144.8	567.6
Senegal	12.7	118.1	n.a.	21.2	196.8	n.a.
Thailand	39.3	158.6	410.1	65.6	264.4	515.9
Ukraine	17.7	70.3	277.9	29.4	117.2	324.8

Source: Authors.
Note: n.a. = not applicable.
a. Full package represents the two prevention interventions, ART, and needle exchange programs and opioid substitution therapy.

as discussed previously, several categories of costs were excluded from this analysis. Second, unit costs are based on findings from the published literature. These likely represent areas where a policy exists conducive to conducting HIV outreach and preventive interventions among high-risk groups, which may not represent the costs needed in areas where the environment is not as favorable. Third, the unit costs for peer outreach were calculated assuming a mature program operating at a relatively efficient scale. Thus, costs for 30 percent or even 60 percent coverage may not have capitalized on these economies of scale, and unit costs are underestimated here. In addition, diseconomies of scale may affect costs as coverage approaches 100 percent. The relation between scale at the level of the service delivery center and at the population coverage level, however, is not well studied.

Table A.5 compares the estimated resources needed with the last available data on HIV/AIDS spending in countries (UNAIDS 2010 progress reports submitted by countries, http://www.unaids.org/en/dataanalysis/monitoringcountryprogress/2010progressreportssubmittedbycountries/). These data are, in some cases, gross estimations of current spending on HIV/AIDS, but they are indicative of the level of current government effort. In Brazil and Kenya, spending on MSM needed to reach 60 percent coverage is less than 10 percent of current spending; in Thailand, needs

Table A.5 Estimated Resources Needed Compared with Current HIV/AIDS Spending Estimates

Country	*Two prevention interventions at 60% coverage (US$, millions)*	*Full package at 60% coverage (US$, millions)*	*Estimated HIV/AIDS budget in last year available (US$, millions)*	*Year of budget*	*Two prevention interventions as a percentage of budget*	*Full package as a percentage of budget*
Brazil	37.1	73.1	715	2008	5	10
India	81.5	283.5	429[a]	2009	19	66
Kenya	1.2	8.9	687	2009	0.2	1
Peru	23.3	91.9	52	2009	45	176
Russian Federation	44.2	738.6	n.a.	n.a.	n.a.	n.a.
Senegal	1.3	12.1	n.a.	n.a.	n.a.	n.a.
Thailand	6.5	67.7	236	2009	3	29
Ukraine	6.4	100.6	79.4	2007	8	127

Source: Authors.
Note: n.a. = not applicable.
a. Estimated from six-year budget.

for MSM and IDUs represent about 30 percent of current spending. In Ukraine, the costs for IDUs drive the estimated needs to greater levels than all of current spending; prevention interventions for MSM alone are much more modest. In Peru, the model may have overestimated the amount of additional resources needed because current efforts have achieved an estimated 44 percent coverage of MSM, and ART access is relatively high (Adam et al. 2009); adding another 15 percent coverage is not likely to increase the need for resources to as high a level as indicated in table A.4. If lower-range figures are used, then the two prevention interventions for MSM at 60 percent coverage represent 9 percent of current spending; adding ART increases this amount to 28 percent of current spending. Results for India seem to be driven by the relatively low level of current per capita HIV/AIDS budgets.

Table A.5 demonstrates that, although spending per MSM may be high, the effort needed to reach high coverage levels is, in general, relatively modest when placed in the context of overall HIV/AIDS budgets. The exceptions are those countries where scale-up of interventions for IDUs is needed. These modest financial needs should be compared with the potential for the disproportionate (to the size of the population of MSM) impact on the HIV/AIDS epidemic these interventions can realize.

Although these findings indicate that investments in MSM are feasible with only modest increases in HIV/AIDS budgeting, these findings should be interpreted on a magnitude-of-order scale. National and local assessment and planning are essential to determine the levels of resources needed and that can be effectively deployed within a given period.

References

Adam, P. C. G., J. B. F. de Wit, I. Toskin, B. M. Mathers, M. Nashkhoev, I. Zablotska, R. Lyerla, and D. Rugg. 2009. "Estimating Levels of HIV Testing, HIV Prevention Coverage, HIV Knowledge, and Condom Use among Men Who Have Sex with Men (MSM) in Low-Income and Middle-Income Countries." *Journal of Acquired Immune Deficiency Syndromes* 52 (Suppl. 2): S143–51.

Bedimo, A. L., S. D. Pinkerton, D. A. Cohen, B. Gray, and T. A. Farley. 2002. "Condom Distribution: A Cost-Utility Analysis." *International Journal of STD and AIDS* 13 (6): 384–92.

Bender, M. A., N. Kumarasamy, K. H. Mayer, B. Wang, R. P. Walensky, T. Flanigan, B. R. Schackman, C. A. Scott, Z. Lu, K A. Freedberg, et al. 2010. "Cost-Effectiveness of Tenofovir as First-Line Antiretroviral Therapy in India." *Clinical Infectious Diseases* 50 (3): 416–25.

Chandrashekar, S., L. Guinness, L. Kumaranayake, B. Reddy, Y. Govindraj, P. Vickerman, and M. Alary. 2010. "The Effects of Scale on the Costs of Targeted HIV Prevention Interventions among Female and Male Sex Workers, Men Who Have Sex with Men and Transgenders in India." *Sexually Transmitted Infections* 86 (Suppl. 1): i89–94.

Constella Futures, Centre for Development and Population Activities, White Ribbon Alliance for Safe Motherhood, and World Conference of Religions for Peace. 2006. "HIV Expenditure on MSM Programming in the Asia-Pacific Region." Background paper produced for the International Consultation on Male Sexual Health and HIV in Asia and the Pacific titled "Risks and Responsibilities" held in New Delhi, India, September 22–26. U.S. Agency for International Development, Health Policy Initiative, Task Order 1, Washington, DC.

Dandona, L., S. G. Kumar, G. A. Kumar, and R. Dandona. 2009. "Economic Analysis of HIV Prevention Interventions in Andhra Pradesh State of India to Inform Resource Allocation." *AIDS* 23 (2): 233–42.

Dandona, L., P. Sisodia, T. L. Prasad, E. Marseille, R. M. Chalapathi, A. A. Kumar, S. G. Kumar, Y. K. Ramesh, M. Over, M. Someshwar, and J. G. Kahn. 2005. "Cost and Efficiency of Public Sector Sexually Transmitted Infection Clinics in Andhra Pradesh, India." *BMC Health Services Research* 5: 69.

Dowdy, D. W., M. D. Sweat, and D. R. Holtgrave. 2006. "Country-Wide Distribution of the Nitrile Female Condom (FC2) in Brazil and South Africa: A Cost-Effectiveness Analysis." *AIDS* 20 (16): 2091–98.

Freedberg, K. A., N. Kumarasamy, E. Losina, A. J. Cecelia, C. A. Scott, N. Divi, T. P. Flanigan, Z. Lu, M. C. Weinstein, B. Wang, et al. 2007. "Clinical Impact and Cost-Effectiveness of Antiretroviral Therapy in India: Starting Criteria and Second-Line Therapy." *AIDS* 21 (Suppl. 4): S117–28.

Fung, I. C., L. Guinness, P. Vickerman, C. Watts, G. Vannela, J. Vadhvana, A. M. Foss, L. Malodia, M. Gandhi, and G. Jani. 2007. "Modelling the Impact and Cost-Effectiveness of the HIV Intervention Programme amongst Commercial Sex Workers in Ahmedabad, Gujarat, India." *BMC Public Health* 7: 195.

Guinness, L., L. Kumaranayake, and K. Hanson. 2007. "A Cost Function for HIV Prevention Services: Is There a 'U'-Shape?" *Cost Effectiveness and Resource Allocation* 5: 13.

John, K. R., N. Rajagopalan, and K. V. Madhuri. 2006. "Brief Communication: Economic Comparison of Opportunistic Infection Management with Antiretroviral Treatment in People Living with HIV/AIDS Presenting at an NGO Clinic in Bangalore, India." *Medscape General Medicine* 8 (4): 24.

Long, E. F., M. L. Brandeau, C. M. Galvin, T. Vinichenko, S. P. Tole, A. Schwartz, G. D. Sanders, and D. K. Owens. 2006. "Effectiveness and Cost-Effectiveness of Strategies to Expand Antiretroviral Therapy in St. Petersburg, Russia." *AIDS* 20 (17): 2207–15.

Mathers, B. M., L. Degenhardt, H. Ali, L. Wiessing, M. Hickman, R. P. Mattick, B. Myers, A. Ambekar, and S. A. Strathdee for the 2009 Reference Group to the UN on HIV and Injecting Drug Use. 2010. "HIV Prevention, Treatment, and Care Services for People Who Inject Drugs: A Systematic Review of Global, Regional, and National Coverage." *Lancet* 375 (9719): 1014–28.

Over, M., E. Marseille, K. Sudhakar, J. Gold, I. Gupta, A. Indrayan, S. Hira, N. Nagelkerke, A. S. Rao, and P. Heywood. 2006. "Antiretroviral Therapy and HIV Prevention in India: Modeling Costs and Consequences of Policy Options." *Sexually Transmitted Diseases* 33 (10 Suppl.): S145–52.

Soderlund, N., J. Lavis, J. Broomberg, and A. Mills. 1993. "The Costs of HIV Prevention Strategies in Developing Countries." *Bulletin of the World Health Organization* 71 (5): 595–604.

Terris-Prestholt, F., L. Kumaranayake, S. Foster, A. Kamali, J. Kinsman, V. Basajja, N. Nalweyso, M. Quigley, J. Kengeya-Kayondo, and J. Whitworth. 2006. "The Role of Community Acceptance over Time for Costs of HIV and STI Prevention Interventions: Analysis of the Masaka Intervention Trial, Uganda, 1996–1999." *Sexually Transmitted Diseases* 33 (10 Suppl.): S111–16.

UN Population Division. 2010. World Population Prospects: The 2008 Revision Population Database. United Nations Population Division, New York, NY. http://esa.un.org/unpp/index.asp. Last accessed September 20, 2010.

APPENDIX B

Extension of the Cost Analysis to Additional Selected Countries

Using the data presented in Adam and colleagues (2009), an attempt was made to extend the costing exercise to 48 countries in addition to the eight countries presented in this book. This exercise has substantial problems:

- Data needed to classify all the countries by their epidemic scenario are not available. Thus, some countries were assigned to an epidemic scenario based on the authors' opinions of the likely situation in that country.
- Data on the prevalence of HIV among men who have sex with men (MSM) are missing for 25 countries (indicated with shaded cells in table B.1). This figure was estimated by applying the ratio of prevalence among MSM to the general population in a neighboring country or among countries in the same epidemic scenario to the HIV prevalence in the general population of the country in question. Obviously, this method is not reliable for determining HIV prevalence among MSM and highlights the need for further research on HIV/AIDS in relation to MSM.
- Nine of the 24 countries where interventions for injecting drug users (IDUs) should be included in the cost have an unknown number of IDUs. The full costing exercise could not be completed for these countries.

- Although Adam and colleagues (2009) give ranges for the prevalence of MSM among adult men in each country, in many cases this range is quite broad (for example, 1 percent to 8 percent). Thus, estimating the number of MSM in each country can be a fairly arbitrary exercise.
- Unit costs could not be estimated for one country (Cuba) because of lack of reliable data on its gross domestic product.

With these limitations, full data were available for 19 (40 percent) of the 48 countries, indicating that the results of any global assessment are likely to be strongly based on assumptions and therefore lack reliability. With these limitations in mind, however, the final nine columns of table B.1 present the results of the costing exercise for the 46 countries included as the cost per individual for MSM.

The results are, generally, in line with the results presented for the eight example countries used in this book. Costs for the two prevention programs are generally estimated to be under US$50 per individual for MSM even at full coverage except in two high-middle-income countries (Chile and Lithuania). Costs for the two prevention programs plus ART are generally under US$300 per individual for MSM, except for high-middle-income countries, with the exception of Guyana, where high HIV prevalence indicates a high need for ART. This result may be the product of applying too high a risk of HIV infection among MSM compared to the general population in Guyana, but without further data this supposition is difficult to confirm. Finally, the results show that the two interventions for IDUs can add substantially to costs. Although these results are far from robust, they may provide very rough benchmarks on the amount of resources needed.

Table B.1 Results of the Analysis for 46 Selected Countries

Country	Indicator prevalence of MSM (%)	Assumed prevalence of MSM (%)	Estimated number of MSM	Number of IDUs	Epidemic scenario	Number of MSM needing ART	Cost per individual for MSM (2010 US$): 30% coverage: Two MSM-targeted prevention interventions[a]	30% coverage: Two prevention interventions + ART	30% coverage: Full package[b]	60% coverage: Two MSM-targeted prevention interventions[a]	60% coverage: Two prevention interventions + ART	60% coverage: Full package[b]	Full coverage: Two MSM-targeted prevention interventions[a]	Full coverage: Two prevention interventions + ART	Full coverage: Full package[b]
Argentina	1–8	3	369,870	n.a.	1	31,328	15	63	n.a.	31	126	n.a.	51	210	n.a.
Armenia	1–8	3	28,080	1,997	2	177	9	11	27	18	22	54	29	37	90
Bangladesh	7–8	7.5	3,707,475	30,349	4[c]	5,813	5	5	7	10	11	14	17	18	23
Belarus	1–8	3	99,690	75,414	2[c]	1,276	11	17	205	22	33	410	36	55	683
Bolivia	1–8	3	80,250	n.a.	1	11,909	9	59	n.a.	19	117	n.a.	31	196	n.a.
Bosnia and Herzegovina	1–8	3	39,840	n.k.	2[c]	86	10	11	n.k.	20	21	n.k.	33	35	n.k.
Bulgaria	1–8	3	79,380	n.k.	2[c]	89	13	13	n.k.	26	27	n.k.	43	45	n.k.
Cambodia	3.5–4.5	4	164,120	n.k.	4	8,961	6	22	n.k.	11	45	n.k.	19	75	n.k.
Chile	1–8	3	166,020	n.a.	1[c]	9,300	16	48	n.a.	32	96	n.a.	53	160	n.a.
China	1–4	3	14,611,800	3,461,050	4	439,815	9	21	75	18	41	150	30	69	251
Colombia	1–8	3	434,010	n.a.	1	58,939	11	66	n.a.	22	132	n.a.	36	220	n.a.
Costa Rica	1–8	3	44,610	n.a.	1[c]	1,225	14	28	n.a.	27	55	n.a.	45	92	n.a.
Côte d'Ivoire	1–3	2	107,660	n.a.	3[c]	14,157	7	47	n.a.	13	95	n.a.	22	158	n.a.
Ecuador	1–8	3	122,280	n.a.	1	12,925	11	52	n.a.	21	103	n.a.	35	172	n.a.
El Salvador	1–8	3	59,760	n.a.	1	3,305	11	33	n.a.	22	66	n.a.	36	111	n.a.
Georgia	1–8	3	42,570	78,750	2	1,579	9	22	425	17	44	850	29	73	1,417
Ghana	1–3	2	134,360	n.a.	1	23,513	7	43	n.a.	13	86	n.a.	22	143	n.a.
Guatemala	1–8	3	97,830	n.a.	1	7,875	10	39	n.a.	20	78	n.a.	33	130	n.a.
Guyana	1–8	3	7,260	n.a.	3[c]	4,020	7	187	n.a.	14	375	n.a.	23	624	n.a.
Haiti	1–3	2	53,820	n.a.	3[c]	3,493	5	23	n.a.	9	47	n.a.	15	78	n.a.
Honduras	1–8	3	57,840	n.a.	1	3,968	10	33	n.a.	19	66	n.a.	32	110	n.a.
Indonesia	3.5–4.5	4	3,037,120	213,043	4	191,339	8	29	44	16	58	88	26	97	147
Kazakhstan	1–8	3	150,750	100,838	2[c]	1,161	12	16	195	25	33	389	41	54	649
Kyrgyz Republic	1–8	3	49,740	24,417	2[c]	400	7	9	108	14	18	215	23	31	359
Lao PDR	3.5–4.5	4	65,480	n.k.	4	2,475	6	17	n.k.	12	35	n.k.	20	58	n.k.

(continued next page)

Table B.1 *(continued)*

Country	Indicator prevalence of MSM (%)	Assumed prevalence of MSM (%)	Estimated number of MSM	Number of IDUs	Epidemic scenario	Number of MSM needing ART	Cost per individual for MSM (2010 US$)								
							30% coverage			60% coverage			Full coverage		
							Two MSM-targeted prevention interventions[a]	Two prevention interventions + ART	Full package[b]	Two MSM-targeted prevention interventions[a]	Two prevention interventions + ART	Full package[b]	Two MSM-targeted prevention interventions[a]	Two prevention interventions + ART	Full package[b]
Lebanon	1–3	2	25,220	n.a.	5[c]	4,856	14	126	n.a.	27	252	n.a.	45	420	n.a.
Lithuania	1–8	3	33,720	4,999	2[c]	2,081	25	76	128	50	152	257	83	254	428
Macedonia, FYR	1–8	3	21,420	n.k.	2[c]	234	10	14	n.k.	20	29	n.k.	33	48	n.k.
Malaysia	3.5–4.5	4	343,200	278,550	4[c]	58,660	14	109	338	27	219	677	45	364	1,128
Mauritania	1–3	2	19,280	n.a.	3[c]	454	7	14	n.a.	13	28	n.a.	22	46	n.a.
Mauritius	1–3	2	8,680	n.a.	3[c]	407	12	37	n.a.	24	74	n.a.	40	123	n.a.
Mexico	1–8	3	974,160	n.a.	1	174,569	15	116	n.a.	31	232	n.a.	51	387	n.a.
Moldova	1–8	3	38,880	3,483	2	463	8	12	30	16	24	61	27	39	101
Mongolia	1–4	3	26,490	n.k.	4[c]	300	7	11	n.k.	15	22	n.k.	25	37	n.k.
Montenegro	1–8	3	5,850	n.k.	2[c]	356	5	6	n.k.	10	12	n.k.	16	19	n.k.
Nepal	7–8	7.5	584,700	29,800	4	19,646	5	8	18	10	16	36	17	26	59
Nigeria	1–3	2	761,480	n.a.	3	71,960	7	36	n.a.	13	72	n.a.	22	121	n.a.
Panama	1–8	3	31,680	n.a.	1	2,351	15	55	n.a.	29	109	n.a.	49	182	n.a.
Papua New Guinea	1–3	2	35,760	n.a.	3[c]	1,589	7	21	n.a.	13	42	n.a.	22	69	n.a.
Philippines	3.5–4.5	4	1,045,880	16,000	4[c]	2,086	8	8	11	15	17	23	25	28	38
Romania	1–8	3	224,070	n.k.	2[c]	5,240	14	27	n.k.	28	55	n.k.	47	92	n.k.
Sri Lanka	7–8	7.5	493,650	n.k.	4[c]	4,571	8	11	n.k.	16	23	n.k.	27	38	n.k.
Tunisia	1–3	2	70,180	n.a.	5[c]	6,594	8	46	n.a.	17	91	n.a.	28	152	n.a.
Turkey	1–3	2	497,680	n.a.	5[c]	1,803	13	15	n.a.	26	30	n.a.	44	51	n.a.
Uzbekistan	1–8	3	253,260	84,210	2[c]	1,524	8	10	77	16	19	154	26	32	257
Vietnam	3.5–4.5	4	1,127,040	147,636	4	48,914	7	21	47	14	41	94	24	69	157

Source: Table adapted from Adam et al. 2009.

Note: n.a. = not applicable, n.k. = not known (but likely to be of substantial enough size to warrant an intervention). Numbers in shaded cells indicate these are authors' estimations, as described in the text.

a. The two prevention interventions are distribution of condoms and lubricant and community-based peer outreach.

b. Full package represents the two prevention interventions, ART, and needle exchange programs and opioid replacement therapy.

c. Epidemic scenario could not be calculated because of lack of data; authors' assessment used to assign country to a scenario.

Reference

Adam, P. C. G., J. B. F. de Wit, I. Toskin, B. M. Mathers, M. Nashkhoev, I. Zablotska, R. Lyerla, and D. Rugg. 2009. "Estimating Levels of HIV Testing, HIV Prevention Coverage, HIV Knowledge, and Condom Use among Men Who Have Sex with Men (MSM) in Low-Income and Middle-Income Countries." *Journal of Acquired Immune Deficiency Syndromes* 52 (Suppl. 2): S143–51.

Index

Boxes, figures, notes, and tables are indicated with *b*, *f*, *n*, and *t* following the page number.

J

K

L

M

T

U

ECO-AUDIT

Environmental Benefits Statement

The World Bank is committed to preserving endangered forests and natural resources. The Office of the Publisher has chosen to print ***The Global HIV Epidemics among Men Who Have Sex with Men*** on recycled paper with 50 percent post-consumer waste, in accordance with the recommended standards for paper usage set by the Green Press Initiative, a nonprofit program supporting publishers in using fiber that is not sourced from endangered forests. For more information, visit www.greenpressinitiative.org.

Saved:

- 9 trees
- 4 million British thermal units of total energy
- 840 pounds of net greenhouse gases (CO_2 equivalent)
- 3,785 gallons of waste water
- 482 pounds of solid waste

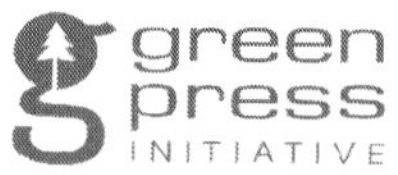